CASE STUDIES
IN PSYCHOTHERAPY

Dedication

To Karen Harrington
You are my future.

CASE STUDIES
IN PSYCHOTHERAPY
SEVENTH EDITION

Editors

Danny Wedding
Raymond J. Corsini

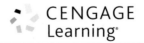

Australia • Brazil • Japan • Korea • Mexico • Singapore • Spain • United Kingdom • United States

CENGAGE
Learning®

**Case Studies In Current Psychotherapy,
Seventh Edition**
Editors: Danny Wedding, Raymond J. Corsini

Publisher: Jon-David Hague

Editorial Assistant: Amelia Blevins

Media Editor: Elizabeth Momb

Brand Manager: Elisabeth Rhoden

Market Development Manager: Kara Kindstrom

Manufacturing Planner: Judy Inouye

Rights Acquisitions Specialist: Roberta Broyer

Text Researcher: PreMedia Global

Production Management and Composition: Teresa Christie, MPS Limited

Copy Editor: S.M. Summerlight

Art and Design Direction: Carolyn Deacy, MPS Limited

Cover Designer: Kathleen Cunningham

Cover Image: Bendy Poppies, 1995

(colour photo) © Norman Hollands / Private Collection / The Bridgeman Art Library

For product information and technology assistance, contact us at
Cengage Learning Customer & Sales Support, 1-800-354-9706

For permission to use material from this text or product,
submit all requests online at **www.cengage.com/permissions**
Further permissions questions can be e-mailed to
permissionrequest@cengage.com

Library of Congress Control Number: 2013932881

ISBN-13: 978-1-285-17523-2

ISBN-10: 1-285-17523-9

Cengage Learning
200 First Stamford Place, 4th Floor
Stamford, CT 06902
USA

Cengage Learning is a leading provider of customized learning solutions with office locations around the globe, including Singapore, the United Kingdom, Australia, Mexico, Brazil, and Japan. Locate your local office at **www.cengage.com/global**

Cengage Learning products are represented in Canada by Nelson Education, Ltd.

To learn more about BROOKS/COLE, visit **www.cengage.com /brookscole**

Purchase any of our products at your local college store or at our preferred online store **www.CengageBrain.com**

Printed in the United States of America
1 2 3 4 5 6 7 17 16 15 14 13

In Memory of Four Giants in the World of Psychotherapy

Carl Rogers
(1902–1987)

Rollo May
(1909–1994)

Joseph Wolpe
(1915–1997)

and

Albert Ellis
(1913–2007)

CONTENTS

DEDICATION   ii

CONTRIBUTORS   ix

FOREWORD   xi

ACKNOWLEDGMENTS   xiii

PREFACE   xv

1 PSYCHOANALYTIC PSYCHOTHERAPY
The Case of Simone / *Jeremy D. Safran*   3

2 ADLERIAN PSYCHOTHERAPY
The Case of Roger / *Harold H. Mosak and Michael Maniacci*   12

3 CLIENT-CENTERED THERAPY
Client-Centered Therapy with David: A Sojourn in Loneliness / *Marjorie C. Witty*   33

4 RATIONAL EMOTIVE BEHAVIOR THERAPY
A Twenty-Three-Year-Old Woman Guilty About Not Following Her Parents' Rules / *Albert Ellis*   59

5 BEHAVIOR THERAPY
Covert Sensitization for Paraphilia / *David H. Barlow*   79

6 COGNITIVE THERAPY
An Interview with a Depressed and Suicidal Patient / *Aaron T. Beck*   88

7 EXISTENTIAL PSYCHOTHERAPY
"If Rape Were Legal . . ." / *Irvin Yalom*   103

8 GESTALT THERAPY
First or Nowhere? / *Sally Denham—Vaughan*   115

9 INTERPERSONAL PSYCHOTHERAPY
A Case Study for the New IPT Therapist / *Marie Crowe and Sue Luty*   139

10 FAMILY THERAPY

The Daughter Who Said No / *Peggy Papp* 149

11 CONTEMPLATIVE PSYCHOTHERAPIES

Using Mindfulness Effectively in Clinical Practice: Two Case Studies / *Tory A. Eisenlohr-Moul, Jessica R. Peters, and Ruth A. Baer* 173

12 POSITIVE PSYCHOTHERAPY

Strength-Based Assessment in Clinical Practice / *Tayyab Rashid and Robert F. Ostermann* 193

13 INTEGRATIVE PSYCHOTHERAPIES

Integrative Therapy with Mr. F. H. / *Larry E. Beutler* 204

14 MULTICULTURAL PSYCHOTHERAPY

Alma / *Lillian Comas-Díaz* 215

INDEX 219

CONTRIBUTORS

Ruth A. Baer

David H. Barlow

Aaron T. Beck

Larry E. Beutler

Lillian Comas-Díaz

Marie Crowe

Sally Denham-Vaughan

Tory A. Eisenlohr-Moul

Albert Ellis

Sue Luty

Michael Maniacci

Harold H. Mosak

Robert F. Ostermann

Peggy Papp

Jessica R. Peters

Tayyab Rashid

Jeremy Safran

Marjorie C. Witty

Irvin Yalom

FOREWORD

Observing an expert perform a skills-based task has always been the most effective way for an apprentice to learn a complex procedure. For this reason, witnessing and studying the work of those who have mastered their craft have always been at the heart of the apprenticeship system. This method of training is more effective when it has been preceded by instruction that allows novices to place their observations into a meaningful conceptual context. This book, which presents case studies conducted and written by experts in specific therapeutic modalities, corresponds to the apprenticeship aspect of a training program. The primary text, *Current Psychotherapies*, parallels these case studies chapter by chapter. Although a reading of that text is not necessary for a fruitful reading of these case studies, it can heighten understanding of what the therapists are doing by presenting the theoretical and applied underpinnings of their systems.

All clinicians personalize the systems that they have studied and chosen to use. Their therapy reflects their personal life histories, the scripts, values, attitudes, and dispositions that form (mostly at a tacit or implicit level) the weft of that elusive fabric we call the psyche. None of us can entirely escape the conditions that have made us who we are, and our experiences inevitably get enmeshed in the treatment plan and the procedures that we use with our clients. For this reason, the therapist, as a person, becomes the primary instrument of therapy. The techniques become secondary.

Most of you who will read these case studies are motivated by an interest in improving your clinical skills. A first reading will excite a sense of profound admiration for the clinicians who worked the marvels of "therapeutic outcome" described in the studies. Their virtuosity should not discourage you from aspiring to their level of expertise. One must keep in mind that these cases are not examples of their least accomplished performances. The editors chose them precisely because they are instructive of the highly evolved clinical skills these therapists possessed at an advanced point in their careers. Although these clients challenged their resources to the utmost, they were clients who were apt, and suitable, for the treatments these therapists were prepared to provide.

Becoming a skilled clinician is like becoming skilled at any other complex human activity. It is the work of the "long-distance runner." It is building a repertoire of techniques and broad strategies that fit a consistent theoretical paradigm, honing various clinical skills, and learning to recognize the appropriate moments to use them. It is the work of fashioning coherent treatment plans for particular individuals who will be facing us filled with hope and anxiety. It is becoming a therapist with a therapeutic personality—the privileged instrument of every successful therapy, polished by the inevitable stresses, frustrations, and failures of life and of our profession—for not every therapeutic relationship turns out as we had hoped it would.

This book raises questions that go far beyond the boundaries of psychotherapy as that discipline is generally construed. The concerns and the personages that are depicted in these cases implicitly evoke issues of cultural anthropology, social psychology, hermeneutics, psychopedagogy, developmental psychology, and cognitive science.

Psychotherapeutics has borrowed the terms *etic* and *emic* from cultural anthropology. The former, etic, characterizes a nomothetic or universal approach to framing theories of personality development; the latter refers to principles that are more culture sensitive and culture bound. An emic approach refrains from generalizing principles beyond the group in which they have been found to be valid. In the limiting case, it treats each individual as possessing his or her own "culture."

Inclusion of the case on meditation reflects the editors' recognition of the richness that non-Occidental philosophies and approaches to healing can bring to the Western therapist. Of course, this East-West conceptualization of the culture specificity of any therapy is not a true dichotomy. Like any other psychological, anthropological, or sociological variable, culture specificity lies on a continuum. All the case studies in this book can be placed somewhere on that continuum.

Readers of this book will no doubt experience an approach-avoidance dilemma with several, if not most, of the therapies described here, for there are drawbacks and benefits for each system. The editors make no apology for that and expect both the practitioner and the trainee to struggle with the issue of choice. The decisions you make about therapy will be quite personal. Some prefer a predominantly intrapsychic approach to therapy; others a more contextual, social engineering approach. Some like the freedom of a time-unlimited model; others a time-limited, even very brief, model. Some will prefer didactic and directive methods; others will be inclined to the Socratic, client-centered approaches. Some will veer to etiological and history-focused exploration; others will prefer teleological, motivational, or even exclusively present-focused perspectives. Some will prefer a reductionistic model; others a holistic model that involves exercise, nutrition, physical fitness, medical exams, and heavy social penetration of clients' ambient worlds. Some of you will prefer the highly cognitive; others the principally affect-centered. You will find examples of all of these among the 14 case studies of this volume.

The following case studies will be rich ore to exploit, but in mining them, you will inevitably transform them. These studies are like rushing streams, of which the Greek philosopher Heraclitus spoke, into which you can dip your foot (or even plunge). You cannot, however, do the same thing twice, not because the case history will change, but because *you* will have changed at a second reading. Be that as it may, you have a banquet table set before you. The chapters were a pleasurable and useful read for me. I have no doubt they will also be for you.

Frank Dumont
Professor Emeritus
McGill University

ACKNOWLEDGMENTS

We are grateful to dozens of colleagues and friends who have taken time to discuss psychotherapy with us and to share their ideas about how it can best be taught. Sometimes, these conversations took hours and went on late into the evening; at other times, a friend would make a casual comment that would later shape our decisions about which cases to include in *Case Studies in Psychotherapy*. Although *Current Psychotherapies* chapter authors usually selected the case study used to supplement their chapters in *Case Studies in Psychotherapy*, we sometimes solicited outside advice and opinions, and we are indebted to the following individuals who helped in a variety of ways with the preparation of this book.

Bernard Beitman
University of Missouri–Columbia

Juris Draguns
Pennsylvania State University

Ken Freedland
Washington University

Glenn Good
University of Florida

James Hennessy
Fordham University

Lockie Johnson
Saba University School of Medicine

Judy Kuriansky
Columbia University

Tony Marsella
University of Hawaii

Richard Nelson-Jones
Cognitive Humanistic Institute, Chiang Mai, Thailand

Tom Oltmanns
Washington University

Paul Pedersen
University of Hawaii

Chris Pearce
California School of Professional Psychology

Paul Priester
University of Wisconsin–Milwaukee

Morgan T. Sammons
California School of Professional Psychology

Sombat Tapanya
Chiang Mai University

Robert Woody
University of Nebraska–Omaha

Christoph Zepeda
California School of Professional Psychology

PREFACE

Psychotherapy is a difficult calling. Its practice requires creativity as well as intelligence, ingenuity as well as training, and hard work as well as good intentions. It is easy to do badly but exceedingly difficult to do well. Its ranks include both charlatans and grand masters. Psychotherapy involves skills that are almost never completely mastered, and it provides opportunities for, and indeed demands, lifelong learning.

Unfortunately, the very features that make psychotherapy so fascinating also make it difficult to teach or explain. Those of us who presume to instruct others in this arcane craft realize that modeling is our most powerful tool, and it is often more heuristic to *show* students what we do rather than tell them what we do. However, all of us realize the limits of our own training: There are myriad clients with multiple problems, and their needs are protean.

One way to deal with the limits of our own experience and training is to expose students to role models through case histories such as those collected in this volume. Each case in *Case Studies in Psychotherapy* is written by an experienced psychotherapist, and each parallels a chapter in the tenth edition of the companion volume, *Current Psychotherapies*.

Hundreds of thousands of students have used *Current Psychotherapies* to learn about the theoretical underpinnings and fundamental methods of a dozen or so therapeutic systems, and the cases in the current volume have been carefully selected to expand and supplement the information in the parent text. This seventh edition includes new cases to illustrate psychoanalysis, client-centered therapy, positive psychotherapy, and contemplative approaches to psychotherapy. These cases illustrate the clinical work of some of the leading figures in the world of psychotherapy.

The serious student of psychotherapy can benefit greatly by reading *Case Studies in Psychotherapy* in tandem with the core chapters in *Current Psychotherapies*. I'm convinced students who make this investment will appreciate more fully both the beauty and the art of psychotherapy.

Danny Wedding
dwedding@alliant.edu

CASE STUDIES
IN PSYCHOTHERAPY

Editors' Introduction

This case study illustrates many of the concepts described in more detail in the Safran and Kriss chapter on psychoanalysis in Current Psychotherapies. *It is also an excellent introduction to long-term psychotherapy (Dr. Safran worked with Simone for four years, typically seeing her three times each week).*

The case shows a therapist and patient working together to resolve transference and countertransference issues, and it illustrates the key psychoanalytic concept of recapitulation of the past in the present. Simon's relationship with her parents is explored in depth (including the "sexual energy" exchanged between father and daughter), and Dr. Safran is able to help his patient understand how the "hole or emptiness inside her" might relate to her bulimia. The case also shows how the therapist and patient worked through termination issues, and it illustrates the ways in which psychoanalysts use dreams in therapy.

It will be useful for you to consider what recommendation you would make if you were a claims reviewer for an insurance company and you were asked to justify the need for four years of treatment for this young woman. Should there be limits to treatment or should it be open ended with termination set by the therapist and patient? How often do psychotherapy patients present with a history of childhood sexual abuse? Were Simone's beliefs about the likelihood of her becoming pregnant through immaculate conception genuine delusions?

It will be especially useful for you to compare and contrast the way Dr. Safran approaches this case with the approaches advocated in other chapters in Current Psychotherapies. *Is psychoanalysis the treatment of choice for bulimia? Do this patient's other problems justify four years of psychotherapy, or is psychoanalytic treatment best conceptualized in terms of personal growth rather than symptom reduction? Does the fact that Simone continued to periodically binge after termination suggest that treatment wasn't effective, or is relapse almost inevitable in cases such as this?*

1 | THE CASE OF SIMONE

Jeremy D. Safran

Simone was a young African American woman with whom I worked for four years. During this period, I saw her three times per week. At the time she began treatment, she was 26 years old. Simone initially sought treatment because of a "general feeling of emptiness" as well as a moderate problem with bulimia, which involved both binging and purging. She was working in a health-food store on a part-time basis and was primarily supported financially by her father. In college, Simone had majored in fine arts, but she was not doing anything related to her college education in the time she was in treatment with me. She was extremely attractive, intelligent, articulate, and well dressed. From the beginning I was struck by her lively and playful manner and her sense of humor. I also began to notice early on a tendency on her part to vacillate between states of narcissistic grandiosity during which she denied any needs or self-doubts, and (less frequently) states of openness and vulnerability during which she was able to admit to feeling extremely alienated and lonely.

Simone was brought up in a middle-class family in the suburbs. She attended a relatively affluent, predominantly white school. When I asked what the experience of being one of the only black children in the school was like for her, she denied any feelings of discomfort or of not belonging. She told me that most of her friends throughout her life had been white and that she had never given it much thought. During the course of treatment, we explored whether being in treatment with a white therapist had any significance for her. At first she denied that this was the case, in the same way that she denied having any feelings about being the one of the few African Americans in a predominantly white school. Gradually over time, however, we were able to explore this issue in greater depth.

Simone had two older brothers and one younger sister. Her father had an MBA and was a business executive when she was growing up. Her mother was a nurse. Simone's father left her mother when Simone was 6. Her father and mother had maintained an on-and-off again relationship over the years, and her mother had always maintained the hope of reuniting with him.

When Simone was a child, her father's presence was unpredictable. He would periodically (e.g., once every one or two months) come home to spend a weekend and then invariably leave early after having a fight with her mother. Simone described poignant memories of running down the road after his car crying. She maintained that initially

Excerpt from Jeremy D. Safran, *Psychoanalysis and Psychoanalytic Therapies* (pp. 122–134), copyright 2012 by the American Psychological Association. Reprinted by permission of the publisher.

she would be excited when she knew that her father would be visiting. Eventually she stopped feeling any excitement (as a form of self-protection) and then transitioned into a third state in which she felt no feelings but pretended to be excited to avoid alienating her father.

Simone's father continued to maintain a relationship with her as she grew older and even now would periodically contact her, take her out for lunch or dinner, make plans to see her again, and then inevitably disappear from her life again. When Simone spoke about her father, I often had the feeling that there was a semi-incestuous quality to the relationship. It was difficult for me to put my finger on why I felt this way. Simone never acknowledged a literal sexual boundary violation in their relationship (and it seemed to me quite possible that there never was one), but the way she discussed their relationship often had a type of romantically charged quality to it. She conveyed a sense of awkwardness and shame about their interactions, and her perception was that her father also felt awkward—"as if he was on a date." Another factor contributing to my speculation that there may have been some time of sexual boundary violation in Simone's childhood was that she sometimes spoke about experiencing a type of "disgusting energy" emanating from her that drove people away. (My experience has been that the feeling of being disgusting in some fundamental way is not unusual for clients who have been sexually violated as children.) The possibility of a sexual boundary violation having taken place in Simone's childhood was not a topic that was ever fully explored in work together. I speculated to myself, however, that a boundary violation of this type may have affected her ability to have romantic relationships with men. I also wondered to myself whether some type of sexual trauma with her father or another man in her childhood may have affected her way of relating to me and her difficulty in accepting support and nurturance from me.

Simone maintained that when she was a child her mother had been highly erratic, alternating between episodes of intense anger and periods of fragility and dependency on her. Simone remembered learning to be vigilant to shifts in her mother's mood in order to avoid triggering an outburst. She also remembered learning to take care of her mother emotionally—a way of being that had become characteristic for Simone. She described her mother as emotionally needy and dependent and felt extremely judgmental of her. This critical perspective on her mother contrasted with an idealized view of her father, who she viewed as independent and with whom she identified.

Simone was extremely shy in school and saw herself as ugly. Her first romantic relationship was at the end of high school. She was involved with a boy for a year but had no sexual relationship with him. When he left school to attend college, Simone became briefly involved with his best friend. On one occasion she had sexual intercourse with him and experienced this as traumatic. When she described the reasons why she had experienced the event as traumatic, it was the first point in our work together that I began to get a sense of some pockets of semidelusional ideation in Simone's thinking that were generally kept well contained. She told me that before this incident she had believed she would give birth to a child through immaculate conception and now this could never happen.

After her relationship with this boy, Simone began to have lesbian relationships and was involved in a lesbian relationship at the beginning of treatment. Before treatment, Simone's longest romantic relationship (subsequent to her first high school boyfriend) had lasted one month. Her typical pattern would be to end romantic relationships when she began to experience her partner as being too "emotionally needy," apparently an inevitability in her mind. When Simone began treatment, she did not see the absence of long-term romantic relationships in her life as a problem or as something she wished to change.

Over the course of treatment, Simone and I spent considerable time exploring the factors contributing to her feelings of emptiness as well as her binging behavior. She fluctuated dramatically (both within sessions and various stages of the treatment) in her ability to look at her own feelings and actions in a self-reflective fashion. At times when she was feeling safer and more open, however, she was able to express a desire to improve the quality of her relationships with people, a wish to be in a long-term romantic relationship, and a curiosity in understanding interfering factors. We explored the way in which her father's unpredictability had contributed to the development of a counter-dependent stance on her part. In addition, we explored the way in which she had identified with her father (and his apparent emotional aloofness) and repudiated the more vulnerable dependent aspects of herself that she associated with her mother (whom she saw as pathetic). We also explored the way in which her binging was connected to a desire to fill an experience of emptiness inside of her as well as the relationship between her dissociation of dependent feelings related both to her feelings of disgust when she experienced romantic partners as needy and her own difficulty in allowing others to relate to her in a nurturing fashion.

At different points in the treatment, Simone revealed additional elements of semi-delusional ideation (e.g., a continuing belief that she would still give birth to the messiah, a belief that certain people she met had special powers, a belief that she could read other people's minds). At such times Simone disclosed information tentatively and with a somewhat self-deprecatingly humorous style as if to say, "I don't take this completely seriously." She vacillated in terms of how trusting of me she felt and how willing she was to reveal beliefs of this type. Her fear that I would not understand or could not fully embrace her beliefs was an ongoing focus of discussion.

Throughout the treatment, Simone was preoccupied with various new age beliefs and ideas. She would spend hours browsing at new age books on bookstore shelves in what seemed a desperate attempt to fill what she described as a "hole" or an "emptiness" inside of her. Inevitably, Simone would leave the store feeling unsatiated—bored with the activity but not fulfilled. In time, we came to understand this activity of hers as similar in function to her binging behavior—that is, a desperate attempt to fill an internal experience of emptiness.

A few months after beginning treatment with me, Simone became involved with a cult, and this involvement continued and intensified over the first two years of her treatment. An important focus of exploration involved her concern that her spiritual interests were incompatible with psychotherapy. In addition, the effects of Simone's dissociated dependency needs emerged more fully in the cult. Although she initially felt quite skeptical of the cult and its leader, over time she became more involved in the cult. The allure of being able to completely surrender to the cult and its leader became more and more apparent to her. The prospect of having somebody completely take charge of her life and tell her what to do and not to do in any given situation was undeniably appealing to her.

As discussed previously, there was a continuous alternation in treatment between periods when Simone seemed quite open and able to engage in an exploratory process and periods when she was highly defended and rejected any attempt on my part to explore underlying feelings or look for deeper meaning. Although these alternating states never completely disappeared, over the course of treatment they became less frequent and intense, and Simone became better able to explore both her internal experience and the meaning of our relationship to her.

At the beginning of treatment, I had the sense that Simone had one foot in treatment and one foot out the door. She would often miss sessions (claiming that she had forgotten) or arrive 15 to 20 minutes late for sessions. For the most part, she would resist any attempt to explore feelings or factors underlying her inconsistent and late attendance, although occasionally she would be more receptive to exploration. I found myself feeling anxious that she would leave treatment precipitously, and I was concerned that any attempt on my part to explore her ambivalence would hasten her departure. I found myself feeling concerned that she would experience my attempts to explore her ambivalence as reflecting my own neediness, and I was more hesitant than I usually am to explore a client's ambivalence about treatment.

Over time, part of our work together involved exploring the way in which her skittishness about commitment to treatment evoked anxious feelings in me that in turn made it difficult to bring myself fully into the relationship and express my own feelings of caring toward her. I began to conceptualize what was taking place as an enactment in which Simone's own anxieties about dependency led to a lack of investment in our relationship, which in turn fueled feelings of anxiety and shame about my insecurity. My own conflicts about dependency and a concern about seeing myself as needy were being triggered by Simone's avoidant style, and they interfered with my ability to constructively explore Simone's contribution to what was taking place between us.

Another more subtle element of my countertransference feeling emerged more clearly over time. When I first met Simone, I experienced her as especially attractive and was impressed by her lively, playful manner and sense of humor. I had found myself looking forward to working with her, and I won't deny that my attraction to her played some role in this. Over time, however, it occurred to me that Simone's physical attractiveness developed a type of abstract, disembodied quality for me. Although Simone continued to have a playful manner, I did not experience it as flirtatious at all, and I was somewhat surprised by what I experienced as a complete absence of any sexual attraction on my part toward her, despite the fact that I continued to find her beautiful in an abstract sense. I wondered to myself whether this aspect of my countertransference might be related to a tendency on her part to desexualize me in her mind in order to make our relationship safe for her. This is not a theme that evolved more fully or that we had time to explore during our work together.

Over time, I became aware of a quality of narcissistic grandiosity in Simone—a belief on her part that she had all the answers and that nobody else, including me, had anything of value to say to her. This attitude is not one that emerged explicitly at first but gradually over time as I became aware of my own countertranference feelings of not being able to say things that she really took in, and I was able to use my feelings as a point of departure for exploring what was going on in our relationship. Gradually, Simone was able to acknowledge that she didn't believe that I might have anything useful to say to her. Ultimately, she was able to articulate an underlying fear that if she did become more receptive, she would become dependent on me and vulnerable to abandonment. Over time, Simone and I were able to collaboratively make sense of her counterdependency and narcissistic defenses in term of her experiences of abandonment as a child, and she became more open to input from me. A central dilemma that emerged for her was the conflict between (1) fearing dependency on others and feeling that nobody (including myself) had anything of value to offer her and (2) desperately wishing that others would be able to introduce their subjectivity in a way that would help her feel less alone.

We explored these themes in a variety of different ways throughout the treatment. To provide one example, I will describe the way in which a dream that Simone reported in the fifth month of our work together led to an exploration of her ambivalent feelings regarding dependency in our relationship and provided hints of her complex feelings about sexuality, men and dependency, and our relationship. She reported this dream shortly after her father had invited her to temporarily move into an apartment he owned and in which he would stay periodically when he came to the city on business trips.

Simone: I'm with some people on a beach and they're playing with a puppy. And they've got the puppy partially submerged under the water . . . maybe to soothe it. But it's not happy. And so I decide to take over. . . . I see a male dog who I think is it's father . . . but it's interesting because this male dog has udders. So I take the puppy and put it on its father's udders and then the puppy seems happy.
Jeremy: What do you make of the dream?
Simone: Well, maybe the dog is actually my father, and maybe it has to do with me moving into his place.
Jeremy: That make sense . . . and I'm also thinking . . . and this is really just playing around with the images . . . so don't take what I'm saying too seriously, maybe the male dog is me.

I say this in a very tentative way so it will be easy for her to dismiss without feeling too dismissive and also in an attempt to gauge how capable she is of acknowledging feelings of intimacy and dependency in our relationship at this point.

Simone: I hadn't thought of that.
Jeremy: How does it feel?
Simone: I don't know . . . I'd have to think about it.

She then goes on to tell me another dream fragment.

Simone: And then in the dream, I see my old adviser from college, Emma . . . she's a woman, but then I look at her shadow and it's the shadow of a man.
Jeremy: What do you make of it?
Simone: I don't know.
Jeremy: I know from what you've told me previously that the last time you visited Emma you felt uncomfortable with her because she felt needy to you.

Earlier Simone had told me that Emma symbolizes neediness to her.

Simone: Well it's like the way she was always trying to look after me and offer me guidance, it felt like there as a kind underlying desperation . . . or neediness . . . like maybe she needs to relate to me as a daughter or something.

I wonder to myself if this might be another reference to our relationship. Perhaps Simone experiences my attempts to help her as representing a form of neediness on my part. But I decide not to explore this potential allusion to our relationship because of a concern that she will find it too threatening. Simone continued to talk about the dream at the following session.

Simone: I was thinking about that dream I had about that male dog with the udders . . . and it makes me feel uncomfortable.
Jeremy: Are you willing to explore what feels uncomfortable about it?

This is a form of defense analysis.

Simone: Well there's something yucky about it. I don't really like to think of myself as getting nurtured by you. There's something scary about it.
Jeremy: Scary in what way?
Simone: Well it would mean that I'm dependent on you and that brings up a whole bunch of feelings.

We continue to explore the range of feelings it brings up: fear, yearning, revulsion, fear of abandonment, and so on.

Simone: You're not really a father figure for me . . . it's like you're not really male. It's like you just exist in my head.

Jeremy: Can you say more about me not being male?
Simone: Well you don't give me advice or tell me what to do.
Jeremy: Would you want me to give you advice?
Simone: No.
Jeremy: Why not?
Simone: Because then I would become dependent on you. You're not like my father that way. Things are complicated with him.

At this point, Simone transitions into talking about her complicated feelings about what she refers to as "the sexual energy" between her and her father. She speaks about how her father always makes it clear to people that she is his daughter when he takes her out for dinner—as if to make sure that they don't assume they have a romantic relationship. She speaks about the fact that on occasion she has slept at her fathers' place when he is out of town and that she feels uncomfortable sleeping in his bed because she knows that he "entertains people there."

I speculate to myself that it is important for Simone to desexualize me in her mind because the potential of my playing a paternal role with her is threatening because of the sexual connotations for her. But again, I don't say anything at this point because I feel it would be premature.

The following session Simone spontaneously brought up the possibility that maybe the male dog with udders in her dream *does* represent me. We continued to explore what this possibility meant to her during this session, and the intertwined threads of conflict around dependency, sexuality, and romantic relationships with both men and women continued to unfold and become further illuminated throughout the treatment.

Approximately halfway through treatment, Simone became romantically involved with Jim, a 30-year old African American musician. Jim was the first male Simone had been romantically involved with since her adolescence. Over a period of time, Simone was able to genuinely contact her desire for Jim and her hope that things would work out between them. I never expressed a preference for Simone to become romantically involved with men rather than women, nor was I aware of experiencing such a preference. Although Simone was not able to explain her new interest in a romantic relationship with a man, I speculated to myself that the process of beginning to become more trusting of me, a male therapist, helped her to begin to experience men in general as safer and less likely to abandon her in the same way that her father had. This possibility was not, however, something I felt Simone was ready and able to explore explicitly in treatment, so I did not introduce it.

Ultimately, Jim rejected Simone. My impression was that she experienced this as excruciatingly painful, and she subsequently shut down and began once again to deny her need for him or for anyone else, including me. During this period, she flirted with the idea of leaving treatment and leaving the city to join an ashram associated with the cult she had joined. After a futile and extended attempt on my part to explore what was going on for her, I settled into providing more of a supportive, containing environment for her in which I would by and large attempt to mirror or empathize with the manifest level of her experience. After approximately two months of this, Simone began to become more emotionally open again, more receptive to exploration, and stopped talking about leaving treatment.

Subsequent to this, Simone began dating a number of men and ultimately settled into a relationship with a man named Scott. It was in the context of this relationship that she had sexual intercourse with a man for the first time since her adolescence. She subsequently moved in with Scott in a rather precipitous fashion and lived with him for approximately three months. During this period, she struggled with intensely ambivalent feelings about the increased intimacy and fears of dependency and engulfment.

We spent considerable time in therapy exploring the difficulty she had in negotiating between his needs and her own, and we also explored the parallel between the issue emerging in the relationship with Scott and the transference.

Over time, Simone found living with Scott increasingly intolerable, alternating between feeling that he was too needy and very occasionally acknowledging fears of abandonment and rejection. Eventually, she left him and then moved in with another man who was a member of the cult. At the same time she began to discuss the possibility of leaving treatment again, maintaining that she was feeling better and that she had accomplished the goals she had at the beginning of treatment. Over a period of time, I gently and tentatively explored with her the possibility that her wish to leave treatment was motivated (at least in part) by a desire to avoid the type of intensely ambivalent feelings evoked by the intimacy of our relationship. Gradually, she came to acknowledge that this was true and then began to settle in a phase of treatment during which she remained considerably more trusting and open for an extended period of time.

Although even during this phase Simone continued to vacillate between periods of self-reflection and periods of shutting down and emotional withdrawal from me, the intensity of these swings decreased considerably. During this phase, Simone substantially decreased her binging behavior and became less preoccupied with eating. She began to work on her art for the first time since ending college and was able to experience this as a source of satisfaction. Simone and I continued to explore her feelings of ambivalence about intimacy and her fear of dependency in both our relationship and relationships in general. She also began to talk more openly about feelings of being "different" because most of her friends were not black, and we began to explore ambivalent feelings about being in therapy with a white therapist. We explored the way in which Simone did not feel completely at home in either the white or black worlds and the way this contributed to her general feeling of alienation and isolation.

In the final six months of our work together, Simone became romantically involved with a new man named Jamal, and this relationship developed a more stable quality than her previous relationships had. Although she was not without feelings of ambivalence, she was better able to tolerate her feelings of dependency on Jamal and was less self-critical of her need for him. She began working on a more consistent basis in the health-food store and developed a plan to save up enough money to return to college with the help of her father's financial assistance and take courses.

Two months before ending treatment, Simone began to raise the possibility of termination. This time, however, things had a different feeling about them than they had previously. It was clear to both of us that she had made some important changes in her life. Although it was far from clear what the future would hold in terms of her current romantic relationship or her plans to return to college, there was a mutual sense that she had started on a different path than the one she had been on at the beginning of treatment. We set a termination date in advance, and over the remaining time together we explored both ways in which she had changed over the course of our work together as well as her feelings about termination.

At first, Simone denied any ambivalent feelings about leaving treatment and expressed an eagerness to "do things on her own" now that she no longer needed my help. I wondered to myself whether it might be a bit premature for her to leave treatment and had some concern that she would not be able to maintain the gains she had made. I also wondered whether her plans to terminate were once again related to her fears of intimacy and abandonment and distaste for dependency. At the same time, however, I considered the possibility that my reactions reflected my own reluctance to let go of her and perhaps a certain narcissism on my part and an overestimation of the significance of my own role in her life.

I disclosed some of these feeling to her, and this facilitated an ability on her part to begin to explore some of her ambivalent feelings about leaving treatment. She was ultimately able to acknowledge anxiety about becoming too dependent on me, fears about how her life would go after she left treatment, and, also toward the end, feelings of sadness about ending our relationship. When we ended treatment, I made it clear that she was welcome to contact me any time just to let me know how things were going or to schedule another session if she wished.

I received a letter from her about two years later. In it she told me that things were basically going well in her life. Apparently, she had left Jamal approximately four months after she had terminated treatment with me. Three months later, she had become romantically involved with another man, and they were still in a stable relationship. She was working for a small group as a graphic designer and was finding the work challenging but satisfying. Simone wrote that periodically she would still lapse into periods of binging, especially during difficult periods in her life (e.g., breaking up with Jamal). She wrote that in general, however, her binging was much more in control than it had been when she began treatment. Overall, Simone felt that her treatment with me was helpful, and I concurred. I had a sense that our work together reached a level of depth that allowed her to make significant changes in her life and significant internal changes as well. I also had the sense that there were many themes left unexplored and that Simone could potentially have benefited from more treatment. It seems possible that she may go into treatment again at some future point in her life, and she might even contact me at some point to explore the possibility of further treatment. At the same time, however, I believe that no story ever completely unfolds in any treatment. At any given point in time, a specific client and therapist are only able to go as deep and accomplish what they are both ready and able to accomplish at that time.

Editors' Introduction

This is a teaching case in the best sense: An example of Adlerian therapy conducted in the context of a graduate course in psychotherapy. Dr. Harold Mosak, a skilled Adlerian therapist, accepts the risks involved in permitting public scrutiny of his work, and in relatively few sessions he provides for new insights and behavioral change in a troubled young man.

This case involves a gay man struggling, in part, with issues of sexual identity. Mosak, like many Adlerians, unquestioningly sees this as a personal decision, and he tells his client, "Homosexuality is a choice, not a biological condition." Do you agree? Is it ever ethical for a therapist or counselor to attempt to change sexual orientation in a client, or even to support a client who desires to change? Does Mosak subtly try to shape his client's sexual values? Questions of sexual orientation and behavior inevitably arise with some clients, and you need to come to terms with your own feelings and beliefs about sexuality if you are going to be effective in helping others understand and respond to their feelings about these sometimes vexing issues.

We believe this is a good teaching case because it provides a meaningful springboard for class discussions of the ethical and professional issues associated with treating clients who may be dealing with sexual or gender identity concerns. In addition, the case illustrates the hands-on application of dozens of Adlerian techniques.

Mosak is more direct and focused, therapy is time-limited, and his style is didactic. This is a form of cognitive therapy that focuses on the values, beliefs, and attitudes of the client. Mosak and Maniacci do a masterful job in illustrating the core elements of individual psychotherapy.

2 | THE CASE OF ROGER

Harold H. Mosak and Michael Maniacci

Alfred Adler developed a theory and strategy of psychology and psychotherapy which have proven to be quite relevant to contemporary clinical and counseling practice. *Individual Psychology,* the name Adler gave his system, derives from the Latin *individuum,* and means "indivisible," emphasizing the holistic perspective that Adlerian psychology is built upon. Distinctions such as conscious and unconscious, mind and body, or approach and avoidance are subjective experiences; in reality, they are a part of a unified relational system. Individuals are viewed as being in movement towards subjectively determined goals which, though influenced by heredity and environment, are in the final analysis the result of choices made according to biased apperceptions. These biased apperceptions about self, others, and the world form a self-consistent cognitive and attitudinal set which organizes and directs movement towards the goal, and is called by Adlerians the *style of life.* The goal, though idiographic and individualized for specific people depending upon the particular circumstances in which they grew up and based upon certain choices they made, in general, is always designed to move individuals from a subjective sense of inferiority towards a sense of superiority, perfection, competence, or completion, from a felt minus situation towards a plus situation. Movement can take place in either of two directions: useful or useless. Useful, as defined by Adlerians, is that which moves with others in prosocial, egalitarian ways; useless is that which moves against others in self-centered, uncooperative ways. All behavior, both adaptive and maladaptive, is conceptualized as taking place within a social field. Behavior that is useful is that which is in line with social interest, a potentiality which requires development and encouragement.

Individuals who move in useless ways are not considered sick, but rather discouraged; they have underdeveloped social interest. They have selected goals which they attempt to move towards in self-centered rather than cooperative ways. Cognitively, they have a private logic which construes events and situations according to biased apperceptions that generally are distorted, overgeneralized, or exaggerated perceptions and are not in line with the less dogmatic common sense followed by most others. The main tasks of life are conceptualized as social tasks which require cooperation, not competition. Adler delineated three of these life tasks: work, friendship, and love. Later Adlerians delineated a fourth and a fifth implied in Adler's writings: a selftask and a spiritual task. Maladjustment is characterized by increased inferiority feelings, underdeveloped social interest, and an exaggerated, uncooperative goal of personal superiority.

Adler conceptualized psychotherapy as the awakening of the client's innate social interest. By explaining the client's subjective distress not as sickness but as discouragement

"The Case of Roger" was written specifically to complement Dr. Mosak's chapter in *Current Psychotherapies.*

due to the erroneous meaning given to life, Adler attempted to encourage the client to move towards a more useful, adaptive style of life. Such a change took place by examining how the client grew up and what choices he or she made. The client's family constellation, family atmosphere, family values and earliest recollections were explored in order to understand what particular goals towards which the individual was striving.

Rudolf Dreikurs described Adlerian psychotherapy as consisting of four processes: (a) forming a relationship; (b) investigating the client's life style; (c) interpreting it to the client; and (d) helping the client to reorient towards a more prosocial stance by modifying certain convictions held by the client and putting into practice more cooperative attitudes and behaviors. Though heuristically valuable, these should not be regarded as "phases" or "stages" in actual clinical practice. Interpretation may occur during every phase of the process, and the establishment and maintenance of a positive relationship will require ongoing effort. New material can be investigated throughout the course of treatment, and reorientation is encouraged beginning with the initial interview.

BACKGROUND AND REFERRAL

The case presented here was selected from the audio recordings of an eleven-week graduate psychotherapy course taught by the senior author at the Alfred Adler Institute of Chicago. "Roger" came to the counseling center at the Institute requesting services. After an intake interview, he agreed to participate in front of a class for a pre-established period of ten weeks at no charge.

Coming in shortly after his thirty-sixth birthday, Roger's major complaint was agoraphobia which had grown progressively worse for the past twelve years. Along with the agoraphobia, his intake sheet noted that he drank heavily, was overweight, was dissatisfied with his job (which he had managed to keep only at the expense of considerable anxiety), had multiple specific phobias, and was actively homosexual. Roger requested no treatment for his sexual orientation which he claimed was not a problem, except for the fact that his agoraphobia interfered with making contact with other gay men.

SESSION 1
FORMING A RELATIONSHIP
AND DEFINING THE PROBLEM

The session began with Mosak attempting to clarify the problem.

Therapist: O.K. What brings you to the Institute?
Client: I have a problem. I guess they call it agoraphobia, a fear of going out in the open. It's been getting steadily worse for the past ten or twelve years. Now it's getting to the point where I can hardly exist.
T: Is that why you brought a friend?
C: Yeah, somebody to go with me. . . .

The friend made it possible for Roger to move about outside. Roger went on to explain that his anxiety was not so acute if he knew where he was going; then at least he would know where he could "run and hide" along the way should he start to panic. He dealt with his anxiety by drinking "a fifth of wine" before his trips outside of his house.

C: . . . I think it's basically insecurity. In the past year I've had three different jobs, and I started a new job last week. I was a wreck for about a week before time, worrying about going to this place. I was frightened to death driving there . . . I had my brother take me and pick me up. But now that I've been there about a week I did it myself the past couple of days. But still, I worry all day about leaving work . . . If I hit traffic, I sit there and worry about getting into an accident. I might panic. It scares me.

T: You've said something twice now, and that is your symptom permits you to put other people into your service. You have to get somebody to accompany you down here, and for a week, you had to get your brother to drive you to work. It almost sounds like you feel pretty helpless and have to count on "the big boys" to take care of you.

The therapist is offering a tentative interpretation. Adlerian psychology is a psychology of use, not possession. For example, Adlerians do not say that someone has a bad temper, but rather that someone uses temper to intimidate others. The bad temper serves the individual's purpose. In Roger's case, Mosak reframes the symptom to show how it is used: Roger is putting others into his service and though he may not totally be aware (conscious) of it, he is responsible for it.

T: What have you done about it [*the agoraphobia*] for the past twelve years?
C: Well, try to cope with it the best I can . . . avoid certain things, avoid certain areas, don't go into the woods or take vacations or do things you normally would do.

Adler considered a neurosis an evasion of the tasks of life. Roger has constricted life to the point where it is manageable. He is saying, in effect, that he will only operate where he feels secure.

T: Yeah, but that doesn't overcome it. That's living within the confines of your symptom . . . Have you done anything about trying to overcome the symptom?
C: Yeah, I went to a psychiatrist downtown for a while. He gave me Thorazine and it made me sick. I never went back to him. In fact, he made me nervous . . . He really didn't seem to care about the problem that much. He made a comment, he said: "You seem mainly interested in yourself . . . I think you're an egotist." That kind of bothered me . . . He was flippant with me too—we just didn't hit it off.

The message is clear. Roger is warning his new therapist: Take me and my problems seriously or else I will not return. In effect, he is saying he wants someone to care about him. If he feels others do not care, his mode of action is consistent with his style of life—he becomes "nervous" and avoids them (in this case his former psychiatrist). Roger did not feel understood by his last therapist.

T: If I had a magic wand and could wave it over your head and get rid of this agoraphobia . . . what would be different in your life?

This is known as *The Question*. Adlerians use it to determine the purpose of the symptom and to differentiate somatic from psychogenic disorders. It is also usually indicative of what is being avoided—that is, for what purpose the symptom is generated.

C: It would take away a lot of the fears, frustrations of planning ahead. You see, I have to plan my week . . . I've got to make arrangements with friends to pick me up and drive me back . . . I could just float and enjoy life . . . I had to give up several good [job] positions because I'm afraid to fly.
T: Suppose I could get you to take a plane ride with me to Los Angeles? Suppose I would take care of whatever would happen at the other end?
C: You're on.

Without realizing it, Roger has told Mosak the purpose of his agoraphobia: he wants to be in control. Without his symptoms, he would not have to "plan ahead" and get others to look after him. The symptoms provide him with the excuse to dictate to others and have them in his service.

The rest of the session involved an exploration of the tasks of life. The extent to which individuals function adequately in each of these areas is a barometer of their level of social interest. Roger rated himself in this way:

Work: Poor. He had to arrange for others to be with him. His symptoms were beginning to interfere with his role as a manager in the trucking business. He had to drink every morning to get to the office.

Friendship: His friendships came mostly through his homosexual contacts, which were being affected by his agoraphobia.

Love: He was engaged once, but she broke it off. He had never had intercourse with a woman but he had frequent sexual relations with men. Roger claimed this area was not a problem.

Self: Basically, Roger thought he was a good person, but he was dissatisfied with his weight. He added that he didn't like himself—he felt "ugly inside." He was also worried about becoming alcoholic.

Spiritual: Roger was raised a devout Catholic. He still prayed and lit candles but avoided confession due to his sexual orientation. When he claimed, "*I* don't need confession," Mosak noted that "Even the Pope has a confessor." Roger replied without a hint of humor, "He needs it more than *I* do."

In conclusion, Roger was offered encouragement. He felt that at thirty-six, it was "too late in life" to continue with much else. He expressed openly his discouragement with himself and his inability to move ahead with his life. Mosak mentioned a former colleague who did not start medical school until he was forty-seven. However, Roger only wanted to work on his agoraphobia, and he seriously doubted his ability to overcome it.

The interview concluded with the therapist structuring the next two sessions, a technique especially effective with controllers. Roger would be meeting with a co-therapist who would be gathering the data for a *Life Style Assessment,* a form of investigation which Adlerians use to understand the goals, intentions, and biased apperceptions of clients. While Mosak implicitly made it clear that he was in control of the process, he respected Roger's desire to be in control.

In summary, Roger is a controller who uses passive means of controlling others. At thirty-six, his passive means of controlling (via his agoraphobia) has begun to exact a toll that even Roger can no longer tolerate, and he has begun therapy. He has strong inferiority feelings and underdeveloped social interest, as indicated by his poor overall functioning in the life tasks. Despite his poor self-concept, he still considers himself somewhat superior (he has higher standards than the Pope). The therapist has shown that he understands Roger's problems, that he takes them seriously, and that he is willing to align his goals with the client's, therefore reducing resistance. Most importantly, he has encouraged Roger, who is seriously discouraged, and he has given him hope.

SESSIONS 2–3
THE LIFE STYLE INTERVIEW

The next two sessions were spent with the co-therapist gathering Life Style Assessment data. Adlerians frequently practice *multiple psychotherapy* and have documented its benefits.

The Life Style Assessment is a diagnostic procedure which investigates the client's past and present situation in order to come to an understanding of the particular person's way of construing the world, other people, and ideas about self. Understanding the premises upon which a client operates helps to tailor treatment to the particular client and brings idiographic relevance to the nomothetic principles of Individual Psychology. The primary areas of investigation are the client's family constellation, which includes sibling descriptions, ratings, and an investigation of parental guiding lines and the family atmosphere, and the client's earliest recollections, the earliest memories the client can visualize and report to the therapist. Through this investigation, the therapist and client can arrive at an understanding of the particular client's personal history and current beliefs.

SESSION 4
THE LIFE STYLE SUMMARY

Mosak and the co-therapist spent the fourth session discussing the Life Style Summary with Roger. First the co-therapist read the recorded data to Mosak. Some highlights follow:

> Roger, age thirty-six, is the oldest in his family. He has a sister, Ginger, minus two (i.e., two years younger), a brother Evan, minus six, a brother, Arthur, minus nine and another brother died in childhood after Arthur. Roger described himself as a dreamer who fantasized a lot, had delusions of grandeur, looked at the world through rose-colored glasses, and who was happy through the age of six/seven. He was sexually promiscuous with boys and girls; they played show and tell. He was overweight as were his siblings. He had the usual arguments/fights with his sister—she is described as dumb and slovenly.
>
> Evan was described as being very precocious, very personable. He loved everyone, everyone loved him, both adults and kids . . . He was more masculine than Roger. Arthur was born handicapped and was always overprotected. He was allowed to have his own way.
>
> Evan was most different—more outgoing and more gregarious. Ginger was most like Roger. She was feminine and he could relate to her more.
>
> As a youngster Roger was afraid of his father, who seemed like a tyrant. Roger was the most intelligent and the most industrious and he had higher standards of achievement. Evan was more athletic, rebellious, better looking, more masculine, and made more mischief. Roger was always overweight and he was the last to be picked for sports.
>
> Roger originally hated school and his mother had to keep taking him out of school. He hated other kids and felt inferior. There were no problems with behavior and Roger was smart enough to keep his mouth shut. He was a patrol boy in the fourth and fifth grades and he enjoyed the role. He was "the captain" who liked having other people under him.
>
> Roger's father would have been fifty-seven but he died in 1965. He was a truck driver and Roger didn't like him. The father used to beat Roger's mother and he chased them out of the house with a gun when he was drunk. He was seldom sober and he was always in a rotten mood. He was filthy and he took family possessions and sold them for booze.
>
> The mother is fifty-nine years old and a housewife. She held the family together; she did the cooking and baking. She was always complaining about her ill health and how close she was to dying. She tried to play on everyone's sympathy and she was usually successful. Roger was most like her.

The co-therapist went on to describe the stormy and troubled marriage of Roger's parents. The mother saw herself as a "martyred saint." They had violent fights. Two other paternal uncles lived with them. Both were ex-convicts and one had five marriages, all ending in divorce; the other was an alcoholic. Mosak dictated the following summary.

SUMMARY OF FAMILY CONSTELLATION

Roger is the oldest of four, in a 2-2 family, which makes him the older of two and the only boy in his group. He grew up in a family characterized by poverty and ethnic and marital discord, a family in which all the men acted as arms of the devil. The father was an alcoholic, a tyrant, abusive, and a squanderer of the family's money. Both uncles were thieves. One was moody in the negative sense, and the other was a playboy with five wives. The only positive model was Roger's mother, but she overdid a good thing. She was not only the standard bearer of good; she was also a martyr and a saint. Nevertheless, Mother was also a fearful person who, in spite of her religious faith, didn't believe that God would preserve her. Roger grew up hating his father, and determined that if all men were like his father and uncles, he wasn't going to be like that. He adopted his mother's standards of rightness and like her, opted for sainthood. Nevertheless, he fell short, but even though he acknowledged at times that he was wrong, he was still "righter" than others. He sat in judgment upon the whole world and himself—they were beneath him and he looked down upon them or expressed temper when he had too much of their wrong. He also looked down upon himself since he too was not all he felt he should be. He was fat in a family where being fat was bad. He was sexually active and this was bad. He was having negative feelings and for an observant Catholic, the thought was as sinful as the deed. He rested his feeling of belonging upon his intelligence, trying to be good, trying to be right, and staying out of trouble because that would make him like the men. He wanted to be a real man, and his sexual promiscuity was evidence of his pursuit. But somewhere along the line, Roger became discouraged, because (a) he misdefined masculinity (e.g., Evan was more masculine because he was more athletic), (b) he could not identify with the male role models in his family, and (c) he couldn't resolve the conflict between "goodness" and masculinity. In Roger's mind, one couldn't be good *and* a man simultaneously. He grew up unhappy partly because of the climate in which he grew up, partly because of his exalted standards for himself and others, partly because of his disdain for other people, and partly because of his disdain for himself.

T: Roger, how does that sound as a summary of the way you grew up?
C: Yeah—very much [*noticeably shaken*]. I think you hit it on the head.

They then went on to review the early recollections. The co-therapist read them aloud.

1. I went to first grade, I didn't go to kindergarten. The teacher asked me to do something—I told her to go to hell . . . [Age 5.]
2. I remember sitting in church. I stared at the statue of Christ on the cross. I was told that if you stared at it long enough, you could see Christ come off the cross. I got very excited and agitated—only saints were supposed to be able to do that. I imagined Christ coming towards me . . . [Age 7; Feeling excited.]
3. I remember an aunt of mine. She had come over with presents. I loved her . . . Everybody loved her. She was a very joyful woman. I was in total awe of her . . . [Age 5–6; Feeling awe.]
4. My mother got pregnant. My father was swearing at her and saying something about getting rid of it. He was going to stick his hand up her and pull it out. [Age 7; Feeling scared.]
5. They [the parents] had a couple that used to come over every weekend—a Polish couple. They started fighting. I remember specifically this woman talking about her sex life, that she wanted it, he didn't. The woman was crying in the kitchen . . . The husband telling her that she's a lousy lay anyway . . . [Age 8; Feeling "something I didn't understand—why was it so important."]

Early recollections are those memories which individuals store and use to assist them in moving through life. They reflect how people perceive life currently, and are quite effective as projective techniques. Mosak proceeded to dictate a note about Roger's view of life, self, and others, and noted Roger's "Basic Mistakes" and "Assets."

SUMMARY OF EARLY RECOLLECTIONS

"Nobody should tell me what to do; otherwise I balk. Men and women get along poorly and the conflict generally has to do with sex. I just can't understand what the conflict's all about. Men brutalize women and all women can do is suffer. Women, independent of men, can radiate warmth and joy. I stand in awe of them but I keep my distance and do not get involved with them. If I did want to get involved, it would be too late anyway. I want to be purged of all sin and be in union with God."

BASIC MISTAKES

1. He doesn't see the possibility of good man/woman relationships. Put a man and a woman in a cage and the blood is going to start to flow.
2. Roger idealizes women, feels he can't have them, and distances himself from them.
3. Roger wants to do it his way. "No one has the right to tell me what to do."
4. Roger tries too hard to be perfect because he regards himself as so much less than perfect.

ASSETS

1. He has positive feelings for women.
2. He does try to be better.
3. He uses religion for sanctification rather than downgrading himself.
4. Even though he is confused, he tries to figure things out.
5. He has a vivid fantasy life. He's had excellent training in it.
6. In many ways he comes close (though not in terms of birth order) to Joseph in the Bible: the one who can read omens in dreams, who has great dreams about the sun, moon, and planets.

T: O.K. Roger, that's our summary. [*Roger gets up to leave.*] No—don't get up yet.
C: I thought we were through.
T: No, just with the summary. Now that's how it looks to us. How do you feel about it?
C: I think it's pretty interesting about the women.
T: About the women?
C: Yeah . . . about not really relating to them—putting them on a pedestal. In my life I have a lot of women friends and they're all looked at this way—and none of them are really with men.
T: Yeah, that comes out in your recollection . . .
C: In fact any woman who's close to me doesn't have a relationship with men . . .
T: Yeah, well men are all bastards anyway.
C: Then why am I sleeping with them?
T: Maybe that's so you can look down on them and look down on yourself?

C: [*Sighing—noticeably shaken*] Maybe it's just too much for me to comprehend right now.

T: O.K. We'll talk about that some more later. You said that the reading of the material was getting to you. What was getting to you?

C: . . . Just thinking about things I've tried to avoid thinking about for a long time.

T: Do you feel understood?

C: Right now—more so than I have in a long time.

T: You see, while what we wrote may not be 100% accurate, it's our first guess about you—

C: I'd say it's a good 95%.

T: And on that basis we have some things that we can already start talking about. If something is wrong, we'll modify it. Now next week we're going to talk a little about this, but we're also going to start talking about your present situation, because basically, that's the thing you've got to change. We may refer to some things in your childhood, but basically we're going to be talking about your fears . . . your job, and all those kinds of things you told us about in the first interview.

C: Very good—I'm looking forward to it.

T: Good. See you next week.

C: Thank you. Goodnight. [*Addressing the class*] Goodnight.

Roger, from wanting to talk only about his symptoms, is now examining his way of relating to the world and other people. Through the use of the Life Style Assessment, he is examining his view of life. Even the previously taboo subject of his homosexuality is now open for discussion and was raised by Roger himself. What was once unconscious and never clearly formulated has now been brought to light and presented to him in a way he can grasp and in his own language, using his own metaphors and imagery. He is told before he leaves that he is to be prepared at the next session to discuss his present situation since that is what he has to change.

SESSIONS 5–9
MODIFYING CONVICTIONS

The fifth session opened with Mosak asking Roger what he remembered from the previous session, two weeks ago (Roger had been sick and missed a week).

C: Well, let's see. I think I remember the fact that there were more good points than bad points about myself. Also, the tendency to put women on a shrine . . . and feel that they're untouchable. I also made a comment that I never have women who have anything to do with men totally as friends. . . .

Roger was obviously struck by the fact that the therapist included more "good points" (i.e., assets) than "bad points." Roger is discouraged, and hearing assets included in his Life Style Assessment encouraged him and helped strengthen the therapeutic relationship. He reports that he was impressed by his new understanding of his attitude towards women. Mosak reread the entire Life Style Assessment summaries and discussed some of the points with him.

T: Now, as you hear it a second time today, Roger, what does it sound like?

C: It doesn't sound like anybody I know.

T: It doesn't?

C: No.

T: And yet two weeks ago you gave me a grade of "95." So what's happened in the two weeks?

C: I feel like a different person now.
T: You feel like you've changed.
C: Yeah.
T: Would you identify for me what the change is like or maybe how or what happened?
C: I don't know what happened. First of all I feel a little more sure of myself today. I feel less emotional today, not as embarrassed.
T: What was wrong with the emotional feeling you had?
C: I don't like to show emotion.
T: Why?
C: It's a sign of weakness.
T: Is it?
C: I think so. I try to be rather cold and calculating most of the time.
T: Where did you learn that emotion was a sign of weakness?
C: Well, I don't like to put up with anybody who shows emotion. I don't have the patience for anybody who starts crying in front of me or starts pouring out their heart to me—I don't like it at all.
T: I see. So if you don't show emotion or other people are not permitted to show emotion to you, then you can keep your distance from them?
C: Yeah. It's like somebody saying that they love you—to me it's a negative word. I don't ever use it because it's stupid. Nobody ever really loves anybody.

Mosak raised the issue of Roger's style of relating to people. Hearing one's style of life summarized can have a disorienting effect upon one's self-image and perspective of others and life. Roger grew emotional upon hearing it, and that bothered him. The therapist interpreted Roger's dampening of emotions as a method for keeping distance from others. As Roger went on to point out, getting close to people meant getting hurt, and he wanted no more pain in his life. By "cutting off" his emotions, he attempted to protect himself.

Roger sees life *vertically* rather than *horizontally*—that is, he is concerned with who is better than or on top of whom. People are not equals cooperating for a common cause and working together; they are "out to get you." This is evident in Roger's agoraphobia: if he does not get too far out of his house, people will not get too close to him.

T: So for you the important goal is to be dominant in every relationship. There's a master and a slave and by golly—
C: I like to call the shots.
T: You better be the master.
C: Um hmm, yeah. I'm the leader too . . .
T: Will you do something for me, Roger? While there's no way for us to predict what's going to happen, I'd like you to compose, since you have a great fantasy life, a future autobiography . . . Ten years from now you'll be forty-five years old. What do you think your life will be like?
C: It could go either way. If this therapy-thing works out, I might be quite a fantastic individual . . . have a lover, a beautiful home somewhere, travel a lot . . .
T: Supposing therapy doesn't take, as it were?
C: Well, I think ten years from now I would just be a bum . . . I would just sell everything, have long hair, and look like Jesus Christ walking down the street . . . It might be rather interesting.
T: No problems, but what meaning?
C: It's better to be a king of derelicts than not a king at all.
T: As you just put it, in ten years, if therapy takes you'll be doing something fantastic . . . and if not, you'll be the king of the derelicts.
C: One way or another I'm going to make it.

Roger is exhibiting what Adler called *antithetical modes of apperception.* He'll either be the best or the worst. The strong sense of inferiority and superiority are two sides of the same coin and the basic problem is the meaning Roger has given to life: He must be the best. With that as a prerequisite for relating, he runs into considerable difficulty in life. The goal at this point in treatment is to encourage Roger to begin relating horizontally to others.

T: Roger, you're counting on your mentality [*Roger's term for "intellect"*] to dominate people . . . What if you met your match?

C: . . . Maybe you're my match.

T: What if somebody gets to you through feelings? What then? . . . You see, two weeks ago, we got to you through feeling.

C: I know—that bothered me all the way home.

T: You see, I didn't see you as submissive [*Roger earlier had referred to himself as "submissive" for showing feelings*]. I saw you as feeling. You're the one who attached "feeling equals weakness." I attached to it "feeling equals humanity." By golly, the guy's human.

C: Yeah, but that phase is over.

T: Oh, I don't know—Isn't it possible I might get you again?

C: It's possible.

T: How hard are you going to defend yourself against it?

Roger claimed he did not have to defend himself in therapy, and Mosak pointed out that no, he did not have to but that in fact he *did*. Roger pointed out that he would be "mortified" if he ran into any of the class on the street—he is afraid to look any of them in the face. The therapist drew a parallel between that and his behavior toward others in general: He keeps his distance from others. When asked if anyone in the room really cared about him, Roger flatly, and sincerely, replied, "No."

C: If I threw myself out the window right now, nobody would shed a tear.

T: Do you think any of them would try and stop you?

C: No. Why would they? They might get their names in the paper tomorrow. That's why they would stop me . . . [*They'd be famous.*]

T: Supposing somebody grabbed you [before you jumped out]? What would you feel?

C: Maybe they'd want to go to bed with me, I don't know.

T: But that's the only reason?

C: They'd probably push me out after one night.

T: So it's inconceivable that anybody would really care?

C: People really don't care about people that much. They put on a good front, but basically—

T: Are you speaking about people or are you speaking about Roger?

C: Just in general.

T: Roger—Do I care? [*Mosak is introducing the issue of "love."*]

C: I'd like to think you care. I'm not sure though.

T: What makes me the exception?

C: Financial gain.

T: I don't get one penny for seeing you.

C: I know that—I appreciate that. But, you get [money] from these people in here [the class].

T: I don't get one penny from them.

C: [*Surprised*] I apologize, I didn't know that. [*Apologizes repeatedly.*]

T: So the best you can do is accuse me of being interested in you as a case study . . .

C: [*Still apologizing sheepishly.*]

T: You've got to find some other reason [than financial gain]—that ain't it. What makes me different? Why might I possibly care for you? Because I'll tell you—You try and go out that window and I'm going to grab you.

C: Maybe you don't want the notoriety—bad for business.

T: Yeah, you're right. But on the other hand, maybe I want the fame? . . . My name would get in the paper. [*Long pause*] Why might I possibly care?

C: I was thinking about that—I'm really rather confused . . . I mentioned it to a friend as a matter of fact—I asked "Why is this man even bothering?"

T: That's my question . . .

C: Feelings of being a great humanitarian?

T: Not really. Not by seeing one patient for free . . .

C: Yeah, that's true.

T: What's my game?

C: Maybe you thought it was an interesting case? . . .

T: You know, Roger, after thirty years—

C: Nothing is new—

T: Yeah . . . [I've dealt with about everything.] Why am I bothering?

C: [*Subdued*] Give me a week to think about it.

T: I will. I hope you will.

C: I am going to think about it.

T: Good, because that's a crucial issue . . . it is not only important in terms of your therapy, but it's important for your life. Because if one person can care for you, then you'll have to ask another question, and that is, maybe two can.

C: [*Somewhat choked up*] It's very difficult for me to believe it.

The interview concluded on that note. Roger added that he does listen to what his therapist talks about. He came to the therapy session alone, and has found it easier and easier to move about unescorted outside. He has also been driving to work with greater ease. Roger commented, "I just wanted you to know that." The drinking had decreased noticeably as well. Asked how he accounted for it, Roger replied, "It's an awakening to reality, finding out I am a somebody."

This session, along with the previous one (the Life Style Assessment interview), was a turning point in treatment. Roger, having begun to accept himself as "a somebody," was losing his feelings of inferiority. The less inferior he felt, the easier time he had with healthy, consensual interaction. He no longer had to *safeguard* himself against what he feared would be a horrible fate if he exposed himself and his imperfections to others.

The sixth session began with Roger claiming to have been doing a lot of thinking. "I haven't wasted so much time in my life as I thought," he reported. His gains, from a behavioral standpoint, continued to grow as he attempted more activities independently. Mosak encouraged even more, and used task-setting (i.e., homework) to continue the growth.

T: So my question, Roger, is what can we do—since apparently you do want to live a happier life—to help you live a happier life? . . .

Mosak is using the pronoun "we." He is communicating to Roger that therapy is a collaborative enterprise, and that human interaction can be one of mutual respect and cooperation.

C: Well, can the people here [the class] make suggestions?

T: No, they're only permitted to be observers.

C: Well, can you make suggestions?

T: I can, but I don't think I want to, Roger, because I don't think that would do you any good. And being committed to your welfare I don't think I would want to do anything that wasn't for your good . . .

THE CASE OF ROGER 23

The responsibility for therapy is squarely on Roger's shoulders. The message being communicated is this: We may be in this together, but *you* are in charge of your life and are ultimately responsible for it, for better or worse. Should any action or homework assignment "backfire," Roger will not be able to blame anybody. He will be responsible.

Roger decided to attend the opera—provided that he could sit in the back row. Roger also agreed to go to the Art Institute. Mosak readily agreed and showed "faith" in Roger's ability to do it. Roger wondered why things had become so hard for him to do. "When I was twenty-one, it was easier," he commented.

T: Because at twenty-one, you apparently got discouraged about yourself and at twenty-one you "came out."

C: Yeah, at twenty-one, exactly.

T: Somewhere along that period, you apparently became discouraged.

C: Well, what happened? What caused the total disintegration . . . ?

T: Well, my guess is, that as time went on your confidence in yourself eroded because you weren't going anywhere in life. And then you have a few bad experiences tossed in [*Roger was deeply hurt by his first lover*], and you weave all of those things together, and you say, "Well, what's the use?" And that's the point I would like to turn around. Because I think people function better when they are encouraged than when they're discouraged.

C: I found out an important thing this week . . . I can't stand disappointments or anybody rejecting me. I never realized how deep rooted it was . . . It goes deeper than just lovers, even people, friends—as a consequence I really go overboard with people as far as being overly generous with gifts, entertaining, so forth.

T: You mean you try to buy their approval?

C: Yeah, a little too much so.

T: Why do you think you need their approval so badly?

C: I don't know, I just don't think I could exist without it.

Roger is overcompensating for his perceived inferiority in the eyes of others. His low opinion of himself, combined with his high standards, convinced him that no one would be able to "truly" care for him, therefore, he bought their approval. Mosak placed Roger's goal into perspective.

T: . . . I don't think any of us could exist, Roger, if we didn't have some approval—but do we *have* to have everybody's approval, and do we *have* to have everybody's approval constantly?

C: That's my problem. I need it constantly. I've got to be constantly wanted, constantly sought after . . .

T: Roger, your desire to please and to buy people—that kind of thing—and your fearing their rejection or disapproval of you is really a very ambitious kind of goal. You see, as a Catholic you believe in God, and here is God, the most perfect Being, right? Does everybody love God?

C: [*Very softly*] No.

T: Some people even reject Him?

C: [*Again, very softly*] Definitely.

T: And even the people who love God—do they love God constantly? So here is God, the most perfect Being, willing to take his chances with human beings—but you're not willing to take the same chances that even God takes.

C: Good point.

T: Do you think you might want to take the same chances with humanity God does? . . . And if somebody rejects you . . . there are always atheists!

C: Doesn't make them an atheist if they reject me, does it? [*Laughing.*]

T: Well, in a sense, it does.

C: In my mind it would—Saint Roger is not being venerated. True—[*laughing again*] very true.

T: . . . Perhaps, Roger, you have a place, even if somebody does reject you?

Roger, needing caring and approval, is afraid of rejection, and Mosak confronts him with the unrealistic and unattainable nature of his goals. He even gets Roger to joke about it. If he gets too intimate with people, they have some control over him, and if he gives up control, they are liable to hurt him—and the surest way to hurt Roger is to reject him. Therefore Roger will attempt to control ("dominate," to use Roger's language) his relationships. What he cannot control, he does not want. If he does it too actively, he is afraid of being too much like his father; therefore he will do it passively, like his mother, through fears and suffering (i.e., agoraphobia). Roger assumes that in order for him to be "relaxed" he must be in control. Mosak is attempting to convince him that maybe he can be *more* in control by being *less* in control.

Roger raised the issue of his engagement when he was nineteen. The discussion which followed highlighted the above issues.

C: I was engaged to a young woman . . . we got along beautifully. She would get me aroused—to a point—but not to actual intercourse, and I broke it off with her . . . Her closing statement to me was "You're queer." Now evidently she picked something up. In the two years I was with her there was no rejection. This is before I even came out and knew what a homosexual was.

T: Well, first of all, her calling you a queer, when you had not come out, was certainly rejection. She was telling you that she was plenty mad at you . . . But secondly, my feeling is that she called you a queer not because she sensed anything, but having tried to arouse you over and over and over again and your not responding, she just had to rub your nose in it. She was just plain mad at you because here she is having gone to all that trouble and you're not going to respond. I don't think she sensed anything.

C: Yeah, it does seem to fall into place.

They continued to explore Roger's relationship to men and women. Roger moved back to the topic of his homosexuality. Of the many possible reasons they discussed for it, three were meaningful to Roger: (a) He had a very low opinion of men and rejected the masculine role while growing up; (b) It was easier to be homosexual than heterosexual. There were no commitments, fewer responsibilities, and less intimacy; and (c) Roger was very concerned that a woman would control him, whereas he could control a man more easily. The interview concluded with a discussion about a woman who had been trying to seduce Roger for the past few weeks.

T: What would happen if you succumb to this girl who is out to seduce you?

C: I would be afraid that I would get involved emotionally.

T: And?

C: I don't know what would happen. It just goes against my mentality or grain. I just can't accept it, that's all.

T: So, you apparently are not willing to rule out that it could ever happen?

C: [*Laughing*] You really know how to get to me.

T: [*Laughing with him*] I hope so.

C: I don't believe you. You're right, I didn't say "No." So maybe I'm not ruling out the idea of it ever happening.

T: Apparently not.

The session ended with one additional point about Roger's homosexuality: Homosexuality is a choice, not a biological condition. If Roger is to choose it, he needs to choose it for "good" reasons, and not out of fear and insecurity.

The seventh session opened with Roger in very good spirits. He had spent a half hour standing on a busy downtown street watching people go by and enjoyed it. The discussion led to him asking about the nature of fears.

T: You see, the only people who have difficulties with fears are those that have to be in control. If you feel you have to be in control, there's so much you have to be afraid of because there are so many things that can go wrong.
C: Well why does somebody get that way? . . .
T: They lose their courage . . . You see, courage is the willingness to take a risk, even if you don't know what's going to happen . . . or even if there's a chance it might go against you.
C: I'm not a coward. I mean I'd fight if I had to or defend myself if I had to . . .
T: You're talking about a total coward, in some areas you think of yourself as a coward. When you're afraid to leave your house, alone, you're a coward. Aren't you?
C: Yeah, but I don't want to think of myself as a coward . . .
T: Well, what is a coward?
C: Someone who's afraid of something.
T: [*Laughing*] By that definition, I guess, in some areas, you're a coward.
C: [*Somewhat taken aback*] No one's ever called me that before.
T: Well, I haven't called you that—
C: Well, you're intimating it.
T: No, I haven't called you that—I'm saying *you think* of yourself as a coward.
C: [*Very softly*] A tough front.
T: Did you hear what you just said? A "tough front" implies that that's not what you are. Strip the front away and you've got somebody who's afraid.
C: I come on very strong with people though, I suppose.
T: A lot of cowards do. They hope that nobody will pick them out . . .
C: But I deal with dockmen, you know, truck drivers. Now I can really buffalo them . . .
T: But in intimate relationships—and I'm not talking about sexual relationships—
C: No, no—
T: Between people, you're scared.
C: Well, I don't have any intimate relationships with people . . .
T: Sure, you see yourself as a coward. You're unwilling to risk it.
C: Why does it have to be cowardly because you're unwilling to risk an intimate relationship? Why do you have to have an intimate relationship?
T: You don't have to, but there's a difference between "I choose not to have any," and "I'm afraid to have any."
C: I'll buy that.

The therapist is working in two directions here. First, he is working to assure that the gains made with the agoraphobia will last. By reframing the symptoms as indicative of a loss of *courage,* Roger's ability to rationalize was greatly diminished. Adlerians call this technique "spitting in the soup." He may still choose to do it, but it will certainly not "taste" as good. With the therapeutic relationship well established, Mosak became more *confrontive* in his interpretive style.

The other direction the therapist was taking involved motivating Roger to engage others meaningfully. Given the limited number of sessions, Mosak was working on Roger's attitude of being "tough" with others. He may be tough when he is in control (e.g., at work with subordinates), but intimately, one-to-one, he is a "coward." Again, the distinction is made between *having* to choose something out of fear and *choosing* to do something due to preference: Roger is choosing out of fear. The discussion rapidly turned to Roger's overall distaste for people in general.

T: You told me that you did all kinds of things to sort of buy people's favor. Why would you want to do that for people who are basically stinkers? . . .

C: I think it's more interesting inviting [over to his home] people you dislike . . . you can prove your superiority to them, put them down . . .

T: Yeah, but then, at least I've been taught—and I happen to think there's a large element of truth in it—that people that have to buy their superiority by pushing other people down don't think very much of themselves in the first place.

C: That may be true but it still is a nice feeling—

T: And that, as you say—

C: [Bitterly] Revenge is sweet . . .

T: Instead of having to talk about *them* [the people Roger looks down upon], let's talk about your inferiority feelings . . . What makes you inferior?

C: A combination of things—the area I was born in, the environment, family, we were a bunch of fat slobs. I didn't want anybody to even see them—I'd be ashamed.

T: What's that got to do with you? . . .

C: I always felt I was cheated because I never really had a good family life . . .

T: Well, I'd say to that perhaps, tough. I feel regret that you didn't have a better family life, but, what's that got to do with today, feeling inferior? A lot of people have transcended their early, unhappy family life. . . .

C: It's my perfection again . . . I won't even go out of the house if . . .

T: In other words, to be equal to the rest of us you have to be perfect, without blemish.

C: Well, I have to be above—I like admiration . . . [Emotionally] All my life I've been put down, with people making fun of me—calling me a fat slob, a pig . . . Now I want people to look at me and I want to be wanted, I want them to eat their hearts out to get at me—male or female. I want them to really just lust after me . . .

T: You said something which just threw me there for a moment.

C: What's that?

T: Male or female to lust over me. Why both?

C: Why both? I enjoy a woman who adores me or wants to go to bed with me, especially when I say no. It turns me on . . .

T: It turns you on to turn them on?

C: [Sheepishly] Yeah, sexually.

T: So basically, you want to get revenge on the world for giving you a bad time growing up?

C: It didn't end at growing up. It continued on and on.

T: So you want to hurt the world back?

C: [Remorsefully] People know how to hurt. They know how to stick a knife in you. Nobody knows the private misery people go through because somebody will just say, "My God—you've gained weight. You look like hell," or whatever the case may be . . .

T: So you plan to continue with your fight against the world?

C: No, I'm tired of fighting . . .

T: It sounds like you're preparing to fight for the rest of your life.

C: If need be . . .

They continued to discuss Roger's stance towards others. Adler described neurotics as going through life as if they were in hostile territory, and that is Roger's movement through life exactly. Mosak encouraged him to change his attitude—about himself, especially.

T: Maybe you want to stop fighting?

C: I'm willing, but—

T: But they aren't?
C: But they aren't exactly. I'm more than willing [*passionately*], I'm tired of fighting. I've been fighting for a long time.
T: There's only one way to tell you're tired—not if your mouth says so, but if you put your fists down.

Mosak encouraged him to choose different friends, ones that would not find so many faults and who would not be so ready to "fight." "I would much rather have friends who are going to treat me well," his therapist added.

C: You know what—you're right. This week I went through a whole list of people I know—mentally, and I started cutting them out. And I must agree with you, some of them are real assholes. They always have been assholes and why I've been bothering with them ten, fourteen years I don't know.
T: Good . . . Is it possible you might want to choose someone who isn't an asshole?

Roger agreed to make the effort. Mosak invited him to have an "easier life": Life, as Roger had been living it, must have been awfully tough. Roger conceded he has a "chip" on his shoulder when he meets people. He expects them to be hostile. Mosak *created an image* for Roger to keep in mind when he met new people.

C: Now I'm going to have to think they're a nice person.
T: Why do you have to think that? Just look them over . . . Why don't you just experience them, just get to know them without any preconceptions about whether they're nice or lousy? . . . Have you ever seen two dogs engaged in sniffing behavior? [*Both laugh.*] They look each other over, you know? . . .
C: [*Laughing*] So you want me to go "sniffing"?
T: Yeah, sniffing around, exactly . . .
C: Then I'll have my fear of rejection again . . .
T: So what—you mean everybody has to love you? Remember, even God doesn't have that privilege. If you know you're good enough, you don't have to worry about what they think.
C: It's time to start taking my shrine apart, right? Someone told me that, about my house. He says you're building a shrine to yourself. And at the time I was really upset. Now I realize he was right. [*Long pause*] Completely. That's something I noticed a long time ago, but I was never ready to admit it . . .
T: So even your house reflects your god-like standards.

Mosak and Roger discussed issues which Roger knew all too well but had never clearly formulated or examined. He was confronted with his "god-like" standards, his strong feelings of inferiority, hypersensitivity, and hostile attitude towards others. While sympathetic to Roger's history, the therapist powerfully confronted Roger with his responsibility for *continuing* to feel and act inferior. Roger cannot keep blaming his past. The other crucial issue worth commenting upon is the Adlerian's emphasis upon behavior—if Roger is truly tired of fighting, then he must "put down his fists." Adlerians emphasize the primacy of behavior; individuals must do more than simply "talk a good game." They must make movement.

Roger raised the issue of his relationship with his mother during the eighth session. He was by then functioning with virtually no agoraphobic symptoms. He had attended a play and enjoyed it; he had ceased having a problem with his drinking.

T: Now, Roger, it would seem to me that nobody could make a person feel guilty unless he chooses to feel guilty himself . . . Why do you choose to feel guilty with respect to your mother?

C: Primarily because she's blind and crippled. She uses this as kind of a crutch against me. It's not like she's alone, she has company all the time—people living with her.

T: How does she make you feel guilty? . . . Give me the words.

C: "You left me—you don't care about me" . . . It just goes on and on.

T: . . . What are your lines?

C: I usually don't say anything because I don't want to hurt her feelings.

After clarifying the problem a bit more, Mosak came to the point.

T: I would like to ask a couple of things, Roger. First of all, when your mother says, "You left me, you don't care for me, etc., etc.," do you think she's trying to get you to feel guilty? . . .

C: She loves it.

T: I got a hunch she wants something else.

C: You do?

T: Yeah—and I got a hunch that that's what you're not delivering. Not because you don't want to deliver it, but because you don't even know that that's what she's asking. My guess is she's inviting you to tell her that you love her . . . Maybe she's just looking for some kind of reassurance that you care? . . .

C: That's true, I never say that to her. I'll have to give that a try. This may be exactly it. I think you hit it pretty well.

They went on to discuss why Roger should choose to feel guilty. The primary purpose seemed to be his desire to be perfect. It was related to his god-like goals. Roger felt that there was so much he should do, he felt guilty for doing anything less than would be ideal. This, combined with the fact that Roger was afraid of getting too close to people and showing/expressing his feelings, created a distance which his mother attempted to close by using her suffering and complaining.

Adlerians believe that you cannot change other people's behavior, but you can change your own, and in that way, possibly the situation. Roger could not change his mother's behavior, but he could change his response to it. When he did, something happened which amazed him. Roger told her he loved her and showed some genuine concern, and his mother became "much more liberal," according to Roger. He reported that after one afternoon conversation, their relationship improved.

The interview then turned to Roger's opinion of the way others perceive him. Roger, while admitting he had come a long way, expressed concern over the fact that he was still afraid of opening himself up too much to others. They just would not like him if they knew the "real Roger." Mosak then "broke" one of his own rules: He allowed the class to participate and say what they thought of Roger. Roger was stunned and waited anxiously. The response was overwhelmingly one of interest and genuine concern. Unlike Roger's (admitted) expectations, no one was bored and no one found him in any way disagreeable. When the class was done, Mosak asked Roger what he thought.

C: [Very subdued] I'm very impressed . . . They make me feel very, very good—I feel great . . . They do take me seriously. I never dreamed that I was worth concern . . .

Roger went on with Mosak to discuss why Roger was so surprised. People had seen all his weaknesses, flaws, and imperfections, and still they cared about him. Roger was sincerely moved. The issue the therapist raised was that now Roger might want to do something about his newly discovered knowledge and take a chance with people. Almost immediately Roger stated, "I've met someone who I think cares and I'm trying."

Roger admitted that he really wanted somebody to love him, and he thought he had found somebody to love, a young man. They had spent an entire week living together (it had been two weeks since the last therapy session) and despite Roger's attempts to "buy" the man's affections, the man had refused to be "bought." He seemed to genuinely care. The session ended with Roger stating, "I do care about people." Mosak gave Roger a homework assignment.

T: What would we see if the real you came out of hiding?

C: [*Laughing*] Probably one hell of a mess . . . an emotional wreck, someone who can't really cope . . .

T: [*Speaking of Roger's tendency to secretly become emotional and occasionally cry when alone*] Crying . . . has nothing to do with masculinity—or to make a pun, mess-culinity, since you said you were a mess.

C: That's a good term—I like that.

T: It only has to do with being human. I would like to set you a task. Do you know any people who aren't messes?

C: Yeah.

T: Good. For the next week, I would like you to act as if you were one of those adequate people. Now it's going to be an act, no doubt about it, but it's not phony any more than a person that plays Hamlet is phony even though he's playing a role. I would just like you to try out that role. I would like you to act, for one week, as if you were not a mess. And if you don't know what that means concretely, then when you get into a certain kind of situation where you feel in doubt, you say "How would so-and-so who is adequate behave in this kind of situation?" And then, act that way.

Roger is moving in a healthy, prosocial direction. Social interest is being fostered. As his attitude changes and his motivation is modified, Mosak is including the behavioral component. Roger is accustomed to thinking of himself as a "mess." His strivings for perfection have usually met with feelings of inferiority; hence, subjectively, he feels like a "wreck"—a mess. Though motivation may change rapidly, the behavioral component requires practice and self-training and quite often lags behind the motivational change. The task to act *as if* he were an adequate person introduces modeling principles, especially when Roger is asked to act as if he were someone adequate that he knows. If Roger follows through with the task, he will incorporate the behavioral component more rapidly into his modified life style. In time, it will be difficult to differentiate acting adequate from being adequate.

Roger came into the ninth session and told of a situation that occurred at work. He had been "ranting and raving" about how life is so "rotten" and how "everybody is out to hurt you and nobody cares," when a woman came up to him and said, "I care." He said all he could think about were the therapy sessions. He said he felt "great." He said he smiled, and it changed the whole course of the evening.

The interview moved to a discussion of Roger's *dreams*. Adlerians view dreams as rehearsal for possible solutions to the problems of living. They are teleologic and serve to generate emotions which carry through to the next day and help motivate individuals to behave in certain ways which are consistent with their styles of life. Roger related this dream:

C: I was laying in bed . . . and I opened my eyes and I looked at the end of my bed. There was kind of a cocktail party going on with everybody dressed in 1800s garb. Out of this crowd came a woman—fantastically beautiful—who sat on the edge of my bed and said, "Well, can I help you with your problem—we're going to talk about it." I said, "Go away—this is the result of too many martinis or something." But we talked and she said, "Tell me what's wrong?" and I went on about things we [Mosak and Roger] had talked about. I really felt much better.

T: Much better about what?

C: About myself and life . . .

T: O.K. It [the dream] is your creation: Why did you put a woman at the foot of your bed?

C: I thought about that. [*Laughing*] I don't know why . . .

T: Why a beautiful woman? You could have put an ugly woman there. Roger, are you toying with the notion of becoming heterosexual? Or at least giving it a whirl?

C: [*Sheepishly*] Ah—yeah, I have been thinking about it.

They went on to discuss Roger's surprising admission. He was afraid that if he got involved with a woman, he would be tied down. It never occurred to Roger that he could get involved with a woman without being committed. It related back to Roger's idealizing women: He believed that women would not just "sleep around."

T: Roger, suppose I went down to see my bookie this afternoon and bet on whether in the next six months you would wind up in bed with a woman, should I give or take odds?

C: You should take them.

T: O.K. What odds should I take?

C: Ninety to one [that he won't sleep with a woman].

T: Ninety to one hardly leaves any room, and your [dream] would sort of indicate to me that your odds are better than ninety to one . . .

Mosak and Roger played the "Game of Probabilities." It is a way of investigating the potential movement of an individual in the future. Though Roger is preparing himself psychologically and emotionally for a heterosexual encounter, behaviorally he is hesitant. Mosak and Roger explored different situations in which Roger might be more comfortable being with a woman.

The session ended with Roger summarizing what he learned in therapy: He was less fearful and accepted himself more. He learned to say "no" to people, to stop feeling sorry for himself, and to "function better." Most importantly, Roger said he learned that he was a human being, and that was the most meaningful thing for him. Before he left, he said that his performance at work had improved so much that he was getting a "major promotion." As he left, he warmly said goodbye to the class and the therapist.

Roger never made it back for the last interview. Unexpectedly, his mother became very ill. Roger decided he wanted to be there for her. She died soon after he arrived. The quarter ended at the Institute and Roger decided to attempt to manage on his own.

SUMMARY AND CONCLUSION

Adlerian psychology is a holistic, teleoanalytic theory that stresses the unity of the person and the examination of the individual's goals and movement through life. Behavior that is useful—that is, conducive to healthy, cooperative functioning—is viewed as the ultimate goal of therapy. Such behavior, with its component emotional and psychological factors, is called social interest.

During the course of psychotherapy, Roger moved from a position of viewing others as his enemies, the world as hostile, and himself as inferior, to a position of genuine concern for others and acceptance of himself. His unrealistically high goals of personal superiority, most prominently evident in his choice of agoraphobic symptoms to control and dominate those around him, gave way to a more accepting, caring, and mutually respectful stance as he gained more confidence in himself and as his feelings of inferiority were put to rest. In nine therapy sessions, he reappraised his orientation to life, others, and himself, and emerged a happier, more productive individual. In short, he developed social interest.

Mosak utilized a number of techniques to move Roger towards social interest. He encouraged him and gave him hope. By utilizing a Life Style Assessment, the therapist worked on modifying the client's mistaken attitudes, and not just eliminating symptoms. At various times, the therapist used such tactics as Confrontation, Future Autobiography, Humor, the Game of Probabilities, Acting "As If," Tasksetting, Dreams, Multiple Psychotherapy, Interpretation, "Spitting in the Client's Soup," Placing in Perspective, Creating Images, and The Question.

As Roger's convictions became more adaptive and flexible, his private logic came more in line with common sense. He became more motivated to meet the challenges of life in a useful, cooperative way. Individual Psychology provides the psychotherapist and client with a system and philosophy to encourage such change.

Editors' Introduction

Marjorie Witty wrote this case to accompany her chapter on client-centered therapy in Current Psychotherapies.

The case study documents her treatment of a man with a serious illness—schizophrenia—and illustrates the client-centered rejection of the medical model and its use of diagnostic labels. Dr. Witty's treatment is fundamentally different than the methods most therapists would employ. She acknowledges that medications may help some people with conditions such as schizophrenia, but she sees little value in diagnosing or labeling these individuals and rejects medication as the treatment of choice for most people with this disorder.

Witty also doesn't see much value in labels such as "Doctor," which she views as affectations that only serve to create artificial hierarchies of expertise that separate her from her clients and preclude genuine connection and dialogue. Will you feel comfortable having clients address you by your first name?

Client-centered therapists attempt to apply some core principles to every therapy situation, and they don't tailor their treatment based on age, race, gender, or class. How does this approach differ from the treatment plan that would be developed by a psychoanalyst, behavior therapist, feminist therapist, or multicultural therapist?

It is instructive to see the therapist acknowledging the mistakes she makes along the way and commenting on these mistakes 25 years later. This is a long case study, but you will understand much more about schizophrenia, the limitations of the medical model, and the core client-centered value of respect for the client after reading the case.

3 | CLIENT-CENTERED THERAPY WITH DAVID: A SOJOURN IN LONELINESS

Marjorie C. Witty

HOW I CAME TO WORK WITH DAVID

In 1987, about six years into my doctoral program in counseling psychology at Northwestern University, one of the persons I was interviewing for my dissertation introduced me to a friend of hers whose son had been diagnosed with a severe mental illness. This woman's wish was simply for her son to have some contact with people. She did not have unreasonable expectations from the therapy. She asked me to see David, who was about 28 years old. I agreed and set up an appointment to see him at my office.

Instead of showing up at the scheduled time, David arrived about four hours late, saying that he had been "walking around Chicago." Realizing that regular appointments wouldn't work, I volunteered to see him at his home because I was still attending classes and his family's home was on my way. For about a year, I saw him weekly at his home, each of us seated at the kitchen table. I asked his mother to remind him the night before of my arrival time the next day. Often when I arrived, David would come out to meet me as I drove up. Occasionally, he would comment on how much more of my back seat had been torn apart since my last visit by my beloved German shepherd (ironically named *Patience*).

I have a particularly vivid memory of one of the early sessions in which David's dysfluency was pronounced. As each syllable spun around in my short-term memory, I awaited the next bit and the next, finally resulting in a sentence I could not comprehend. At the end of that taxing session, David took my hand and said with complete fluency, "Thank you for your patience." Because I had not been sure up to that point that he had much awareness of me, I was surprised and touched by his expression of gratitude. From that point on, I was "all in."

David then and today is a person of character and creativity. He paints and has written poetry in both English and Spanish. In the time we worked together, he didn't blame others; he didn't express self-pity or complain about his situation of unrelenting loneliness. What he wanted—and continues to want—is understanding and respect. David also wishes to share his life with others and to enjoy camaraderie with them as can be seen in the following therapy session.

After about a year of our working together, David's parents found a community in Hawaii that provided a haven for persons with severe mental illness. It was near the beach and had a community garden. David agreed to try it, and he ended up spending two years in that program. When it closed, he began working with a social worker in Hawaii who looked out for him and kept in touch with his family. Before he left for this community, I requested permission to tape our two last sessions. Both David and his mother gave permission.

As I undertook this case study, I recontacted them and received permission for this project to use case notes and the transcript of one of the sessions. In the process of contacting them, his mother told me that she had published a book in collaboration with David. From this source I learned about David's life after he left Chicago and was able to read some of his writing.

A CLIENT-CENTERED POSITION ON CASE FORMULATION

Case Studies in Psychotherapy illustrates approaches to conceptualizing clients and the therapeutic methods advocated by the major theoretical orientations. The majority of orientations regard initial and ongoing case conceptualization as essential to the appropriate identification of treatment goals and interventions that are believed to lead to successful outcomes. An outcome may be defined in terms of achievement of insight, the reduction of problematic behaviors or symptoms, compliance with medication and therapy, better scores on objective test measures, higher levels of social adjustment, improved social skills, trauma-management skills, better quality of life, becoming a fully functioning person, and so on. Whether bio-, psycho- or sociogenic causal factors are stressed, case formulation is mostly considered essential to guiding the therapy process. The hegemonic influence of the *medical model*[1] is ubiquitous in the education of counselors, social workers, and psychologists, who learn to view diagnosis as necessary to justify the selection of specific, effective "treatments."

In contrast to the medical model (see Elkins, 2007; Wampold, 2001), the dominant paradigm in clinical psychology—the client-centered vision of the person as a self-determining and self-righting agent—is heretical. Conceptualizations may range from feminist psychology's political analyses of the impacts of social class; disability; ageism; sexism; homo-, bi-, and transphobia; and racism to cognitive behavioral theories' identification of irrational core beliefs, psychodynamic theories' explication of disorders of self and attachment, trauma psychology's elaboration of the impact of varieties of trauma, and biological theories of genetically influenced vulnerabilities. I recently consulted with a therapist about his transgender client and presented a nonpathological understanding of this difference in gender-identity development. At the end of the consultation, he commented, "There *must* be some form of trauma at the root of this!"

It's very hard to pry a therapist away from a unitary theory of causation. All of these formulations share the same essentialist assumption about psychopathology located in the microcosm of the individual soma or psyche, or in the societal macrocosm, or the two in combination. Exceptions to the essentialist assumptions undergirding the medical model are found in the various humanistic theories as well as systems, social constructivist, and narrative or collaborative approaches (Anderson & Gehart, 2006; McNamee & Gergen, 1992).

---

[1]The medical model in psychotherapy is a descriptive schema borrowed from the practice of medicine and superimposed on the practice of psychotherapy. The schema—including its assumptions and terminology—accurately describes the processes and procedures of medical practice and has been highly useful in that field. However, the schema does not accurately describe the processes and procedures of psychotherapy and is problematic when superimposed on that field. In medicine, a *doctor* diagnoses *a patient* on the basis of *symptoms* and administers *treatment* designed to *cure* the patient's *illness*. In psychotherapy, medical model adherents *say* that a doctor diagnoses a patient on the basis of symptoms and administers treatment designed to *cure* the patient's illness. However, when practitioners make this claim, they are superimposing a medical schema on psychotherapy and using medical terms to describe what is essentially an interpersonal process that has almost nothing to do with medicine (Elkins, 2007).

A UNIVERSAL THEORY OF PSYCHOLOGICAL MALADJUSTMENT

Carl R. Rogers's definitive theoretical statement (1959) provides us with a theory of therapy and personality, an account of infant development, a motivational theory based in organismic theory, and a theory of interpersonal relationships. Rogers's theory posits that psychological maladjustment results from incongruence between a person's concept of self and her organismic experiencing. A client-centered therapy relationship restores the client's congruence through experiencing self in the context of the therapist's unconditional regard. Rogers's theory of therapy does not function based on specific diagnoses because his theory of human maladjustment is universally applicable and his therapy offers the same facilitative therapeutic conditions for all persons and all sorts of problems. His theoretical formulation is situated at the universal level of analysis, not at the level of group categorizations. At the same time, Rogers foregrounds the client's phenomenology—reality as uniquely perceived—at the level of analysis where "I am like no other person."

Rogers's theory of psychological maladjustment asserts that persons often suffer with "conditions of worth" (Rogers, 1959, p. 204). This concept simply refers to the child's having internalized attributions about his or her embodied self from parents, teachers, peers, and others who assert that he is "bad," "selfish," "stupid," "ugly," "worthless," "a sissy," or "lazy" and "a coward." These judgments shape the child's picture of him- or herself. Rogers posits that the human being, like any living organism, is an ongoing process of organismic valuing. Picture an infant who tastes peas for the first time and spits them all over himself and his highchair while shaking his head in disgust as if to say, "No peas! No mas!" Organismic valuing refers to "an ongoing process in which values are never fixed or rigid, but experiences are being accurately symbolized and continually and freshly valued in terms of the satisfactions organismically experienced . . . " (Rogers, 1959, p. 210). As we mature, this process becomes more available to awareness and to direct expression in language, but the process is theorized to precede the acquisition of language.

In particular, an infant or child's aggressive behavior, or what is interpreted as "disrespectful" behavior, evokes strong, often punitive conditions of worth; eventually these pleasurable experiences or honest expressions go underground and are ejected from the child's conscious experiencing. When a child's self-concept begins to contradict the flow of organismic experiencing, there is a significant increase in tension, anxiety, and vulnerability that Rogers defines as *incongruence*. Tension between a child's inherent organismic valuing process (righteously hating those who scold and devalue her) and her self-concept (I am a loving child!) leads to distortions in self-perception and inaccurate self-representation. Increasingly, the child denies to awareness all manner of authentic experiences, including those in which she excels or exhibits positive aspects of self. An apt description for this condition is that of having been *colonized* and *alienated* from the truth of one's physical, emotional, and cognitive being.

CLIENT-CENTERED THERAPY RESTORES THE SELF TO CONGRUENCE

While "problem-centered" approaches enjoin the client to identify his or her problems, to set treatment goals, and comply with treatments, the client-centered therapist provides the client an empathic and accepting psychological climate characterized by freedom and safety. In this interpersonal environment, the client can allow herself a wider aperture of experiencing, which often begins with reiterating the introjected attributions composing the self. When, most surprisingly, the therapist does not counter these excoriating self-judgments, the client is free to reconsider their accuracy from within this novel context of acceptance and respect.

In client-centered therapy, the overarching goal is to be of help to the client, however that help is ultimately construed. Beyond this metagoal, the therapist's goals are for herself: to realize her commitment to experience and to implement the therapeutic attitudes outlined in Rogers's theory of therapy (1951, 1957, 1959) and to remain in all ways consistent with the ethical principle of respect for the client and the client's freedom. This stance of principled nondirectiveness (see Grant, 1990) is fundamental to client-centered practice.

Rogers identifies the therapist's congruence as a sine qua non of the process of therapy. If the client does not perceive the honesty and genuineness of the therapist, then she will not be able to believe her perceptions of the therapeutic conditions of empathic understanding and unconditional positive regard. *Congruence* refers to the therapist's genuineness—entering the relationship transparently as oneself without the usual professional façade. It refers to a willingness to be known and to not deceive the client. The therapist aims to empathically understand the client's communications, to respect the person's autonomy throughout the process of therapy, and to prize and accept the client as one who is doing the best he or she can. These therapist-experienced conditions, in concert with the client's inherent motivation to actualize organismic potentials, are viewed as the change-inducing variables. In this environment of freedom and safety, the client determines her own process and content within each session and from week to week over the course of therapy, also determining when she is ready to end the therapy relationship.

Because the therapist is committed to the self-definition and self-determination of the client as an ethical stance, he need not attempt to persuade or reframe or guide the client. He need not press the client to take psychotropic medications or be hospitalized. Occasionally, the client may ask directly for the therapist's thinking on a particular issue. Principled nondirectiveness is logically consistent with the desire to respond honestly to the client's requests and questions. If the therapist has ideas or can accommodate the request, then he may offer a response and check in with the client regarding the helpfulness of the response, and the therapist will be particularly interested in whether his response showed an accurate understanding of what the client was seeking.

You might ask, "But what about the client who continually wants direction and who seemingly wants to remain dependent on the therapist?" Client-centered therapists accept the person where he or she is, without judgments about "immaturity" or applying diagnostic labels such as "dependent personality disorder." If we can ethically meet clients' requests or answer questions or provide various types of accommodations, then our inclination is to accept these requests at face value. We assume that the dependent behavior of the client will most often give way to greater levels of self-regulation when the dependency is not punished or judged to be unacceptable. As Ehrbar comments, "Paradoxically the intent to instill an internal locus of evaluation in the client is directive and is thus inconsistent with client-centered therapy . . . !" (Proctor & Napier, 2004, p.157). Client-centered therapists also acknowledge that there are many resources for growth and support and find it congenial to work in tandem with other therapists or providers should the client wish to experiment with other sources of support.

A CLIENT-CENTERED VIEW OF POWER AND AUTHORITY

As early as 1942, Rogers addressed the issue of whether or not a therapeutic relationship is compatible with authority. He states, "It seems to the writer that the counselor cannot maintain a counseling relationship with the client and at the same time have authority over him. Therapy and authority cannot be coexistent in the same relationship" (Rogers, 1942). One may object that inequality between the client and therapist is inherent by virtue of the structure of one person seeking help from another (Brodley, 2011a; Proctor, 2002). Because of this structural inequality, client-centered therapists attempt to share power and to relinquish power as much as we can. We almost never insist on terms of formal address such as "Doctor," although some clients persist in referring to us with such terms. We also try to identify the sources of expertise involved in answering questions when such expertise is sought. The idea is to make the process of arriving at answers or opinions transparent to the client and to share our rationale along with the logic undergirding our answers to clients' questions.

As the therapeutic attitudes are perceived by the client over time, Rogers hypothesizes that change will occur in fairly predictable directions (Rogers, 1961). Clients usually experience greater self-comprehensibility, self-acceptance, self-authority, and openness to their own and others' experiences. They become more skilled at making decisions and choices that align with their own organismic valuing process. Clients tend to move toward greater compassion and generosity toward others as their own needs and wants are asserted and recognized and satisfied in the process of living. Clients take more risks in order to fulfill the inner guidance of the organism as opposed to conforming to outside demands; in fact, clients in client-centered therapy experience deeper, increasingly existential living (Rogers, 1961).

Rogers's therapy is a *psychological* therapy meaning that the domain of the work is the client's relation to herself being in the-world and being with others. In this respect, the client-centered therapist does not take on responsibility for diagnosing and treating "illnesses" such as eating disorders, depression, panic disorder, PTSD, and the like. Rogers rejected diagnosis as a precondition for therapy (Rogers, 1957; Shlien, 2003). When meeting a client for the first time, he did not want to see the client's previous psychiatric or psychological records, wishing instead to encounter the client without preconceived ideas or diagnoses. Because he believed that the client's perceptions of reality were what counted, clinical assessments were unimportant and irrelevant. He made clear that client-centered practice would not change because the client was diagnosed with a particular disorder or was a "homosexual" or was developmentally disabled or belonged to any other group. Rogers would not have endorsed the idea that our therapy changes according to the client's gender, social class, or race. The therapeutic attitudes do not change in character, although the therapist's *attunement to the individual* may lead to unique and nonsystematic expressions and accommodations. Serendipitously, this attunement promotes the client's understanding of the therapist's communication and intentions. An example of this attunement is my experience with a client whose voice was so soft that I sat on the floor fairly close to her feet in order to hear. I had decided that, given her vulnerability, I did not want to request that she speak louder. There are many examples of these attunements to the client so as to implement the therapeutic attitudes.

ROGERS'S POSITION ON DIAGNOSIS

In his book *Client-Centered Therapy* (1951), Rogers argues from a paper he presented at Harvard in 1948 in which he warned that the shift of the locus of evaluation from the person to the clinician leads to dependency on the presumed expert who is going to apply the curative "treatment." Presciently, he expresses a deep concern about the implications of diagnosis as leading to control of the many by the few.

> One cannot take responsibility for evaluating a person's abilities, motives, conflicts, needs; for evaluating the adjustment he is capable of achieving, the degree of reorganization he should undergo, the conflicts which he should resolve, the degree of

dependence which he should develop upon the therapist, and the goals of therapy, without a significant degree of control over the individual being an inevitable accompaniment. As this process is extended to more and more persons, as it is for example to thousands of veterans, it means a subtle control of persons and their values and goals by a group which has selected itself to do the controlling. The fact that it is a subtle and well-intentioned control makes it only less likely that people will realize what they are accepting. . . . If the hypothesis of the first trend proves to be most adequately supported by the evidence, if it proves to be true that the individual has relatively little capacity for self-evaluation and self-direction, and that the primary evaluation function must lie with the expert, then it would appear that the long range direction in which we are moving will find expression in some type of complete social control. The management of the lives of the many by the self-selected few would appear to be the natural consequence. If, on the other hand, the second hypothesis should be more adequately supported by the facts, if, as we think, the locus of responsible evaluation may be left with the individual, then we would have a psychology of personality and of therapy which leads in the direction of democracy, a psychology which would gradually redefine democracy in deeper and more basic terms. We would have a place for the professional worker in human relations, not as an evaluator of the self, behavior, needs and goals, but as the expert in providing the conditions under which the self-direction of both the individual and the group can take place. The expert would have the skill in facilitating the independent growth of the person (Rogers, 1951, pp. 224–225).

Rogers's psychological therapy involves encountering the client on her own terms, and trying to see the world from her perspective. As Brodley has stated, the only reality relevant to the person's development and healing is reality as perceived by the client herself. In this sense, within the context of therapy, the theory of personality and motivation as formulated by Carl R. Rogers (1959) is as irrelevant as any other biopsychosocial or psychiatric theory! In other words, the therapist is not aiming at convincing the client that he possesses an actualizing tendency or even that his experiences are worthy of respect. In the grand gamble regarding success or failure in therapy, Rogers puts his bets on the client's actual experiencing of the core conditions as a path to a more nuanced, self-differentiating, accepting, and authoritative experience of the organism—hence, a more congruent self.

THE NONDIRECTIVE ATTITUDE

Raskin's description of the nondirective attitude describes what is involved in this approach.

There is [another] level of nondirective counselor response which to the writer represents *the* nondirective attitude . . . in the experience of some, it is a highly attainable goal, which . . . changes the nature of the counseling process in a radical way. At this level, counselor participation becomes an active experiencing with the client of the feelings to which he gives expression, the counselor make a maximum effort to get under the skin of the person with whom he is communicating, he tries to get *within* and to live the attitudes expressed instead of observing them, to catch every nuance of their changing nature; in a word, to absorb himself completely in the attitudes of the other. And in struggling to do this, there is simply no room for any other type of counselor activity or attitude; if he is attempting to live the attitudes of the other, he cannot be diagnosing them, he cannot be thinking of making the process go faster. Because he is another, and not the client, the understanding is not spontaneous but must be acquired, and this through the most intense, continuous and active attention to the feelings of the other, to the exclusion of any other type of attention (Raskin, 1947/2005; Rogers, 1951, p. 29).

Meeting the client on her own ground, giving full attention to the exclusion of any other intention to formulate or diagnose, and experiencing the attitudes of unconditional positive regard and empathic understanding of the client's frame of reference are the only appropriate goals for therapist (Baldwin, 1987). Rogers's therapy is exemplary as a profoundly egalitarian and mutual relational conversation.

Although, in fact, Rogers's sessions contain a high percentage of empathic understanding responses, client-centered practice in its totality over time takes many forms. It is first and foremost a living human relationship in which the therapist offers help (however that may come to be defined); as in any relationship, issues crop up and are addressed. Questions about the therapist are sometimes raised—questions about racial identity, relationship status, sexual orientation, political beliefs, educational degrees, social class, parental status, and so on. The client will only pose these questions if she has not been discouraged or punished for asking—as occurs, for example, when the therapist comments "Well, this therapy is about you and your concerns; not about me." On our side, the therapist may ask questions for clarification; make statements from our own frames of reference; make spontaneous personal expressions of joy, dismay, and sympathy; and sometimes volunteer opinions even when they are not strictly solicited by the client. The practice with each client is, by definition, unique to this pairing. The therapist also has personal boundaries and personal requirements that she may occasionally need to disclose to her clients and that become part of the collaboration. "Please do not wear any scented products or perfumes since I am susceptible to migraine!" "Please leave your firearm in your car when you come to sessions because guns make me nervous." "Yes, you can bring the baby. Let's see how it goes." "Sure, I'll remind you that you wanted to continue to discuss the problem with your husband next week when we meet," and so forth. As a client-centered therapist's practice matures and deepens, we enjoy psychological freedom and spontaneity within an ethical position of nondirectiveness.

CONSISTENCY BETWEEN MEANS AND ENDS

I have frequently heard the view that claims that people who grew up in collectivist, traditional cultures that venerate authority within the family, in the civic sphere, and in religion and politics will not be able to function well in the egalitarian atmosphere of client-centered therapy and that they require more directive approaches.

This contention illustrates a misunderstanding of the principle of nondirectiveness as if the client-centered therapist will reject being perceived as an authority, scold the client for any display of dependency or requests for help, and criticize the client's traditional attitudes—for example, seeing women as inferior to men. On the one hand, if the therapist accepts and embodies the authority position, then he simply reinscribes hierarchical structures of power, using unethical means for an ethical end (Brodley, 2011a; Levitt, 2005; Proctor, 2002; Witty, 2005). On the other, an attempt to "enlighten" the client as to the superiority of egalitarianism contradicts the principle of respect for the client. The answer to persons who are living within such traditional structures and hierarchies is neither to engage them from a stance of expertise and authority nor to attempt to "liberate" them but rather to meet them as one person to another, accepting their inclination and need to elevate and idealize the therapist and to credit our utterances with a great deal of meaning and authority.

If we believe that the process of therapeutic change is a natural response to the therapeutic conditions in concert with the person's own potentials for growth, then in the long run the client's own self-authority is likely to emerge. Her emergent "voice" may bring her into conflict with her family and culture or it may not, but from our point of view there is no ethically acceptable alternative to providing a nondirective moral space that inevitably empowers the person. Maureen O'Hara, who has compared the emancipatory educational project of Paolo Freire with Rogers's views on therapeutic change, states:

> It is a profound contradiction for a liberational educator, community worker, humanistic therapist or workshop convenor to use techniques that, even momentarily, rely on the domination or objectification of another. . . . Freire (1970) decries revolutionary leaders or educators who "massify" the oppressed, practicing manipulation and indoctrination behind some rationalization:
>
>> In fact, manipulation and conquest, as expressions of cultural invasion, are never means for liberation. They are always means of "domestication." True humanism, which serves human beings cannot accept manipulation under any name whatsoever (Freire, 1970, p. 114 cited in O'Hara, 2006, pp. 120–121).

THE THERAPY SESSION

The following verbatim transcript is one of our last sessions before David left for a program for persons with severe mental illness in Hawaii where he was to live for the next six years. David has read and had the opportunity to edit this document, and he has given permission to use this material for publication.

It is important to understand that I had already met with David numerous times prior to this session because the central theme of this session echoes many earlier sessions yet may sound as though I am hearing about these events for the first time. I experienced these sessions as being called on to witness a calamity that had unjustly been visited on an innocent person. As a therapist, one is always a witness to the life and suffering of the client, but in David's case, this implicit stance emerged as the central and fundamental truth of our relationship. I felt that implicitly David called me to believe and bear witness to the fact that he has been deceived, tormented, insulted, violated, and humiliated by voices. He calls my attention to the fact that he has been taken away by the police, pushed into ambulances, and hospitalized and medicated against his will since the voices began.

Note: The client (C) is David; the therapist (T) is Marge.

C1:   Well, the first thing I want to talk about is that I woke up today early—and I'm not—I didn't stay up because I knew I was going to hear the voices, and I didn't see any reason to, you know, make any—uh—great effort. But I did feel good when I woke up, and I—uhm—did get up, and I would have *stayed* up if I hadn't thought I would hear the voices.

T1:   So then what you did was—did you go back to bed? [A tracking response asking for clarification].

C2:   Yeah.

T2:   'Cause you did start hearing the voices?

C3:   Yeah, and this is one of the main things that the voices criticize is that I'm lazy. I'm saying that for the benefit of the tape! [short laugh].

T3:   Mm hm, right [short laugh].

C4:   And uhm. . . .

T4:   But it's funny because in a way one of the reasons that you're so-called lazy is you get tormented by the voices!

In this response, I interrupted David and made a comment from my own frame of reference, a supportive interpretation that illustrated both my momentary loss of neutrality and desire to defend him from the voices' accusation of laziness. I regard this as a "spontaneous" response but one that, if practiced systematically, would constitute an error of attitude, meaning that I would have slipped into the mistaken practice of trying to influence my client's own self-evaluation in a more exculpatory, self-acceptant direction instead of attempting to understand his expressive communications. In contrast to "reframing" the client's cognitions and evaluations, client-centered therapists try to understand and accept even the most excoriating self-assessments, respecting the client's right to be his own source of evaluation.

C5:   Well, yeah, I either stay up all night or I am so disoriented when I fall asleep that I guess I have to admit that I usually miss when the sun comes up. Uhm—I'm—I'm—uh—t—ti—tired of waking up late.

T5:   It's frustrating to have your routine disrupted so much so that you can't seem to get on a regular schedule. Is that your point?

A better, more accurate response here would have been simply "You're tired of waking up late." Client-centered therapists consider the "target of empathic understanding" to be the intentional communication of the client, both the narrative content and the person's implicit relation to the narrative or the "point." In this response, I erred a bit on the general side, deriving a point from what was implied rather than staying with his exact expression. Even when the client accepts a response—which David does here and, as in this case, it is wide of the mark—it is incumbent on the therapist to listen to her own response with an eye to its accuracy.

C6:   Yeah, and it's my problem. And like I said, I think that's the main thing that the voices and other people are critical of. They think it's some kind of fault, but all that I have to say about it is that it says on my birth certificate that I was born at 11 o'clock in the morning, so if I was born at 11 why shouldn't I just sleep till 11?

T6:   Mm hm.

C7:   And I know it's kinda stupid to believe that when you're born has any significance, but I feel that it's a comfortable thing to wake up late, and I've proven in the past that I'm capable of getting up in the morning, but that happens in situations where there is some *reason* to get up.

T7:   Mm hm, where there's something that you want to do or go some place you want to go.

C8:   I had a hard time getting up at Gould's farm, but . . . but, I mean, Gould's farm was a complete, uhm, shambles. I mean, that uh—the voices were—were—were happening the whole time.

T8:   Mm hm.

C9:   Uh—I—I—think I've shown pretty well in my life—not overall—but pretty well, that when there's something to do, or the situation is pleasant, or somehow you're coming off of—uhm—some kind of uh—pa—passage, that I—I can wake up at, but uhm, I—I'm—I'm not sure. I think that the voices, especially the ones on the TV, because those are, you know, more real, you know, I think there's no question that they're threatening me.

T9:   Mm hm. I wanted to uh check with you. Does this machinery bother you at all? The tape recorder? I mean, does it feel like you're hearing anything from it? Cause I didn't want . . .

C10:   No, I don't think I've ever been taped before.

T10:   Uh huh, just let me know if it bothers you.

David's reference to the voices on the TV that were threatening him caused me immediate concern regarding whether he was being bothered by the tape recorder. Mostly I had not taped our sessions, so I wanted to know immediately if it was bothering him, although in my checking this out with him, I missed an opportunity for an empathic response.

C11:   Yeah.
T11:   But anyway.
C12:   I can't remember being taped before.
T12:   Yeah, well, let me know, but your point is that for some reason the voices that you hear over the TV are more real, and they're more threatening. Is that right then?

Client-centered therapists' responses are deliberately tentative in tone, even when the declarative form is used. This tentativeness signals to the client that I am not privy to his meanings and must make an effort to get it right. If I don't, I want to be corrected. As clients settle into the relationship and trust the therapist (perhaps in part because of this careful effort), they become much freer to spontaneously correct the therapist's errors of accurate understanding.

C13:   Um—uh—uhm—uhm—placable as it seems, you know, that—that—this is—this is—really, you know, something that see—that seems to be happening.
T13:   Mm hm. I made a mistake. In other words, you didn't say that they're more threatening but that you feel that they're threatening *you*.
C14:   I could have sworn they said something to that effect last night. And it didn't uh—uh—didn't go very well with my—you know—functioning.
T14:   Mm hm.
C15:   It is destructive, and I don't know why it's necessary. I mean, there's no, no . . .
T15:   It's destructive to your functioning.

Client-centered therapists make a practice of openly acknowledging mistakes in empathic understanding when they occur as I do in T13. This practice is a natural outgrowth of respect for the client as an equal participant in the conversation. As this transparency persists over time, by sharing how one arrived at an answer to a question or the logic and reasoning behind a tentative interpretation, the client develops a tacit or explicit understanding that the therapist's goal is to understand the client's communications, not to improve, correct, or educate. It is also important to note that David is aware of the destructive impact of the voices. Many persons categorized or labeled as "psychotic" or "schizophrenic" are believed to have little or no insight into their own "illness" or their situation in general. Here David is expressing his opinion that the effects on him are destructive and unnecessary.

C16:   There's no question that—that you know I have certain needs. I like to have a cigarette when I wake up in the morning, but if I wasn't hearing the voices, I don't think I would have turned into a chain smoker. I—I—I know that the voices are using some of my ideas against me, and I don't think that's very good. And . . .
T16:   It's like you're explaining to me that these voices really screw you up in a lot of ways, right? Because you smoke more, and it interrupts your sleeping habits, right? And it really makes it hard for you.

In this response the opening phrase "It's like you're explaining to me . . . " is an example of my reflecting the client's agency or intentionality in this moment. This practice contrasts with the simplistic instruction to listen for "feelings." Although occasionally clients use explicit feeling words, probably most often they are "describing," "explaining," "regretting," "wondering how . . . ," "frustrated by," and so on. By reducing these expressions to simple feeling words, the therapist substitutes "round" terms for precise meanings expressed by the client. In David's next sentence, for example, he is asserting a descriptive truth of his experience with the voices.

C17:   Yeah, well, I mean, both of them are chauvinists, there's no question about that.
T17:   And what does that mean?

This question for clarification was understandable but probably a mistake; I should have simply reiterated his term and allowed him to clarify if he wished to do so. In working with clients who have various kinds of expressive difficulties (including those who must work with a therapist who doesn't share their mother tongue, children, and those with articulation problems) the therapist must balance her desire for a high degree of understanding with the desire to free the client to give his narrative unimpeded. It is frustrating to be constantly stopped and asked to clarify small points of meaning, so in work with clients whose expressions may be ambiguous, I sometimes prefer to let the ambiguity stand in order to respect the client's own rhythm and pace of expression.

C18:   Well, they're—very bu—bullish, you know.
T18:   Did you mean like macho?
C19:   Yeah.
T19:   Mm hm.
C20:   So.
T20:   Unpleasant, very unpleasant, and kind of dictatorial.

As stated previously, this clarification of the meaning of the word *chauvinists* risked pushing David off of track.

C21:   Yeah. They—they—they—just—you know—kind of—I don't know—ruined the basic struggle that I was going through. And they just kind of—ruin—ruined it when I think I was—when I think I was going to make a turn anyway.

From the beginning of the session, David gives more and more evidence of the interference from the voices as he attempts to get his sleep schedule going and other attempts at organizing himself in terms of when he awakens and begins his day. He goes on to clarify the hostile and undermining quality of the voices and now, asserts the disastrous effects they have "when I was going to make a turn anyway." He describes this calamity that he experienced and continues to experience and how it commenced years before.

T21:   Not sure if I follow you. Do you mean that you were going along in your life, struggling with various things, and then when the voices came into your life, they ruined that?
C22:   Well, it's just that I think I was—I was at a point, you know—when I was—when the voices first happened, that I was getting a better orientation, and really, you know, that was—that was significant enough because I was—whatever would have happened without the voices would have been significant enough because Lords house [residential care home] is is a real—uh, you know, funky place. I mean, not that it's dirty or anything, but it—it—it—um, it's just uhm, got a kind of a very uh—un—uh—mo—un—pa—un—un—un—pa—very—un—un—functioning group of people. That's—that's about the size of it, and most of the people don't do anything, you know. And that . . .
T22:   It's upsetting to be around a lot of people who are just kind of doing nothing.

Although my response captured the last parts of David's statements, I missed the most important point, which was his assertion that he had been in the process of "getting a better orientation" when the voices first started, and that that was significant.

C23: So, it's—it's a spa—special type of uhm, situation which is just very weird you know, because it doesn't fit in with the neighborhood. The neighborhood is mostly Spanish. And it—it do—doesn't fit in with the other elements of like, uhm, middle class and stuff.

T23: So it's like you felt kind of out of place there, I mean because Lords House didn't fit in.

In this response, as I look at it now, I think that even though David did not explicitly state that he felt out of place, I gave myself the license to make an empathic guess as to why it was important to him regarding the fact that the residential care home itself did not "fit in with the neighborhood." This represents the focus on the client's relation to his narrative content. I follow and teach this instruction in doing this form of therapy the principle of trying to understand the client's "point."

C24: Yeah.

T24: Didn't fit in.

C25: Is that this? [David gestures toward my right.]

T25: I don't know. Oh! It's the radiator—I bet—that you're hearing, yeah.

C26: Oh. See I'm—I'm drp—I'm pretty sure that there was one day when—when the voices had kept me up all night and that day I think was the day when the voices became uh—uh—a real uh—mess, you know? And uh, came across in a very su—s-s-s-ertive way.

T26: A very assertive way?

C27: Yeah.

T27: Now, this is three years ago? [Actually, it occurred probably around nine years earlier.]

C28: Yeah.

T28: I see. In other words, you're talking about the point at which it seemed like the voices really created a mess in your life?

In this response, I extrapolate from his earlier statement in C26 "and that day I think was the day when the voices became uh—uh—a real uh—mess, you know?" saying "it seemed like the voices really created a mess in your life." This changes his meaning from the "voices became a real mess" to "the voices really created a mess in your life." My response is an error of accuracy. This is a common mistake I have long observed in teaching client-centered therapy, so it is humbling to find myself making it here. In this category of "mistake," students stay close to the stated expression but actually extrapolate a meaning that weaves the individual bits together so as to give them more sense instead of sticking with a statement that they actually don't understand. I think it is much better to stay with the client in hopes that he will elaborate his statement or spontaneously clarify it. If the client fails to do so, then the therapist may ask for clarification. The intent of this practice is not to be pedantic or persnickety or obsessively detailed. The intention is one of respect. This entails not speaking for the client, not putting words in the client's mouth. Making the client's ambiguous statements less ambiguous is an unintentionally paternalistic behavior. It misrepresents to the client a clarity he does not yet have in his expression and risks confusing or misleading him about what he was trying to express. To state that you didn't follow or in some cases restate verbatim what you do not understand empowers the client by giving him the opportunity to clarify his statement and perhaps elaborate further on his point. As Nat Raskin pointed out, it is faithful to the principle of the client as an architect of both the content and process of the therapy (Raskin, 1988). In these small ways, the client-centered therapist's moment-to-moment practice embodies an attitude of principled nondirectiveness (see Grant, 1990).

C29: Well, they started on their kind of uhm—bas—basic—uhm—buh—ba—brain thing. They—they seemed to have some kind of kind of motive or plan, and that's when they sort of started. And it all has to do with trying to gain my trust at first, and then revealing that—that uhm—kind of uh—special uh, knowledge that they had about—about—about my past. So—so I guess, you know, they tried to get my trust at first, and they succeeded and then—then—uh, then after the weekend was over, I went on this big walk around Chicago. And I mean if the voices had been a normal experience, just a sort of a temporary you know, thing, then the voices would have stopped after I went on that walk around Chicago. Uhm, you know, it would have just been one weekend which was weird, but—but they didn't stop. And when I got back, then—then—uh—it—uhm—continued.

This series of statements is given with a heaviness and sense of fatalism and of remembering something very painful.

T29: In a way it's like what you're describing is that somehow they got your trust in the beginning.

C30: Yeah.

T30: And then they turned on you, right? By revealing special knowledge about your past.

C31: Yes, yeah.

T31: So the feeling is one if you were kind of conned or betrayed.

C32: Yeah, that—that they kind of exci—excited—these kind of potentials in my mind, and I guess the reason I trusted them was because I—felt that I—I was—uhm—uhm—pretty powerful myself.

T32: You mean at that time in your life you felt powerful yourself, so they didn't seem threatening to you at that point so you could afford to trust them.

C33: Right, I—I—what I was saying was that I—I had a day in between this night when I stayed up all—all night. I had a day in between and I got up early on the day when this started . . . Oh, God . . . (Pause) . . . I mean, that's what—that's what I think. Because after I stayed up all night, I went to sleep, and I'm pretty sure that I slept. Because the day on Saturday when the whole thing came about—uhm—uhm—that was a full day, and that—that uh—that's my belief anyway—is that I had a good night's sleep, and I woke up early and I was just kind of, might say, innocent at that point.

David's utterance of "Oh, God" was one of the most emotional statements he made in this session.

T33: Not sure I follow the sequence, are you saying that you stayed up through a whole night . . .

C34: Yeah, listening to the voices, I sat in a chair.

T34: And then you went to bed the next day and slept pretty well. And then you woke up and . . .

C35: And I had that day in between, which is you know, just your basic day.

T35: Where you didn't hear them?

C36: Not really, no.

T36: And then they came back?

C37: Yeah. That's what I think because—because I—I am sure I have the time orientation to some extent.

T37: At least well, you're trying to remember things that happened several years ago.

C38: Yeah.

T38: Right, and you're trying to tell me what how it came on.

C39:   Yeah, what—see—I don't think that I would have accepted the voices so openly if it hadn't seemed like a natural occurrence upon waking up, whereas really, the other night I stayed up all night and didn't go to sleep until the morning, so . . .

T39:   I guess I understand this point that you mentioned that when you woke up, you felt kind of innocent, or I guess just open.

C40:   Right.

T40:   Right. And then you started hearing the voices, and it seemed kind of benign, like well, you could afford to trust them, or it wasn't anything problematic at that point, so you're describing to me how you came to take them in, right, or "allow" them in.

C41:   Right.

T41:   Mm hm.

David is taking pains to describe the sequence of events that occurred years past that led to the "invasion" of the voices. He comments that he wouldn't have "accepted the voices so openly" had they not been coincident with his waking up. His narrative in this session makes clear that the voices are a "mess," and that they ruined his functioning and that they are "destructive." I have no inclination to counter David's reality, to reframe his experience as the "onset of illness," or persuade him that the voices should be viewed as unworthy of his attention. As with any other client, I take David's account at face value within the context of the therapy session.

Do I think he "has" schizophrenia or some psychotic thought disorder? Does he experience "auditory hallucinations?" These questions about diagnoses and symptoms are irrelevant to our conversation. Within humanistic psychology as a whole, intense debates between the advocates of biological causation and diagnoses and those who reject the discourse of disease reflect resistance to the current hegemony of the psychiatric establishment and its pharmaceutical sponsors. However, the debate has no bearing on who I am with David and what I am ethically committed to in my relationship with him (Sanders, 2007; van Blarikom, 2006). This stance is not taken to avoid involvement and place the burden on the families of the person with "mental illness" (although that is most often where it falls in our society). My point is that within the context of my therapy relationship with the client, my ethic is solely one of obligation and responsibility to my client. In extreme circumstances, I may decide to intervene, which would constitute a necessarily paternalistic response. Such interventions that are driven by obligation to the professional code of ethics cannot be automatically justified as in the client's best interests. When parents of other clients with a diagnosis of severe "mental illness" have implored me to pressure the client to either take medication or go into the hospital, I have reiterated the significance of the client having one person who will be committed to her only. To join the coalition between the psychiatrist and the parents and family members would mean that the client no longer can trust me to respect her own choices and not take power over her.

C42:   And the problem is that nobody else seemed to notice it, except this guy, Perry.

T42:   Nobody seemed to notice what, that . . .

My own implicit belief that the voices were internal to David is exposed here in that I completely fail to understand his statement. Understandably, if I heard a voice I didn't recognize, I would ask someone near me if they also heard it.

C43:   The voices.

T43:   Uh huh.

C44:   Kenny might have noticed them, but I mean what can you say about Kenny, he's just kind of a real creep.

T44:   Alright, these people that were living with you then at Lords?

C45:   Yeah.

T45:   I see. And you think that they might have also heard what you were hearing.

C46:   Yeah. But uhm—uhm—uhm—I think not nearly to the extent that I was. Uhm—uh, because you know they, I tried to explain that th—this is you know—a ver—fault of—falling—fa—falling into a kind of a—you know, uhm—dream reality, uhm, but the problem is it's *real*, and you see, my parents believe that it's schizophrenia, and the psychiatrist believes that it's schizophrenia, and uh, I guess my sisters believe that it's schizophrenia, but I have no question that it's real.

To me, this is a remarkably lucid description. David's experience has been one of "falling into a kind of dream reality, but the problem is it's *real*," and *no one believes his assertion*. Instead, he is urged to translate his experience into "consensual reality," which does not feel true. He isn't sick or "schizophrenic"—he is being intruded upon, shamed, and threatened. These psychologically meaningful experiences do not correspond to David's understanding of "illness." I can understand why he is affronted by others' assertions about his "schizophrenia" in that his ability to articulate what has happened is fully intact. His ability to argue from his own perception of reality is fully engaged and clear. His assessment of the impact of the voices is reasonable and coherent.

One might argue that all of the typical signs of "severe mental illness" that David reports—hearing voices who have hostile intent, feeling that his privacy has been invaded, that he is threatened by the radio and TV, that his own thoughts are somehow being broadcast against his will—are, if deliberately depathologized, common experiences in our culture. I also wish to avoid "normalizing" his experiences as merely a form of "distress," which I believe euphemizes the severity and catastrophic nature of his condition. I have no doubt that David's life has been one of almost constant affliction, the etiology of which is still contested and caused by many factors in combination. Regarding the relevance of the question of etiology, however, Lisbeth Sommerbeck, a Danish psychotherapist who has worked exclusively within the psychiatric context, states:

> As already stated, psychiatric diagnosis is of no issue in client-centered theory and therapy. The conditions necessary and sufficient for facilitation of the client's most constructive potentials are trusted to be the same for everybody, irrespective of diagnosis. Or seen from another angle: the act of (psychiatric) diagnosing would imply that the therapist is in the position of the expert, he *(sic)* would view the client from his (the therapist's) own frame of reference, the locus of evaluation would be in the therapist, and it would be the therapist, not the client, who knew what was wrong with the client. All this has nothing to do with client-centered therapy; it belongs to the medical model, not to the client-centered model (Sommerbeck, 2003, p. 33).

T46:   Do you mean that it's upsetting to have all these people around you in your life, your parents, your sisters . . .
C47:   Yeah.
T47:   Dr. So-and-so—
C48:   See there's been a big change. My parents are being quite sympathetic now, but uh—uhm—th—this is—this is because they both believe that I—I have also shown some some uhm, truth or r—reason and so [doorbell rings]. . . . Well, I guess you have the door.
T48:   Yes, that's probably (. . .). I interrupted you, David, you were, I guess, I don't know. Where were you?
C49:   Something about my parents . . .
T49:   Being sympathetic?
C50:   Right.
T50:   Because something about that you found some truth or . . .

C51: Well, I really couldn't dream these explanations up by myself. I would have had to be experiencing something to come up with these things that I try to explain. Uh, I think that's the main thing.

T51: So it's like you feel like you have more credibility.

C52: Well, they're on my side, you know, and that's not always been the case that they have uhm—given—given—m—me—uhm—you know the uh—the—well, for example, last night, this girl left her checkbook in a taxi and the driver came to the front door to return it and I didn't want to let him in because he was wearing a jacket that looked like a policeman, you know, and I have ridden in police cars and ambulances and stuff quite a few times and . . .

T52: So it scared you.

C53: Right. But see, that's the main thing, though, my parents have not tolerated uhm—ba—bad behavior on my part. They have called or they have taken me to the hospital, and uhm—in—in that sense, you know, this "whooya tooya" business and stuff and it is really facetious because I I have—uhm—been uh—uhm—tolerated by my parents uh only after I have been hospitalized thirty times. So that proves you see that we have gone along with the uhm—system, and for the voices, and I especially mean the voices on the TV and on the radio and on the street, to say "whooya tooya" I don't think they have the right to do that because my parents have not patted me on the back and you know, expressed their love, you know, they have taken dramatic steps, you know, to get—get this—uh—fever out of—out of my head.

T53: Is the point, David—it's like you feel pissed off at the voices because you feel like you haven't had an easy time of it. Nobody's coddled you. In fact, your parents have had you hospitalized and taken away in cars and things like that, and so it's been very hard on you, and then to have the voices mock you is very upsetting, or just angers you?

C54: Right, yeah, one time I was at a flea market with my sisters and my mom, and the voice on the radio says 'that's why we're mocking you!' and what she's referring to is, is this, kind of, rattling I do with my fingers, uh, I mean, I—I uh—I didn't decide to break my fingers. They just got broken in accidents.

T54: But you're being held responsible for your fingers rattling, when it's not your fault, that is, it was accidental that your fingers have been broken in accidents.

C55: Right. I guess. I mean I have read *To Kill a Mockingbird*. Sometimes I feel that that uhm, that this Boo Radley [a reference to a character in *To Kill A Mockingbird*] that stays in the house all the time, and has some strange affection for little kids, you know, it's kind of one part—part of things that I deal with, so, anyway. I uhm—I uhm—met—met—mad. . . . I guess uhm that I—I uhm—ma—make uh—fe—focus on certain thoughts, you know, I think that that's what I'm supposed to do and I don't know if I'm suppo—supposed to look at the negative side of things.

T55: And you're confused about the fact that your attention tends to focus on certain thoughts that are negative, but you're not sure if you should be paying attention to those things?

C56: I—uhm—I'm just—really upset because the voices insist on certain thoughts, and I uhm, especially in the last week or so I've been, I've been accepting these things, and real—really becoming very stupid. So, anyway. It is . . .

T56: Is it that you feel kind of demoralized right now, kind of defeated because you've been accepting some things that make you feel stupid?

C57: Yeah. And of course smoking.

T57: Smoking, you've been smoking and that bothers you too?

C58: Yeah. So uh I guess that—that the sa—sem—sss—sensation of—of you know puh—pulling the—somehow I'm really focusing on—on this thing of "trees and tracks and trying and trips and treking and tra—tra—trap—trafficking" and I can't get these things out of my mind. These t- t- tru—truism and stuff.

T58: You mean it's just like a bunch of words all beginning with "tr," and you just can't get your mind off that groove, kind of, is that it?

C59: Yeah.

T59: And it's annoying to you?

C60: Well, I—I sought—sought. . . . I heard the voices say one—one time something about CIDOC [Centro Intercultural de Documentacion] in Mexico, and they seemed to be saying that they didn't treat me right at CIDOC and eh—a foc—focus on—on that situation is—is not really relevant. I mean I was 18. I did the whole thing by myself. I caught the bus. I didn't get lost. I didn't lose anything—except my passport—which it turns out that I didn't lose anyway, and I went to the embassy to try to get a new one, and I climbed the mountain, Mount Popo, [Popocatepetl] and—and I went on lots of long walks and there's no question that in Chicago I've walked as much as the next guy. And, it is you know at—you said something about mocking. Well I've made that relation before in my mind, you know, with the word *mark*, and with *To Kill a Mockingbird*—Mockingbird, you know, and now the voices are saying just a minute ago, "That's Jimmy boy!" and "Tom's great compromise is down the drain!" you know, and that you know I—I have made that association before, I have really—really—don't need to be in intracted—tracted by that.

T60: I'm not sure what happened. Did—you don't feel that I was trying to stimulate some sort of association, did you, by my . . . ?

I think, in retrospect, I was anxious in this segment when he stated that "you said something about mocking." When he ended with his statement that he "really—really—don't need to be intracted," I took his meaning too personally.

C61: No, you were just saying—

T61: I was basically just trying to understand how the voices were treating you, what the relation was.

Here, I should have let David complete his statement because it seems as though he probably did understand my motives and did not make an assumption that I was up to anything.

C62: Right. So anyway, I mean, I think that was just a normal part of the conversation, because I said first, something about going to a flea market and the lady says "That's why we're mocking you."

T62: Well, I'm not exactly sure what the sequence was, but I certainly didn't intend anything by using that term. But what you're telling me is the voices are somehow—or you make these associations between the term *mocking* and *mark* and *To Kill a Mockingbird*, right? And it's kind of disturbing, that bunch of associations.

C63: Right, uhm, that's the kind of stuff that the voices prey on. And I—I know that.

T63: That's the kind of grist for their mill, almost.

C64: Yeah, I know that. You know yesterday I was just thinking about moccasins, you know, eh I—I really don't—don't see it as mocking, I see it as "my cousin," "moccasin." That's all there is to it. But the voices—voices don't make the association either, so why should I? Heh. That—that is just as significant as pair of socks, right? Heh. And uhm—I uhm am—in—am—kind of uhm in—in fo—focusing—and I don't know if that means that I should make associations 'cause that means that I'm trying to focus, you see, and I think that, you know, to build some kind of personal inference around it, is not what I'm trying to do. And I I think that it—it's—it—intractable anyway.

T64:   David, I'm not sure I followed much of what you just said, but it—I guess part of what I understood was you're confused in a way of what to pay attention to in your mind? It's like you want to focus, but you don't—

C65:   It's just "Monkey see! Monkey do!" The voices—the voices continue making assertions, and I—I—I just want to say something back, but I guess I'm too eh—exc—exssss—eh—eh I think it's—it's excluding, you know, I can't—I can't forget, you know, that, you know, I have done some things which were, you know, mistakes, that they weren't, you know, what was lucky, you know.

T65:   You feel I guess some remorse, you rememb . . . [tape flip] you can't quite forget about those, or you can't put them out of your mind, even though they're in the past.

A more accurate response might have been "You'd really like to argue back against the voices but then you think about some mistakes you've made and it kind of undermines you from opposing them."

C66:   Just uhm, all I know is last year when I was completely out of control, I wrote something about "Jimmy boy" and "times of great compromises of certain compromises or uncertain times." And that was meaningful to me because I have this tendency to want to share . . .

T66:   Share with other people.

C67:   Right. And it's—sh—it's—it's nothing wrong with that, and that's what the voices are preventing. And that's about all I have to say.

T67:   It's like the voices are preventing you from sharing your life or your thoughts with other people and that makes you mad.

C68:   Right, right. They're preventing me from using my basic wits now. I don't expect to be any anybody special. I just expect to feel camaraderie with other people, that's all.

T68:   It's not like you want to be a star or a special person, but you'd like . . .

C69:   I have no respect for stars. I think they're all idiots.

T69:   But you would like to feel a sense of camaraderie with other people.

C70:   Right, there's no question that America's a bunch of—a bunch of real asinine bastards trying to get their trip together. And I could care less. The voices have totally ruined my trip.

T70:   And you're pissed off at them because they've ruined your life.

I should have used his term *trip* instead of the word *life*. I am not sure that *trip* is as far-reaching as the word *life*.

C71:   Well, huh, nobody's ever going to get their trip together, so that's just too fucking bad. Michael—Michael Jackson is supposed to be everybody's hero and the guy's even vainer than I am.

T71:   When I mentioned the term *stars*, it seems to me you then started—it reminded you of your antipathy toward a lot of these rock stars—is that what happened?

C72:   Yeah.

T72:   Uh huh.

C73:   I mean, you know, when you're 15 years old, you know, and somebody's saying something about like "leper messiah, he sucked up into his brain," you know—you know, same to you! I mean it—it's not—it's—not music, okay?

T73:   David, I am going to need to stop in a minute.

C74:   Okay.

Assessment of the Session

A close look at this session shows a large number of tracking or empathic following responses along with "true" empathic responses. An empathic "following" response is a tracking response in which the therapist is simply verbally noting what he or she is being told. An example of a simple tracking response is seen in T37. Wilczynski, Brodley, and Brody's "Rating System for Nondirective Client-Centered Interviews—Revised" (2008) defines a *true* empathic response as one in which the therapist *experiences* an inner understanding of the client's communication. An example of a true empathic response is T70 where I say, "And you're pissed off at them because they've ruined your life."

There are mistakes in the session in which I interrupt or distract David, although I do not feel—as I read the transcript—that those mistakes led to any significant effect in this session. I believe that my behavior in the session was largely consistent with the stance of principled nondirectiveness. For instance, when I make clear to David that I am not following him completely or when I explicitly check by asking him "Is that your point?" the implicit message is that I value being corrected; that his account of reality is of the utmost importance. Hopefully, the client who experiences consistent, effortful, empathic responding concludes correctly that your intention is simply to understand, that you value getting his expressed meaning accurately and that you actively *want* to understand. Serendipitously, the empathic understanding response form that is given by the therapist to check her own understanding also conveys the therapist's unconditional positive regard.

There was a series of client statements and my responses at beginning at C29 through T41 where the momentum of the session subtly quickened and where I felt we were very much in contact with each other. I felt my responses were on target and that David experienced my accurate empathic responses with enthusiasm and relief and greater connection. Clearly, this client is fully capable of representing his experience in the session, of using the "affordances" offered in the therapy situation (Bohart, 2004). I think it is possible that David experienced at *least some temporary comfort in being believed, understood, and accepted. Brodley who worked for* five years in an institution with persons with diagnoses of schizophrenia remarked that these clients tended to "clear up" in the process of being carefully understood at least for the duration of the session. This point is important as it points to the possibilities for greater comprehensibility and support if it were possible to provide a consistent climate of the therapeutic conditions. Currently, there is an international group called *Intervoice* as well as English, German, and Danish groups for "voice hearers" that function as a source of support for persons who have to cope with voices (Romme, Escher, Dillon, Corstens, & Morris, 2009, p. 77). The point here is that there is an array of interpersonal options for assistance and care.

Rogers's motivational theory consists of the axiom of the actualizing tendency, which is the directional life force characteristic of all life forms. A client-centered therapist (as Rogers outlined in his "Attitude and Orientation of the Counselor" in 1951) tentatively, and later with more experience, more confidently, holds the hypothesis that the client before him has the capacity for development, self-regulation, and growth—the capacity to make choices. Even when those choices may turn out to be deleterious or harmful to the person, this process of self-determination progresses toward greater self-differentiation, awareness, and behavioral regulation and, through learning from one's mistakes, better decisions.

When an unafflicted client is working with us, the therapist enjoys great satisfaction in observing the pace of personal change, the increasing self-authority, greater capacity for independent action, and stronger internal sense of self as the locus of evaluation. When we answer the call of the other, the one who is greatly afflicted, one whose basic expression is enigmatic or disorganized or dysfluent, the tendency to abandon the belief in the growth hypothesis arises out of fear of our own inadequacy and fear for the client.

This fear is not irrational. Functioning as a client-centered therapist in today's clinical culture is a great challenge. Graduate students are encouraged to undertake a suicide assessment the moment the client expresses a wish for death as a relief from suffering. In these crisis situations, a therapist needs to possess a high degree of self-confidence and a confidence in the client and be willing to risk his or her professional safety to stay with a client who is experiencing frightening chaotic inner events—voices that are experienced as intrusive or insulting, threatening to the client, or demanding that the client act against others close to them. Rogers has stated that at these times of crisis, what is needed is not to abandon the hypothesis. Instead, it is the time in which faith in the client's inner resources for change and self-direction is most needed.

A PHENOMENOLOGICAL UNDERSTANDING OF LIVING A LOST LIFE

Client-centered therapists seek to understand the client's immediate, moment-to-moment communication. Over time, these moments of understanding allow us to build a more elaborated and complex understanding of the client's frame of reference. This two-way process of communication and reception is a dynamic one that implies we are always tentative and willing to revise our grasp of meanings. I believe we can assume that the person seeks to be understood, even when the client is noncommunicative. Involuntary clients—such as those persons who are incarcerated or institutionalized or children and adolescents who are remanded to therapy by authorities—may be exceptions.

As the therapy relationship persists over time, I experience the growth of my own understanding generated by the process of empathic responding through having the understandings endorsed by the client, or, conversely, by being corrected. The client's take on things and use of particular words and phrases takes shape in my mind as I construe her communications in terms of my own personal framework of meanings, memories, emotional history, and the conscious and unconscious assumptions I bring to the interaction from my own "location" in the social world. From my own social and cultural location, I strive in this instance to encounter David, a man who has lost his life as he knew it.

In this session and throughout our therapy relationship, David recalls and reiterates the devastation which he has experienced; the intrusion of voices, the loss of his self-determination through forced hospitalizations, and forced injections of neuroleptic medications. His affliction and the inadequate approaches to meeting his needs have led to his loss of not only the potentials for growth and development but also the fundamental experience of a comprehensible self. As he has aged, David is left behind unable to operate on his world and so instead succumbs to a passivity so common in our mental-health system where the medications are heavily sedating and there are no opportunities for meaningful contribution to the public world.

When reading Jonathan Lear's book *Radical Hope* (2006), I was struck by the similarity between the catastrophic loss experienced by the Crow nation and the analogous loss of one's personal world. In the book, *Plenty Coups*, the last great Crow chief, gives this account:

> I have not told you half of what happened when I was young. . . . I can think back and tell you much more of war and horse stealing. But when the buffalo went away, the hearts of my people dropped to the ground, and they could not lift them up again. After this nothing happened. There was little singing anywhere (Lear, 2006, p. 2).

Lear proceeds to conduct an ethical inquiry into the impact of a radical loss of the whole framework of meaning within which the Crow people understood their lives. "After this nothing happened" meant that all of the large and small acts of living—making ready for battle, decorating one's horses for battle, planting one's coup stick, displaying scalps won in battle—were no longer possible except as *enactments* of past exploits. Being a Crow warrior whose life was given meaning through constant warfare and the building up of courageous character in war became impossible once the buffalo were gone and the Crow were forced to adopt a settled agricultural life.

This book illuminated for me, although the situations are radically different, the profundity of "normal" loss as opposed to the loss of the whole framework of meaning. After the voices came, it is not too much of an exaggeration to say that David lost his life as he knew it. The avenues to a larger world of relationships and experiences—his social visibility as a person who counted to others—vanished as he could no longer inhabit those contexts. As Lear explains, losing one's structure of meaning—one's traditions, one's culture—also entails losing moral definitions and evidence that one is living a courageous life.

> One would experience a rip in the fabric of one's self. If we think of the self as partially constituted by its most basic commitments, then in jettisoning those commitments one would be disrupting one's most basic sense of being (Lear, 2006, p. 65).

Just as David lost his visibility and position in society, his circle of friends, the chance for affection and sexual love, children and family, the chances for interesting work and new learning, his family lost the beautiful, creative, brilliant child they had loved and nurtured. And we, as a society, lost all the possibilities for creative, productive engagement David might have offered to us.

For the individual labeled and diagnosed as suffering from severe "mental illness," no matter the source or etiology of the affliction, imagine the suffering of experiencing the ongoing torment of insulting voices that threaten you or talk nonsense and find that no one believes you. Attempts to convince David that what he was so vividly experiencing was not "real" but was "schizophrenia" were undoubtedly well intentioned but only left him even further estranged. This experience-distant response offers no real explanation and no help. This radical disjuncture between David's perceived reality and "consensual reality" constitutes invalidation of his personhood. It is a way of being cancelled. You are no longer respected as a person who has the right and the capacity to tell truth. You don't count—only the "illness" counts—and that transit to the land of the sick justifies almost total control of your decisions.

Stolorow captures the alienation and estrangement that accompanies emotional trauma and attributes a person's reaction to the trauma in terms of his loss of everyday certainties that he terms *absolutisms*.

> When a person says to a friend, "I'll see you later" . . . these are statements . . . whose validity is not open for discussion. Such absolutisms are the basis for a kind of naïve realism and optimism that allow one to function in the world, experienced as stable and predictable. It is in the essence of emotional trauma that it shatters these absolutisms, a catastrophic loss of innocence that permanently alters one's sense of being-in-the-world. Massive deconstruction of the absolutisms of everyday life exposes the inescapable contingency of existence in a universe that is random and unpredictable and in which no safety or continuity of being can be assured. Trauma thereby exposes "the unbearable embeddedness of being" (Stolorow & Atwood, 1992, p. 22). *As a result, the traumatized person cannot help but perceive aspects of existence that lie well outside the absolutized horizons of normal everydayness. It is in this sense that the worlds of traumatized persons are fundamentally incommensurable with those of others, the deep chasm in which an anguished sense of estrangement and solitude takes form* (Stolorow, 2011, p. 145, my emphasis).

We could say that not only is David's world "fundamentally incommensurable with those of others" but also it is very likely that few others realize that anything so devastating has occurred. Most of us have no reference for this experience of finding the world you have known slowly vanishing—and being replaced with an incomprehensible moonscape inhabited by hostile whisperers who never stop.

The institutions of our culture have failed persons who undergo these experiences, making social control the goal instead of supporting the development of self-regulation and self-determination. David has stated that the medications have never stopped his voices and that they make him "stupid." His mother observes that at this point in his life, at age 53, his previous brilliance, creative intelligence, and psychomotor mastery as a superior swimmer and athlete have greatly diminished, certainly in part because of decades of neuroleptics. A new vision of care is needed; in this, European countries such as the United Kingdom, Denmark, the Netherlands, and France are more advanced than the United States (see Romme et al., 2009).

An environment that might be closely organized around and attuned to each person who is currently "severely mentally ill" is both imaginable and fundable if our society changes its priorities. Clients would have access to personal assistants and caregivers whose mission would be devotion to the emotional and physical health and security of the person and to take seriously and at face value his communications regarding his day-to-day fluctuations in mood and energy. Group sessions might be arranged to help the person respond to hostile or threatening voices; ceremonies of protection could be performed. His or her belongings and possessions would be guarded against theft or carelessness. The person would be given opportunities to earn money in many different ways and to avoid work when overwhelmed without censure or disappointment from the community. Spiritual practices, artistic opportunities, and ways in which the person might help others and give care to others would dignify the person's life.[2]

Principles of respect, acceptance, and appreciation of the afflicted person would govern these communities, all of which is obvious but extremely hard to realize in a culture that wants to distance itself from the "alien" and in which the "gold standard" life is defined by earning power and conspicuous consumption. However, it is clear that more collectively oriented cultures in which people live together in larger compounds and have opportunities for participation result in longer lives and better recovery (van Blarikom, 2006, pp. 161–162). A deep moral and political shift will need to occur in our culture to realize this humane model of care. Most important would be the freedom of the person to experiment with possible modes of healing. There would be no more coercive practices, unwanted injections, forced hospitalization except under extreme circumstances (such as committing violent crimes). Many who work in institutions may bridle at this idea, asserting that that is what already happens and that these unfortunate practices are necessary to protect the person and others. Perhaps in some cases this may be true. In many, it is not (Szasz, 1997).

A PRACTICE OF HOPE

I hope a reading of the transcript offered here robustly displays the selfhood of this client. David articulates what he perceives to have occurred in his life—the destructiveness and devastation he has endured. In most of our sessions, his interactions with me satisfy the first of Rogers's necessary and sufficient conditions, which is two persons are in contact (Rogers, 1957). Contrary to many descriptions of persons who are diagnosed with schizophrenia, David resembled the majority of the clients I have worked with over the last 38 years: he participated in therapy voluntarily; he desired to communicate and be understood; his frame of reference was, to a large extent, accessible. In spite of some

---

[2]Although there have been attempts at creating such communities, they are works in progress, and it is interesting that the more successful programs have found that the model of *individual placement and support* (IPS, or treatment tailored to the client's own preferences and interests) has better outcomes than other models such as *psychosocial rehabilitation* (PSR) (Mueser et al., 2004, p. 485).

expressions and language that I was not able to understand, I did not need to apply "process diagnoses" (Warner, 1998, 2006); nor did I see David as *pre-expressive*, which Prouty describes as a person who is not yet in contact and does not indicate any desire to communicate (Prouty, 1994). I am in agreement with Warner's statement regarding the ongoing debate over etiology of severe mental illness.

> As with client-centered work in general, this model of client-centered work with "thought-disordered" psychotic experience doesn't depend on resolving issues of etiology. Whether the cause of psychotic experience is primarily biological, . . . primarily developmental/familial . . . or some mixture of the two, the human impulse to communicate and to process experience remains. A client's having a safe space in which to sort through thoughts, feelings and choices maximizes the person's potential for having a positive sense of self and confidence in relating to others in the world (Warner, 2002, p. 470).

Although "schizophrenia" has been reported by many researchers, anthropologists, and native healers, persons who have been so categorized do not constitute a clearly delineated group. As is apparent from stories such as Georgina Wakefield's account of her son's affliction, *Living with Christian* (2010), and the accounts of other people who hear voices, in many cases persons adapt, sometimes with support of medication, to these voices and to living with immense difficulties of this affliction. David has not had the advantages that persons living in Europe have had where groups organized for "voice hearers" are given vital support (Romme et al., 2009). By contrast, David's story is a long, solitary struggle to cope with the physical and social sequelae of living with this condition.

Carl Rogers grew up with experiences in agriculture. From an early age, he was sensitized to the processes of life and never ceased to be inspired by the natural world. In his book *A Way of Being*, Rogers illustrates the growth tendency in recalling his root cellar from childhood:

> The actualizing tendency can, of course, be thwarted or warped, but it cannot be destroyed without destroying the organism. I remember that in my boyhood, the bin in which we stored our winter's supply of potatoes was in the basement, several feet below a small window. The conditions were unfavorable, but the potatoes would begin to sprout—pale white sprouts, so unlike the healthy green shoots they sent up when planted in the soil in the spring. But these sad, spindly sprouts would grow two or three feet in length as they reached toward the distant light of the window. The sprouts were, in their bizarre, futile growth, a sort of desperate expression of the directional tendency I have been describing. They would never become plants, never mature, never fulfill their real potential. But under the most adverse circumstances, they were striving to become. Life would not give up, even if it could not flourish. In dealing with clients whose lives have been terribly warped, in working with men and women on the back wards of state hospitals, I often think of those potato sprouts. So unfavorable have been the conditions in which these people have developed that their lives often seem abnormal, twisted, scarcely human. Yet, the directional tendency in them can be trusted. The clue to understanding their behavior is that they are striving to move toward growth, toward becoming. To healthy persons, the results may seem bizarre and futile, but they are life's desperate attempts to become itself. This potent constructive tendency is an underlying basis of the person-centered approach (Rogers, 1980, pp. 118–119).

A poem David wrote strikes a similar chord of life still striving and ultimately not lost. He said at one point, many years into his affliction, "I still have hope that my life will be interesting."

REFERENCES

Anderson, H., & Gehart, D. (Eds.). (2006). *Collaborative therapy: Relationships and conversations that make a difference.* New York: Routledge/Taylor Francis Group.

Baldwin, M. (1987). Interview with Carl Rogers on the use of self in therapy. In M. Baldwin & V. Satir (Eds.), *The use of self in therapy* (pp. 45–52). New York: Haworth Press.

Bohart, A. C. (2004) How do clients make empathy work? *Person-Centered and Experiential Psychotherapies, 3*(2), 102–116.

Bohart, A. C. & Tallman, K. (1999). *How clients make therapy work.* Washington, DC: American Psychological Association.

Brodley, B. T. (2011a). Ethics in Psychotherapy. In K. A. Moon, M. Witty, B. Grant, & B. Rice (Eds.), *Practicing client-centered therapy: Selected writings of Barbara Temaner Brodley* (pp. 33–46). Ross-on-Wye, UK: PCCS Books.

Brodley, B. T. (2011b). The nondirective attitude in client-centered therapy. In K. Moon, M. Witty, B. Grant & B. Rice (Eds.). *Practicing client-centered therapy: Selected writings of Barbara Temaner Brodley* (pp. 47–62). Ross-on-Wye, UK: PCCS Books.

Brodley, B. T. (2011c). Client-centered values limit the application of research findings: An issue for discussion. In K. Moon, M. Witty, B. Grant & B. Rice (Eds.), *Practicing client-centered therapy: Selected writings of Barbara Temaner Brodley* (pp. 63–70). Ross-on-Wye, UK: PCCS Books.

Brodley, B. T. (2011d). The actualizing concept in client-centered theory. In K. A. Moon, M. Witty, B. Grant, & B. Rice (Eds.), *Practicing client-centered therapy: Selected writings of Barbara Temaner Brodley* (pp. 153–170). Ross-on-Wye, UK: PCCS Books.

Cooper, M., O'Hara, M., Schmid, P., & Wyatt, G. (Eds.). (2007). *The handbook of person-centered psychotherapy and counseling.* New York: Palgrave McMillan.

Cooper, M., Watson, J. C., & Holldampf, D. (2010). *Person-centered and experiential therapies work: A review of the research on counseling, psychotherapy, and related practices.* Ross-on-Wye, UK: PCCS Books.

Ehrbar, R. D. (2007). Taking context and culture into account in the core conditions: A feminist person-centered approach. In G. Proctor & M. Napier (Eds.), *Encountering feminism: Intersections between feminism and the person-centred approach* (pp. 154–165). Ross-on-Wye, UK: PCCS Books.

Elkins, D. N. (2007). The medical model of psychotherapy: Its limitations and failures. *Journal of Humanistic Psychology, 49*(66), 66–84.

Elliott, R., & Freire, E. (2010). The effectiveness of person-centred and experiential therapies. In M. Cooper, J. C. Watson, & D. Holldampf (Eds.), *Person-centred and experiential therapies work: A review of the research on counseling, psychotherapy, and related practices* (pp. 1–15). Ross-on-Wye, UK: PCCS Books.

Freire, P. (1970). *The pedagogy of the oppressed.* New York: Continuum.

Grant, B. (1990). Principled and instrumental nondirectiveness in person-centered and client-centered therapy. *Person-Centered Review, 5,* 77–88.

Grant, B. (2004). The imperative of ethical justification in psychotherapy: The special case of client-centered therapy. *Person-Centered and Experiential Psychotherapies, 3*(3), 152–165.

Lear, J. (2006). *Radical hope: Ethics in the face of cultural devastation.* Cambridge, MA: Harvard University Press.

Levitt, B. E. (2005). Non-directivity: The foundational attitude. *Embracing non-directivity: reassessing person-centered theory in the 21st century* (pp. 5–16). Ross-on-Wye, UK: PCCS Books.

McNamee, S,. & Gergen, K. (Eds.). (1992). *Therapy as social construction.* Thousand Oaks, CA: Sage.

Mueser, K. T., Clark, R. E., Haines, M., Bond, G., Essock, S. M., Becker, D. R., Wolfe, R., & Swain, K. (2004). The Hartford study of supported employment for persons with severe mental illness. *Journal of Consulting and Clinical Psychology, 72*(3), 479–490.

O'Hara, M. (2006). The radical humanism of Carl Rogers and Paolo Freire. In G. Proctor, M. Cooper, P. Sanders, & B. Malcolm (Eds.), *Politicizing the person-centred approach* (pp. 115–126). Ross-on-Wye, UK: PCCS Books.

Proctor, G. (2002). *The dynamics of power in counselling and psychotherapy: Ethics, politics and practice.* Ross-on-Wye, UK: PCCS Books.

Proctor, G., & Napier, M. (2004). *Encountering Feminism: Intersections between feminism and the person-centred approach.* Ross-on-Wye, UK: PCCS Books.

Prouty, G. (1994). *Theoretical evolution in person-centered/experiential therapy: Applications to schizophrenic and retarded psychoses.* Westport, CT: Praeger.

Raskin, N. J. (1947/2005). The nondirective attitude. *The Person-Centered Journal, 12,* 1–2.

Raskin, N. J. (1988). Responses to person-centered vs. client-centered? *Renaissance, 5,* 3–4.

Rogers, C. R. (1942). *Counseling and psychotherapy.* Boston: Houghton Mifflin.

Rogers, C. R. (1951). *Client-centered therapy: Its current practice, implications, and theory.* Boston: Houghton Mifflin.

Rogers, C. R. (1957). The necessary and sufficient conditions of therapeutic personality change. *Journal of Consulting Psychology, 21,* 95–103.

Rogers, C. R. (1959). A theory of therapy, personality, and interpersonal relationships as developed in the client-centered framework. In S. Koch (Ed.), *Psychology: A study of a science. Vol. III: Formulations of the person and the social context* (pp. 184–256). New York: McGraw-Hill.

Rogers, C. R. (1961). *On becoming a person.* Boston: Houghton Mifflin.

Rogers, C. R. (1980). *A way of being.* Boston: Houghton Mifflin.

Romme, M., Escher, S., Dillon, J., Corstens, D., & Morris, M. (2009). *Living with voices: 50 stories of recovery.* Ross-on-Wye, UK: PCCS Books.

Shlien, J. M. (2003). *To live an honourable life: Invitations to think about client-centred therapy and the person-centred approach.* Ross-on-Wye, UK: PCCS Books.

Sommerbeck, L. (2003). *The client-centred therapist in psychiatric contexts.* Ross-on-Wye, UK: PCCS Books.

Stolorow, R. (2011). The phenomenology, contextuality, and existentiality of emotional trauma: Ethical implications. *Journal of Humanistic Psychology, 51*(2), 142–151.

Stolorow, R. D. & Atwood, G. E. (1992*). Contexts of being: The intersubjective foundations of psychological lilfe.* Vol. 12. Psychoanalytic inquiry book series, Hillsdale, NJ: Analytic Press Inc.

Szasz, T. (1997). *Insanity: The idea and its consequences.* New York: John Wiley & Sons.

van Blarikom, J. (2006). A person-centered approach to schizophrenia. *Person-Centered and Experiential Psychotherapies, 5*(3), 155–173.

van Blarikom, J. (2007). Is there a place for illness in the person-centered approach? A response to Sanders. *Person-Centered and Experiential Psychotherapies, 6*(3), 205–209.

Wakefield, G. (2010). *Loving Christian: One family's journey through schizophrenia.* Ross-on-Wye, UK: PCCS Books.

Wampold, B. E. (2001). *The great psychotherapy debate: Models, methods, and findings.* Mahwah, NJ: Erlbaum.

Warner, M. S. (2002). Luke's dilemmas: A client-centered/experiential model of processing with a schizophrenic thought disorder. In J. Watson, R. Goldman, & M. S. Warner (Eds.), *Client-centred and experiential psychotherapy in the 21st century: Advances in theory, research, and practice* (pp. 459–472). Ross-on-Wye, UK: PCCS Books.

Warner, M. S. (1998). A client-centered approach to therapeutic work with dissociated and fragile process. In L. Greenberg, J. Watson, & G. Lietaer (Eds.), *Handbook of Experiential Psychotherapy,* New York: Guilford.

Warner, M. S. (2006). Toward an integrated person-centered theory of wellness and psychopathology. *Person-Centered and Experiential Psychotherapies, 5*(1), 4–20.

Weil, S. (1951). Reflections on the right use of school studies with a view to the love of God. *Waiting for God* (pp. 105–116). New York: Harper & Row.

Wilczynski, J., Brodley, B. T., & Brody, A. F. (2008). A rating system for studying nondirective client-centered interviews—Revised. *The Person-Centered Journal, 5*(1,2), 34–57.

Witty, M. C. (2005). Nondirectiveness and the problem of influence. In B. Levitt (Ed.), *Embracing non-directivity: Reassessing person-centered theory and practice in the 21st century* (pp. 228–247). Ross-on-Wye, UK: PCCS Books.

Editors' Introduction

Albert Ellis was trained as a psychoanalyst but found he was not getting the results he wanted so, in characteristic style, he created his own system, known as rational emotive behavior therapy (REBT). REBT is the precursor of many of today's cognitive and cognitive-behavioral therapies.

Ellis's style was inimitable, as anyone knows who heard him speak or who had the good fortune to observe him in a therapy session. He was direct, forceful, confident, and convinced of the correctness of his views.

In the case that follows we have an opportunity to observe Ellis working with a young woman whose thinking is clearly irrational and who presents the type of problem with which REBT therapists seem to excel. We also see Ellis making mistakes in therapy, acknowledging his mistakes, and critiquing his own work.

The reader will find it interesting to contrast Ellis's style with Aaron Beck's treatment of a depressed clinical psychologist in Chapter 6. Ellis was known as a master clinician, and Beck has the same reputation. However, as these two cases clearly demonstrate, their therapy styles are different, and REBT therapists approach clients in a somewhat different way—e.g., Ellis maintains that human "musts" almost always precede the "automatic thoughts" that cognitive therapists believe to be at the heart of human suffering. Also note that Albert Ellis is much more forceful, active, and direct than Aaron Beck, who is more likely to use Socratic dialogue and gentle, probing questions. Which therapist would you prefer if you were the client?

How much do you know about the imbroglio involving Albert Ellis and the Albert Ellis Institute? Do you have a position on the decisions that were made on both sides?

How do you think your own personality will influence your decision about which therapeutic approach to adopt? Do you believe some clients are a better fit for cognitive therapy, while others are a better fit for REBT or behavior therapy? If so, why?

4 | A TWENTY-THREE-YEAR-OLD WOMAN GUILTY ABOUT NOT FOLLOWING HER PARENTS' RULES[1]

Albert Ellis

Martha, a twenty-three-year-old woman, came for help because she claimed she was self-punishing, compulsive, afraid of males, had no goals in life, and was guilty about her relationship with her parents.

SEGMENTS FROM THE FIRST SESSION

C-1:   Well, for about a year and a half since I graduated from college, I've had the feeling that something was the matter with me. I seem to have a tendency toward punishing myself. I'm accident-prone. I'm forever banging myself or falling down stairs, or something like that. And my relationship with my father is causing me a great deal of trouble. I've never been able to figure out where is the responsibility and what my relationship with my parents should be.

T-2:   Do you live with them?

C-3:   No, I don't. I moved out in March.

T-4:   What does your father do?

C-5:   He is a newspaper editor.

T-6:   And your mother is a housewife?

C-7:   Yes.

T-8:   Any other children?

C-9:   Yes, I have two younger brothers. One is twenty; the other is sixteen. I'm twenty-three. The sixteen-year-old has polio, and the other one has an enlarged heart. We never had much money, but we always had the feeling that love and security in life are what count. And the first thing that disturbed me was, when I was about sixteen years old, my father began to drink seriously. To me he had been the in-fallible person. Anything he said was right. And since I moved out and before I

From Ellis, A. (1974). *Growth through Reason* (pp. 223–286). Hollywood: Wilshire Books. Reprinted by permission of the author.

[1]In this early case of REBT, I stress the cognitive and philosophic techniques commonly used in this therapy. From the beginning, however, REBT has been highly behavioral, especially in its use of *in vivo* desensitization or exposure with clients like Martha, who are afraid to risk failure and rejection. REBT makes use of operant conditioning, stimulus control, relapse prevention, and many other behavioral methods. It is also very forceful, emotive, and experiential, and uses many affective methods such as shame-attacking exercises, rational emotive imagery, forceful coping statements, and vigorous disputing of clients' irrational beliefs.

moved out, I've wondered where my responsibility to my family lies. Because if they would ask me to do something, if I didn't do it, I would feel guilty about it.

T-10:   What sort of things did they ask you to do?

C-11:   Well, they felt that it just wasn't right for an unmarried girl to move out. Also, I find it easier to lie than to tell the truth, if the truth is unpleasant. I'm basically afraid of men and afraid to find a good relationship with a man that would lead to marriage. My parents have never approved of anyone I have gone out with. In thinking about it, I wonder whether I, subconsciously maybe, went out of my way to find somebody they wouldn't approve of.

T-12:   Do you go with anyone now?

C-13:   Yes, two people.

T-14:   And are you serious about either one?

C-15:   I really don't know. One is sort of serious about me, but he thinks there's something the matter with me that I have to straighten out. I have also at various times been rather promiscuous, and I don't want to be that way.

T-16:   Have you enjoyed sex?

C-17:   Not particularly. I think—in trying to analyze myself and find out why I was promiscuous, I think I was afraid not to be.

T-18:   Afraid they wouldn't like you?

C-19:   Yes. This one fellow that I've been going with—in fact, both of them said I don't have a good opinion of myself.

T-20:   What do you work at?

C-21:   I'm a copywriter for an advertising agency. I don't know if this means anything, but when I was in college, I never could make up my mind what to major in. I had four or five majors. I was very impulsive about the choice of college.

T-22:   What did you finally pick?

C-23:   I went to the University of Illinois.

T-24:   What did you finally major in?

C-25:   I majored in—it was a double major: advertising and English.

T-26:   Did you do all right in college?

C-27:   Yes, I was a Phi Beta Kappa. I graduated with honors.

T-28:   You had no difficulty—even though you had trouble in making up your mind— you had no difficulty with the work itself?

C-29:   No, I worked very hard. My family always emphasized that I couldn't do well in school, so I had to work hard. I always studied hard. Whenever I set my mind to do anything, I really worked at it. And I was always unsure of myself with people. Consequently, I've almost always gone out with more than one person at the same time, maybe because of a fear of rejection by one. Also, something that bothers me more than anything is that I think that I have the ability to write fiction. But I don't seem to be able to discipline myself. Instead of spending my time wisely, as far as writing is concerned, I'll let it go, let it go, and then go out several nights a week— which I know doesn't help me. When I ask myself why I do it, I don't know.

T-30:   Are you afraid the writing wouldn't be good enough?

C-31:   I have that basic fear.

T-32:   That's right: it is a *basic* fear.

C-33:   Although I have pretty well convinced myself that I have talent, I'm just afraid to apply myself. My mother always encouraged me to write, and she always encouraged me to keep on looking for something better in everything I do. From the time I started to go out with boys, when I was about thirteen or fourteen, she never wanted me to get interested in one boy. There was always something better somewhere else. "Go out and look for it." And if somebody didn't please me in all respects, "Go out and look for somebody else." I think that this has influenced the feeling that I've always had that when I might be interested in one person, I'm always looking for someone else.

T-34:   Yes, I'm sure it probably has.

C-35:   But I don't know what I'm looking for.

T-36:   You seem to be looking for perfection. You're looking for security, certainty.

Generally, in doing psychotherapy, I first obtain a moderate degree of background information to identify a symptom that I can concretely use to show her what her basic philosophy or value system is and how she can change it. I thus asked her, in T-30, "Are you afraid the writing wouldn't be good enough?" because I assume, on the basis of rational emotive behavior theory, that there are only a few reasons why she is not writing, and that this is probably one of them. Once she admits she has a fear of failure in writing, I emphasize that this is probably her general or basic fear—so that she will begin to see that her fear of failure is all-pervasive and may explain some other dysfunctional behavior she has mentioned. In T-36, I flatly tell her that I think she's looking for perfection and certainty. I hope she will be somewhat startled by this statement. I intend eventually to show her that her writing fears (and other symptoms) largely stem from her perfectionism. As it happens, she does not appear ready yet to take up my hypothesis; so I bide my time, knowing that I will sooner or later get back to forcing her to look at some of the concepts behind her disturbed behavior.

C-37:   The basic problem is that I'm worried about my family. I'm worried about money. And I never seem to be able to relax.

T-38:   Why are you worried about your family? Let's go into that, first of all. What's to be concerned about? They have certain demands which you don't want to adhere to.

C-39:   I was brought up to think that I mustn't be selfish.

T-40:   Oh, we'll have to knock that out of your head!

C-41:   I think that that is one of my basic problems.

T-42:   That's right. You were brought up to be Florence Nightingale.

C-43:   Yes, I was brought up in a family of sort of would-be Florence Nightingales, now that I analyze the whole pattern of my family history. . . . My father became really alcoholic sometime when I was away in college. My mother developed a breast cancer last year, and she had one breast removed. Nobody is healthy.

T-44:   How is your father doing now?

C-45:   Well, he's doing much better. He's been going to AA meetings, and the doctor he has been seeing has been giving him pills to keep him going. He spends quite a bit of money every week on pills. And if he misses a day of pills, he's absolutely unbearable. My mother feels that I shouldn't have left home—that my place is with them. There are nagging doubts about what I should—

T-46:   Why are there doubts? Why *should* you?

C-47:   I think it's a feeling I was brought up with that you always have to give of yourself. If you think of yourself, you're wrong.

T-48:   That's a *belief*. Why do you have to keep believing that—at your age? You believed a lot of superstitions when you were younger. Why do you have to retain them? Your parents indoctrinated you with this nonsense, because that's *their* belief. But why do you still have to believe that one should not be self-interested; that one should be self-sacrificial? Who needs that philosophy? All it's gotten you, so far, is guilt. And that's all it ever *will* get you!

C-49:   And now I try to break away. For instance, they'll call up and say, "Why don't you come Sunday?" And if I say, "No, I'm busy," rather than saying, "No, I'll come when it's convenient," they get terribly hurt, and my stomach gets all upset.

T-50:   Because you tell yourself, "There I go again. I'm a louse for not devoting myself to them!" As long as you tell yourself that crap, then your stomach or some other part of you will start jumping! But it's your *philosophy,* your *belief,* your sentence to *yourself*—"*I'm* no god-damned good! How could I do that lousy, stinking thing?" *That's* what's causing your stomach to jump. Now, that is a false sentence. Why are you no goddamned good because you prefer you to them? For that's what it amounts to. *Who* said you're no good—Jesus Christ? Moses? Who said so? The answer is: your parents said so. And you believe it because they said so. But who the hell are they?

C-51:   That's right. I was brought up to believe that everything your parents say is right. And I haven't been able to stop believing this.

T-52:   You haven't *done* it. You're *able* to, but you haven't. And *you're* now saying, every time you talk to them, the same crap to yourself. And you've got to see you're saying this drivel! Every time a human being gets upset—except when she's in physical pain—she has always told herself some bullshit the second before she gets upset. Normally, the bullshit takes the form, "This is terrible!"—in your case, "It's terrible that I don't want to go out there to see them!" Or people tell themselves, "*I shouldn't* be doing this!"—in your case, "*I shouldn't* be selfish!" Now, those terms—"This is *terrible!*" and "*I shouldn't* be doing this!"—are assumptions, premises. You cannot sustain them scientifically. You *believe* they're true, without any evidence, mainly because your parents indoctrinated you to believe that they're true. . . . Not only believe it, but *keep* indoctrinating yourself with it. That's the real perniciousness of it. That's the reason it persists—not because they taught it to you. It would just naturally die after a while. But you keep saying it yourself. It's these simple declarative sentences that you tell yourself every time you make a telephone call to your parents. And unless we can get you to see that you are saying them, and contradict and challenge them, you'll go on saying them forever. Then you will keep getting pernicious results: headaches, self-punishment, lying, and whatever else you get. These results are the logical consequences of an irrational cause, a false premise. And it's this premise that has to be questioned.

As soon as Martha, in C-45, says that she has nagging doubts whenever she thinks of herself first, I try to show her that this idea is only an opinion, that it cannot be empirically justified, and that it will lead to poor results. I am herewith being classically rational emotive: not only explicating but attacking Martha's self-defeating premises and values, and trying to actively teach her how to attack her basic mistaken views.

C-59:   I get so mad at myself for being so illogical.

T-60:   There you go again! You are not only saying that you *are* illogical, but that you *shouldn't* be. Why *shouldn't* you be? It's a pain in the ass to be illogical; it's a nuisance. But who says it's *wicked* for you to be wrong? *That's your parents'* philosophy.

C-61:   Yes, and also there's the matter of religion. I was brought up to be a strict, hard-shelled Baptist. And I can't quite take it any more. This has been going on for—(*Pause*) Well, the first seeds of doubt were sown when I was in high school. Nobody answered my questions. And I kept asking the minister, and he didn't answer my questions. And when I went to college, I started reading. I tried very hard, the first two years in college. I went to church all the time. If I had a question, I'd ask the minister. But pretty soon I couldn't get any answers. And now I really don't believe in the Baptist Church.

T-62:   All right, but are you *guilty* about not believing?

C-63:   Not only am I guilty, but the worst part about it is that I can't tell my parents that I don't believe.

T-64:   But why do you have to? What's the necessity? Because they're probably not going to accept it.

C-65:   Well, they didn't accept it. I was going to get married to a Jewish fellow as soon as I graduated from college. And, of course, the problem of religion came up then. And I didn't stand up for what I believed. I don't know; rather than have scenes, I took the coward's way out. And when I spend Saturdays and Sundays with them now—which is rare—I go to church with them. And this is what I mean by lying, rather than telling the truth.

T-66:   I see. You're probably going to extremes there—going to church. Why do you have to go to church?

C-67:   I always hate to create a scene.

T-68:   You mean you always sell your soul for a mess of porridge?

C-69:   Yes, I do.

T-70:   I don't see why you should. That leaves you with no integrity. Now it's all right to do whatever you want about being quiet, and not telling your parents about your loss of faith—because they're not going to approve and could well upset themselves. There's no use in throwing your irreligiosity in their faces. But to let yourself be forced to go to church and thereby to give up your integrity—that's bullshit. You can even tell them, if necessary, "I don't believe in that any more." And if there's a scene, there's a scene. If they commit suicide, they commit suicide! You can't really hurt them, except physically. You can't hurt anybody else except with a baseball bat! You can do things that they don't like, that they take too seriously, and that they hurt themselves with. But you can't really hurt them with words and ideas. That's nonsense. They taught you to believe that nonsense: "You're hurting us, dear, if you don't go along with what we think you ought to do!" That's drivel of the worst sort! They're hurting themselves by fascistically demanding that you do a certain thing, and then making themselves upset when you don't do it. You're not doing the hurting—they are. If they get hurt because you tell them you're no longer a Baptist, that's their doing. They're hurting themselves; you're not hurting them. They'll say, "How can you do this to us?" But is that *true?* Are you doing anything to them or are *they* doing it to themselves?

C-71:   No, I'm not.

T-72:   But you *believe* that you're hurting them. It's crap! . . .

T-104:   . . . What you had better do is relatively simple—but it's not easy to do. And that is—you've already done parts of what needs to be done. You have changed some of your fundamental philosophies—particularly regarding religion—which is a big change for a human being to make. But you haven't changed enough of your philosophy; you still believe some basic dogmas. Most people—whether Jew, Catholic, or Protestant—believe certain dogmas. The main dogmas are that we should devote ourselves to others before ourselves; that we must be loved, accepted, and adored by others, especially by members of our own family; and that we must do well, we must achieve greatly, succeed, do right. And you firmly believe these major ideas. You'd better get rid of them!

C-105:   How do I do that?

T-106:   By seeing, first of all, that every single time you get upset . . . you told yourself some superstitious creed—some bullshit. That, for example, you're no good because you aren't successful at something; or that you're a louse because you are unpopular, or are selfish, or are not as great as you should be. Then, when you see that you have told yourself this kind of nonsense, you have to ask yourself the question, "*Why* should I have to be successful? *Why* should I always have to be accepted and approved? *Why* should I be utterly loved and adored? Who said so? Jesus Christ? Who the hell was he?" There is no evidence that these things *should* be so; and you are just parroting, on faith, this nonsense, this crap that most people in your society believe. And it's not only your parents who taught it to you. It's also all those stories you read, the fairy tales you heard, the TV shows you saw. They all include this hogwash!

C-107: I know. But every time you try to overcome this, you're faced with it somewhere else again. And I realize—I've come to realize—you know, the thing that made me try to straighten myself out was that I know I've got to learn to have confidence in my own judgment.

T-108: While you've really got confidence in this other crap!

C-109: Yes, I'm very unconfident.

T-110: You have to be—because you believe this stuff.

I continue actively teaching and depropagandizing Martha. Not only do I deal with the irrational philosophies that she brings up, but I prophylactically mention and attack others as well. I keep trying to expose to her a few basic groundless ideas—such as the ideas that she must be loved and must perform well—and to show her that her symptoms, such as her self-sacrificing and her lack of self-confidence, are the natural results of these silly ideas. . . .

C-127: . . . I also want to find out—I suppose it's all basically the same thing—why I have been promiscuous, why I lie—

T-128: For love. I get the impression you think you're such a worm that the only way to get worth, value, is to be loved, approved, accepted. And perhaps you're promiscuous to gain love, because it's an easy way: you can gain acceptance easily that way. You may lie because you're ashamed. You possibly feel that they wouldn't accept you if you told the truth. These are very common results; anybody who desperately needs to be loved—as you think you do with your crummy philosophy—will be promiscuous, will lie, will do other things which are silly, rather than do the things she really wants to do and rather than gain her own self-approval.

C-129: That's what I don't have; I don't have any.

T-130: You never tried to get it! You've been working your butt off to get other people's approval. Your parents' first, but other people's second. That's why the promiscuity; that's why the lying. And you're doing no work whatever at getting your own self-acceptance, because the only way you get self-respect is by not giving that much of a damn what other people think. There is no other way to get it; that's what self-acceptance really means: to thine *own* self be true!

In my response, T-130, I epitomize one of the main differences between REBT and most other "dynamic" systems of psychological treatment. Whereas a psychoanalytically-oriented therapist would probably have tried to show Martha that her promiscuity and lying stemmed from her early childhood experiences, I believe nothing of the sort. I assume that her childhood lying, for example, was mainly caused by her own innate tendencies toward crooked thinking—which in turn led her to react inefficiently to the propaganda her parents may have imposed on her. What is important, therefore, is her own reactivity and not her parents' actions. I also believe, on theoretical grounds, that the reason for Martha's present promiscuity and lying is probably her current need to be inordinately loved; and she freely seems to admit (as she also previously did in C-19) that my educated guess about this is true.

If I were proved to be wrong in this guess, I would not be perturbed but would look for another hypothesis—for example, her promiscuity might be a form of self-punishment, because she thought she was unworthy on some other count. As a rational emotive behavior therapist, I am willing to take a chance on being wrong with my first hypothesis because, if I am right, I usually save my client a good deal of time. Moreover, by taking a wrong tack, I may well help myself and the client get to the right tack. If, however, I try the psychoanalytic, history-taking path, to arrive at the "real" reasons for my client's behavior, (a) I may never find what these "real" reasons are (for they may not exist, or years of probing may never turn them up); (b) I may still come up with the wrong reasons; and (c) I may sidetrack the client so seriously that she may never discover what her basic disturbance-creating philosophy is and therefore never do anything about changing it. For a variety of reasons, then, I took a very direct approach with Martha.

C-131: You have to develop a sort of hard shell towards other people?

T-132: Well, it isn't really a callous shell. It's really that you have to develop your own goals and your own confidence so much that you do not allow the views and desires of others to impinge that much on you. Actually, you'll learn to be kinder and nicer to other people if you do this. We're not trying to get you to be against others, to be hostile or resentful. The less vulnerable you get to what others think of you, actually the more sensitive, kindly, and loving you can often be. Because you haven't been really loving, but largely maintaining a facade with your parents. Underneath, you've been resentful, unloving.

C-133: I can be loving, though.

T-134: That's right. But you'd better be true to yourself first; and through being true to yourself then you'll be able to care more for other people. Not all people, and maybe not your parents. There's no law that says you have to love your parents. They may just not be your cup of tea. In fact, it looks like in some ways they aren't. Tough! It would be nice if they were: it would be lovely if you could love them and have good relationships. But that may never really be. You may well have to withdraw emotionally from them, to some extent—not from everybody, but probably from them somewhat—in order to be true to yourself. Because it seems to me they act like leeches, fascists, emotional blackmailers.

C-135: Yes, that's the term: emotional blackmailers. This I know; this has been evidenced all through my life. Emotional blackmail!

At every point, I try to show Martha that she does not have to feel guilty with withdrawing emotionally from her parents, nor for doing what she wants to do or thinking what she wants to think. I do not try to get her to condemn her parents or to be hostile to them. Quite the contrary! But I do consistently show her that they have their own problems in logical thinking and that she'd better resist their emotional blackmailing. As it turns out, she seems to have always known this; but my actively bringing it to her attention will presumably help her to act, now, on what she knows and feels. I am thereby helping her, through frank and therapist-directed discussion, to get in touch with her real feelings and to follow them in practice.

T-136: Right. And you've been accepting this blackmail. You had to accept it as a child—you couldn't help it, you were dependent. But you don't *still* have to accept it. You now can see that they're blackmailing; and now you can calmly resist it, without being resentful of them. Then their blackmail won't take effect. They'll probably foam at the mouth, have fits, and everything. Tough!—so they'll foam. Well, there's no question that you can change. We haven't got any more time now. But the main problem—as I said awhile ago—is your philosophy, which is an internalizing, really, of their philosophy. And if there ever was evidence of how an abject philosophy affects you, there it is: they're thoroughly miserable. And you'll be just as miserable if you continue this way. If you want to learn to *change* your philosophy, this is what I do in therapy: beat people's crazy ideas over the head until they stop defeating themselves. That's all you're doing: defeating yourself!

I keep utilizing material from Martha's own life to consistently show her what is going on in her head, philosophically, and what she'd better do about changing her thinking. This first interview with Martha indicates how REBT, right from the start, encourages the therapist to talk much more about the client's value system than about her symptoms and how it uses the information she gives to highlight her own disturbance-creating ideas and to attack them. I think that this session also shows that although I do not hesitate to contradict Martha's assumptions at several points, I am essentially supportive in that I keep showing her (a) that I am on her side, (b) that I think I can help her, (c) that I am fairly sure what the real sources of her disturbances are, and (d) that if she works at seeing these sources and at doing something to undermine them, the chances are excellent that she will become much less upsettable. My "attack," therefore, is one that would ordinarily be called "ego-bolstering." Or, in REBT terminology, it is one that is designed to help Martha fully accept rather than severely condemn herself.

To this end, I consistently have what Carl Rogers calls "unconditional positive regard" for Martha, for I accept her in spite of her difficulties and inanities, and believe that she is capable of overcoming her crooked thinking by living and working primarily for herself. I also show that I am on Martha's side, not because I personally find her attractive, bright, or competent, but because I feel that every human has the right to choose to live primarily for himself or herself.

SEGMENTS FROM THE SECOND SESSION

This session takes place five days after the first session. Martha has already made some progress, has calmed down considerably, and is now in a better condition to work on some of her basic problems.

T-1:   How are things?

C-2:   Things are okay. I went to visit my parents on Monday night. And every time I was tempted to fall prey to their emotional blackmail, I remembered what you said, and I was able to fight it.

T-3:   Fine!

C-4:   My mother is having a rough time yet, because of having her breast removed. She hardly says anything. She's really in a fog. She gets confused, and she uses the confusion to give her a hold on the family. She was putting on a martyr act the other night; and usually I would have given in to her, but I said, "Quit being a martyr! Go to bed." She just looked at me as though I was a strange creature!

T-5:   And you didn't get upset by it?

C-6:   No, I didn't get upset by it. I had the feeling that I was doing the right thing. And that was, I think, the major accomplishment in the past few days.

T-7:   Yes; well that was quite a good accomplishment.

C-8:   Now if there are any bigger crises that will come, I don't know how I'll face them; but it looks like I can.

T-9:   Yes; and if you keep facing these smaller crises as they arise—and they tend to be continual—there's no reason why you shouldn't be able to face the bigger ones as well. Why not?

C-10:   I guess it's a case of getting into a good habit.

T-11:   Yes, that's right: getting ready to believe that no matter what your parents do, no matter how hurt they get, that's not your basic problem. You're not deliberately doing them in; you're just standing up for yourself.

As often occurs in REBT, although this is only the second session, Martha is already beginning to implement some of the major ideas that were discussed during the first session and is beginning to change herself. I deliberately support her new notion that she can handle herself with her parents, and I keep reiterating that she does not have to react to their views and behavior by getting upset. I thereby am approving her new patterns and rewarding or reinforcing her. But I am also repetitively teaching—taking every opportunity to reassert that she can think for herself and does not have to react negatively because her parents or others view her unfavorably. . . .

C-40:   In school, if I didn't do well in one particular thing, or even on a particular test—and little crises that came up—if I didn't do as well as I had wanted to do . . .

T-41:   You beat yourself over the head?

C-42:   Yes.

T-43:   But why? What's the point? Are you supposed to be perfect? Why shouldn't human beings make mistakes, be imperfect?

C-44:   Maybe you always expect yourself to be perfect.

T-45:   Yes. But is that *sane?*

C-46:   No.

T-47:   Why do it? Why not give up that unrealistic expectation?

C-48:   But then I can't accept myself.

T-49:   But you're saying, "It's shameful to make mistakes." Why is it shameful? Why can't you go to somebody else when you make a mistake and say, "Yes, I made a mistake"? Why is that so awful?

C-50:   I don't know.

T-51:   There *is* no good reason. You're just *saying* it's so. Recently I wrote an article for a professional publication, and they accepted it, and they got another psychologist to write a critique of it. He wrote his critique—a fairly savage one—and he pointed out some things with which I disagree, so I said so in my reply. But he pointed out some things which he was right about; where I had overstated my case and made a mistake. So, I merely said about this in my rejoinder, "He's right; I made a mistake here." Now, what's the horror? Why shouldn't I make a mistake? Who am I—Jesus Christ? Who are you—the Virgin Mary? Then, why shouldn't you be a fallible human being like the rest of us and make mistakes?

C-52:   It might all go back to, as you said, the need for approval. If I don't make mistakes, then people will look up to me. If I do it all perfectly—

T-53:   That is an erroneous belief; that if you never make mistakes everybody will love you and that it is necessary that they do. That's a big part of it. But is it true? Suppose you never did make mistakes—would people love you? Maybe they would hate your guts because you were so perfect, wouldn't they?

C-54:   And yet, not all the time. There are times—this is rare, I grant you—but sometimes I'll take a stand on something that other people don't like. But this is rare!

T-55:   Yes, but what about the times when you know you're wrong? Let's take those times—that's what we're talking about. You know you're wrong, you made a mistake, there's no question about it. Why are you a louse at *those* times? Why is it shameful to admit your mistake? Why can't you accept yourself as a fallible human being—which we all are?

C-56:   (*Pause*) Maybe I have the idea that if I keep telling myself how perfect I am, I won't realize how imperfect I am.

T-57:   Yes, but why shouldn't one accept the fact that one is imperfect? That's the real question. What's shameful about being imperfect? Why must one be an angel—which you're trying to be?

C-58:   Probably there's no good reason.

T-59:   No. Then why don't you look at *that?* There's no good reason. It's a definitional thing, saying "To be good, to be perfect, to be a worthwhile human being, I must be perfect. If I have flaws, I'm no damned good." And you can't substantiate that proposition. It's a senseless proposition; but you believe it. The reason you believe it is your society believes it. This is the basic creed of your silly society. Certainly, your parents believe it. If they knew one-sixtieth of your errors and mistakes—especially your sex errors!—they'd be horrified, wouldn't they?

C-60:   Yes.

T-61:   You have the same silly horror! Because *they* think you ought to be a sexless angel, you think you ought to be.

C-62:   (*Silence*)

T-63:   You've accepted their idiotic judgments—the same judgments that have driven your father to drink and made your mother utterly miserable. They both have been miserable all your life. That's what perfectionism leads to. A beautiful object lesson there! Anybody who is perfectionistic tends to become disturbed, unhappy—ultimately often crazy. The gospel of perfection!

C-64:   That's what I have to work on. Because I don't want to get like they are.

T-65:   No, but you are partly like they are already—we had better change that. It isn't a matter of getting—you've already got! Let's face it. You don't do the same kind of behavior as they do, but you hate yourself when you don't. You make the mistakes; they don't make them. But then you say, "I'm no good! How could I have done this? This is terrible! I'm not Florence Nightingale. I go to bed with guys. I do bad things. I make blunders. How awful!" That's the same philosophy that they have, isn't it? And it's an impossible philosophy, because we'd really literally have to be angels to live up to it. There *are* no angels! Not even your parents!

I make a mistake when I tell Martha that she believes she is worthless largely because her parents and her society teach her to believe this. I fail to note that practically all humans seem to be born with a tendency to believe this sort of drivel; that they must be pretty perfect and are no good if they are not; and that therefore their parents and their society are easily able to convince them that this is "true."

Clinically, however, I felt when I talked to Martha that she was already prejudiced against her parents' views and that she might therefore see the perniciousness of her own ideas if I emphasized how similar they were to those of her parents. As a rational emotive behavior therapist, I am a frank propagandist, since I deliberately use appeals that I think will work with a given client. But I only propagandize in accordance with what appears to be the empirical reality that some people do define themselves as worthless slobs. I do not propagandize only to win Martha's approval, but to dramatically (emotively) bring to her attention the realities of life.

Rational emotive behavior therapists are sometimes accused of foisting on their clients their own prejudiced views of the world. Actually, they base their views on the facts of human existence and the usual nature of people. And they teach individuals with disturbances to look at these facts and to realistically accept and work with them. They may teach through dramatic or emotive methods in order to put a point over more effectively, taking into consideration that clients generally hold their wrong-headed views in a highly emotionalized, not easily uprootable manner.

C-66:   (*Pause*) I guess that's this great fear of failure. That might have been what was keeping me from concentrating on writing, which I really want to do. I'm afraid that I might make a mistake, you know.

T-67:   Yes, that's the other grim tragedy. Two things happen if you have a terrible, grim fear of failure. One is, as you just said, you get anxious, unhappy, ashamed. Two, you don't live; you don't do the things you want to do. Because if you did them, you might make a mistake, an error, be a poor writer—and wouldn't that be awful, according to your definition? So you just don't do things. That's your parents again. How could they be happy, when they haven't done anything? And you have been following the same general pattern. You haven't taken it to their extremes as yet, but it's the same bullshit, no matter how you slice it. And in your case you're afraid to write; because if you wrote, you'd commit yourself. And if you committed yourself, how horrible *that* would be!

C-68:   I've done a lot of thinking since the last time I saw you. And I've gone at the typewriter with a fresh burst of enthusiasm. I'm really anxious to get to my writing—I want to get home from work so I can write. Nothing big has happened, but I feel as though if I concentrate on it and keep feeling this way, all I have to do is to keep working at it.

T-69:   And one of two things will happen. Either you'll become a good writer, with enough work and practice; or you'll prove that you're not—which would be a good thing, too. It would be far better to prove you're not a good writer by working at it than not to write. Because if you don't write, you may go on for the rest of your life hating yourself; while if you really work solidly day after day, and you just haven't got it in this area, that's tough. So you won't be a writer—you'll be something else. It would be better to learn by that experience.

C-70:   That's right. Because—I don't know—I felt so different, sitting at the typewriter and working at it, that it got to be enjoyable.

T-71:   It will!

C-72:   But it was painful before.

T-73:   It was painful because you were *making* it painful by saying, "My God! Look what would happen if I failed! How awful!" Well, anything would become painful if you kept saying that.

C-74:   Another thing that bothers me, I guess—it's the whole pattern of behavior; the way everything has been in my life. It's a sort of—"Go ahead and do it now, and then something will come along and take care of it." Like my parents always said, "We'll go ahead and do this, even though we don't have the money for it, and it'll come from somewhere."

T-75:   Right: "In God we trust!" . . .

C-84:   . . . And when I tell myself, "Don't be silly; you can't do it, so don't," I'm tempted to go ahead and do it anyway.

T-85:   Yes, because you're telling yourself stronger and louder: "It'll take care of itself. Fate will intervene in my behalf. The Lord will provide!"

C-86:   And I get mad at myself for doing it—

T-87:   That's illegitimate! Why not say, "Let's stop the crap!" instead of getting mad at yourself? How will getting mad at yourself help?

C-88:   It doesn't. It just causes more tension.

T-89:   That's exactly right. It doesn't do any good whatsoever. Let's cut out all the self-blame. That's doesn't mean cut out all criticism. Say, "Yes, I am doing this wrongly, so how do I not do it wrongly?"—instead of: "I am doing it wrongly; what a louse I am! I'm no good; I deserve to be punished!"

I persist at showing Martha that she can take chances, do things badly, and still not condemn herself. At every possible turn, I get back to her underlying philosophies concerning (a) failing and defining herself as a worthless individual and (b) unrealistically relying on the world or fate to take care of difficult situations. She consistently describes her feelings, but I bring her back to the ideas behind them. Then she seems to accept my interpretations and to seriously consider working against her disturbance-creating ideas. My persistence and determination may importantly induce her to tentatively accept my explanations and to use them herself.

C-90:   When I am particularly worried about anything, I have very strange dreams. I have dreams that I can't describe, but I have them several times a week.

T-91:   There's nothing unusual about that. They're probably anxiety dreams. All the dreams say—if you told me what they are, I could show you right away—the same kind of things you're saying to yourself during the day. They're doing it in a vague and more abstract way. But that's all they are, just repetitious of the crap you're telling yourself during the day. In dreams, our brain is not as efficient as it is when we're awake; and therefore it uses symbols, vague representations, indirectness, and so on. But the dreams tell us the same crap we think during the day.

C-92: I had a dream last week that disturbed me. I dreamed that I ran off somewhere with my boss, and his wife found us in bed; and I was so upset over that—I really was. Because I never consciously thought of my boss in a sexual way.

T-93: That doesn't mean that that's what the dream represented, that you thought of your boss in a sexual way. There's a more obvious explanation of the dream. All the dream is really saying is: You did the wrong thing and got found out.

C-94: I never thought of that.

T-95: That's all it was saying, probably. And what's one of the wrongest things you can do in our society? Have intercourse with your boss and have his wife find out! That's all. It probably has little to do with sex at all; and you're probably not going around unconsciously lusting after your boss.

C-96: No, I don't think I am.

T-97: No. But it would be the wrong move, if you did have sex with him; it might, of course, jeopardize your job. So that's all you're saying in your dream: if I do the wrong thing, I'm no goddamned good; I may lose my job; I may get terribly penalized; and so on. That's what you say all day, isn't it? Why should you not translate it into dreams at night? It's the same crap!

In REBT, dreams are not overemphasized and are often used only to a small extent; for, as I say to Martha, they are hardly the royal road to the unconscious (as Freud believed), but seem to be rather distorted and muddled representations of the same kind of thinking and feeling that the individual tends to do during his waking life. Since they are experienced in symbolic, vague, and ambiguous ways, and since they can easily be misinterpreted (according to whatever biases the individual therapist happens to hold), the REBT practitioner would rather stick with the client's conscious thoughts, feelings, and behaviors and with the unconscious (or unaware) thoughts and feelings that can be deduced from them. Dreams are rather redundant material, and can consume a great deal of therapeutic time if they are taken too seriously. Moreover, long-winded dream analysis can easily (and dramatically!) distract the client from what he'd better do most of all: look at his philosophies of life and work hard at changing them.

The beauty of the REBT approach is that no matter what the client seems to be upset about, the therapist can quickly demonstrate that there is no good reason for her upsetness. Thus, if Martha's dream represents (a) her lusting after her boss, (b) her being out of control, or (c) any other kind of mistake, REBT theory holds that she cannot be a rotter and that she therefore need not be terribly anxious, guilty, angry, or depressed. She creates her disturbed feelings, not from the dream events, nor from her foolish motives that may be revealed in these events, nor from the happenings in her real life, nor from anything *except* her own attitudes about these events, motives, or happenings. And I, as her therapist, am concerned much more with her attitudes than with things transpiring in her waking or sleeping life. So if REBT is consistently followed, *any* emotional problem may be tracked down to its philosophic sources (or the ways in which the individual blames herself, others, or the world); and these philosophies may then be challenged, attacked, changed, and uprooted.

C-192: I guess the main thing is to keep in mind that a lot of the thoughts I have—whenever I get a thought like that, I'd better challenge it.

T-193: That's right, to see that it is invalid. First you start with the feeling—the upset. Then you know, on theoretical grounds, that you have an invalid thought, because you don't get negative feelings without first having some silly thought. Then you look for the thought—which is pretty obvious most of the time. You're invariably blaming yourself or saying that something is horrible when it isn't. Then you say, "Why is this horrible? Why would it be dreadful if such-and-such a thing happened?" Challenge it; question it; counter it. That's the process. And if you go through that process, your thoughts can't persist. Because they're your irrational thoughts now. They're no longer your parents' ideas. You have internalized them.

C-194: (*Long pause*) I guess it has to be done.

T-195: Yes. And you will get immense benefit from doing it—as you've already been deriving this week. It felt good when you acted that way, didn't it?

C-196: Since I have been back at the typewriter again, I've been thinking differently. I can see myself falling back, as I used to be able to do, into a clear pattern of thought. I mean, I'm not just thinking in symbols and metaphors, but am able to describe things incisively, or at least have descriptive impressions of things.

T-197: Yes. That's because you're letting yourself go—you're not pouncing on yourself so much.

C-198: Yes, you're right. Not that I've done very much in this last week, but I do feel like I'm loosening up more.

T-199: That's very good progress in one week's time! All you have to do is keep that up—and go a little further.

C-200: And another thing I've done: I haven't called up my father because I felt I had to. And he hasn't called me—so that means something.

T-201: Fine! When would you like to make the next appointment?

Martha's apparent progress represents a common occurrence in REBT. After one or two active-directive sessions, clients frequently report that something they thought they were never able to do before is now in their repertoire. This does not mean that they are truly "cured" of their emotional disturbances. But it often does seem to mean that they are well on the way to resolving at least one or two major aspects of these disturbances.

Even if clients such as Martha are quickly helped, this hardly means that all or most individuals who try REBT encounters are similarly relieved; many of them, of course, are not. I assume, however, that a certain large minority of people can almost immediately profit by the REBT approach; and I assume that a given individual with whom I am talking may be one of this minority. If my assumption proves to be correct, fine! If it does not, I am prepared, if necessary, to doggedly continue with the approach for as many sessions as are desirable—until the client finally begins to see that she is causing her own upsets, that she can observe the specific meanings and beliefs by which she causes them, that she can vigorously and consistently dispute and challenge these beliefs, and that she can thereby become considerably less disturbed.

THIRD SESSION

The third session with Martha was uneventful. Because she was afflicted with some expensive physical ailments and had financial difficulties, she decided to discontinue therapy for a time.

SEGMENTS FROM THE FOURTH SESSION

The fourth session with Martha took place nine months after the third session. She had expected to come back to therapy sooner than she actually did, but she was able to get along nicely and didn't feel impelled to return until she had a specific problem to discuss. She now comes with this problem—her relations with men.

T-1:   How are things with you?

C-2:   Pretty well, I would say. I've been hearing good things about you from some of the people I sent to see you. From Matt, in particular. He thinks that you've helped him immensely.

T-3:   I'm glad that he thinks so.

C-4:   And I see that you're making yourself comfortable, as usual. That's the way I found you last time: shoes off, feet up.

T-5:   Yes; that's the way I usually am.

C-6:   I came to you back in January because I needed some help in writing; and also I didn't know how to handle my parents.

T-7:   Yes.

C-8:   Well, I think I solved those two problems fairly well. I get along very well with my parents now. Not because I'm giving in to them at all. I've sort of established myself as a human being, apart from them completely. And I also found some other work. I was working, as I told you, for an advertising agency. But it didn't have any interest for me at the time. I was terribly bored, and I felt I could write on my own. But I was afraid. Then I got an idea for a novel, and a publisher has taken an option on it, and I've been working on it ever since. It will be published in the spring by the same publisher who has been having such success recently with several young novelists.

T-9:   I see. That's fine!

C-10:   So that's all working out very well. But there's something that is bothering me, that I thought you could help me with. I've been thinking of getting married. I've been thinking of marriage in general, first of all. But before that—maybe I'm not quite sure that I really know how to love anybody. Not that I consider that there's a formula. But I've always, in a way, been somewhat afraid of men. The other thing is that there is someone in particular who would like to marry me. And—maybe I'd better tell you how this all happened.

T-11:   Sure.

C-12:   In trying to analyze it—in trying to figure it out—I guess it all started to go back to my father. My father was a nice guy, but he has been alcoholic since I was twelve; and he has been getting worse since I last saw you. But I was absolutely adoring of my father when I was a little girl. And then I realized he was a human being, and he fell off his pedestal. Now I don't know how much can be attributed to that, but I don't think I ever trusted a man. I guess I was afraid that if I devoted myself to that person completely, sooner or later he would walk out on me. And this has always terrified me, no matter what kind of associations I've had. I always have to keep one step ahead of them.

T-13:   All right; it *would* terrify you if you keep saying to yourself, "They'll find out how worthless I am and leave me!"

C-14:   I guess you're right.

T-15:   And if you get rid of that fear—and as you said yourself, a couple of minutes ago, it is a fear—then you can be pretty sure that you'll love someone. I don't know *whom* you'll love—this person you're talking about, who wants to marry you, or anybody else—but I'm sure you have the *capacity* to love if you're not absorbed in, "Oh, my God! What a louse I am! When is he going to find it out?" See? . . .

C-40:   Another thing that I seem to do: every time I get interested in someone, I find myself looking at other men.

T-41:   Yes, that's possible. But it's also possible that if you think of one man in terms of marrying him and you still get interested in other men, you may not be so sure as yet, in terms of your experience, that it should be the first one. And therefore you'd like to try others. So some of what you feel may be normal, and some of it may be your fear of getting involved. The basic problem still is getting you to be unfearful—to realize yourself that you don't have to be afraid of anything . . .

C-42: Well, I would like to overcome this. I don't want to be afraid of them—that they might leave me.

T-43: The basic thing they can do, as you said before, is reject you. Now, let's suppose that they do. Let's suppose that you went with this guy, and you really let yourself go with him, and he finally did reject you, for whatever his reasons might be. What could you conclude should this happen?

C-44: I could always suppose that he was the one who had shortcomings, rather than me.

T-45: But let's suppose he doesn't have serious shortcomings, and he rejects you. Let's suppose he's perfect and then he spurns you. Now what does that prove?

C-46: I don't know.

T-47: All it proves is that he doesn't like you for some deficiencies. It proves, assuming that he's objective about your deficiencies, that you have certain defects. But does having these defects prove that you're worthless? Or that you're thoroughly inadequate, that you're no good?

C-48: It doesn't.

T-49: That's exactly right! And yet that's what you automatically think every single time: that it means something bad about you. That's what your parents believe: that if you are deficient and somebody finds it out, that proves that you're worthless, as a total human. Isn't that their philosophy?

C-50: I guess so.

T-51: They've told you that in so many words, so many times—as you told me they did awhile ago. When they found out something about you that they didn't like—such as your not running to their beck and call—you were not just a daughter who didn't like them that much (which is all that was evident); no, you were a louse—no good! They called you every name under the sun. They tried to make you guilty, you told me. Over the phone, they'd call you several times—and so on. Isn't that right? They assume that when someone is deficient in their eyes, that person is a slob. That's their philosophy: that unless you're an angel, you are no good.

C-52: I guess I just carried it with me. I let myself carry it with me.

T-53: That's right. You've let yourself carry it with you—which is normal enough. Most people do. But look at the results! If it had good results, if it really made you happy, we might say, "Go carry it!" But the result is the normal result—or the abnormal result, in your case. You can't give to a man because you're always worrying, "How worthless I am! And how soon will he see it? And before he sees it, maybe I'd better do something to get rid of him." Which is your logical conclusion from an irrational premise, the premise being that if people do find your deficiencies and therefore reject you, you're totally no good. Actually, there are *two* premises here. One, that they'll find your deficiencies and therefore will reject you—which is quite an assumption! Two, that if they do reject you, you're no damned good. These are two completely irrational premises. They're not supported by any evidence.

I try to show Martha that it is not her boyfriend but her own attitudes about herself that are upsetting her, and that no matter how defective she is, and no matter how badly her boyfriend (or anyone else) rejects her, she can still fully accept herself and try to better her relationships. Although I am therefore ruthless about insisting that she acknowledge her deficiencies, I am (in a typical REBT manner) highly supportive about the possibility of her unconditionally accepting herself. In REBT, the therapist generally does not give warm, personal affection (since there is the always existing danger that the client will, in getting it, wrongly think he is "good" *because* the therapist or group cares for him). Instead, the rational emotive behavior therapist (and group) tries to give unconditional acceptance, that is, complete tolerance and lack of condemnation of the client no matter what his or her faults are. I think an incisive reading of these sessions with Martha will show that I am rarely loving or warm to her but that I frequently show full acceptance of her.

C-56:   How do I go about convincing myself that this is wrong?

T-57:   The first thing you'd better do before you convince yourself that this is wrong is to convince yourself—that is, fully admit to yourself—that you very strongly have this belief. You can't very well tackle a belief and change it unless you fully admit that you have it. After seeing this, the second thing is to see the degree—which is enormous and intense—to which you have it. You can at first do this by inference—by observing your behavior and asking yourself what ideas lie behind it. For your behavior itself is not necessarily fearful. It may take the form of your *feeling* in a state of panic, or it may be defensive.

C-58:   Well, my behavior is mostly defensive.

T-59:   All right. Then we have to start with your defensive behavior. Look at it, question it, challenge it, and see—by inference, at first—that it could only be this way if you *were* fearful. For why would you be defensive if you were not, underneath, also afraid of something? If we can get you to see how many times a day you're unduly restricted, defensive—and therefore fearing—until you see the real frequency and intensity of your fears, then at least we get you to see what the cancer really is. You can't really understand the cancer without seeing the depths of it. Okay, we have the first step, then, which is to make you see fully what the depths of your cancerous ideation are. Then, as you begin to see this, the second step is to get you to calmly assess it. The first cancer is your defense and your fear behind it. The second cancer is—and this is the reason why so many people *are* defensive—if you admit to yourself, "My God! What a terribly fearful person I am!" you will then tend to blame yourself for that. In other words, you say on level number one, "My heavens, I'm a wrongdoing person, am therefore terribly worthless, and I'd better not let anyone know this." So you become defensive because your real philosophy is: "What a worthless slob I am because I'm imperfect; I have deficiencies; I have faults." So the first level is to make yourself fearful because of your feelings of worthlessness—the philosophy that human beings who are deficient are no damned good. Then, as a derivative of that first level, you come to the second level: "Because I'm deficient, because I'm fearful, because I'm neurotic, I'm a louse and am worthless for *that* reason. So I'd better deny that I'm really that fearful *(a)* because people will find out about it and hate me and *(b)* because I'll use my fear to prove to myself what a louse I am."

    So first we have to get you to admit the fact that you're fearful, defensive, and so on—that you are a perfectionist who tends to bring on feelings of worthlessness. Then we have to get you to see that by admitting your fear and defensiveness you're not a louse for having these traits; and to get you to see that simply because you have a *feeling* you're worthless doesn't mean that you really *are.* So we have to get you to *(a)* admit that you feel like a skunk; *(b)* objectively perceive—and not blamefully perceive—that you believe you're one; and *(c)* (which is really just an extension of b) start tackling your concept of being a skunk. . . .

C-72:   But actually, your parents bring you up that way. Because you are naughty, you stand in a corner; you don't get your supper; you get spanked; or someone says to you, "That wasn't very nice; that wasn't very good!"

T-73:   That's right. They don't only spank you—that wouldn't be so bad, because then they would just penalize you—but they also say, "You're no good!" And the attitude they take in doing the spanking is an angry attitude; and the whole implication of the anger is that you're worthless. People do this in order to train you when you're a child; and it's a very effective method of training. But look at the enormous harm it does! Incidentally, one of the main reasons we would want you to undo your self-blaming tendencies is that if you do get married and have children, you will tend to do the same kind of thing to them that was done to you—unless you see very clearly what was done to you and what you're doing now to continue it.

C-74:   And also, I'm absolutely terrified of being somebody's mother.

T-75:   Yes, that's right. Just look how incompetent you might be, and how you might screw it up! And wouldn't *that* be awful!

C-76:   You know, I've been asking myself that a hundred thousand times.

T-77:   All right; but those are the times we have to clip. Let's just take that sentence, "Suppose I was somebody's mother and brought my child up badly." That's what you're saying. How are you *ending* the sentence?

C-78:   Wouldn't that be awful! Wouldn't I be terrible!

T-79:   That's right. Now is that a logical conclusion to make from the observed facts? Let's suppose the facts were true—that you did bring up a child badly. Let's suppose that. Would it still follow that you'd be a worthless slob?

C-80:   No, it wouldn't. Because I'd be defining—that's what it is—I'd be defining *worthless* in terms of whatever it is I lack, whatever it is that I do badly in.

T-81:   That's right. The equation you'd be making is: my deficiency equals my worthlessness. That's exactly the equation—and it's a definition. Now is it a *true* definition?

C-82:   No.

T-83:   It's a true or an accurate definition if you *make* it true—if you *insist* that it's true.

C-84:   But it's not necessarily a correct one.

T-85:   That's right. And what happens when you make that definition?

C-86:   Then you feel worthless, because you define yourself as worthless.

T-87:   Yes, pragmatically, you defeat yourself. If it were a definition that led to good results, that might be fine. But *does* it lead to that?

C-88:   No. Because you tend to look at everything negatively, rather than—I hate to say positively, because it sounds like "positive thinking," and that's not it.

T-89:   Yes, let's say it makes you look at things negatively rather than looking at them without prejudice.

C-90:   Yes, without prejudice.

From responses T-77 to T-89, I resort to a questioning dialogue, instead of my previous use of straight lecturing and explaining. I keep asking Martha various questions about what she's telling herself, what results she is thereby getting, and whether the things she is saying to herself and the definitions she is setting up about her behavior are really accurate. She shows, by her answers, that she is following what I have previously explained and that she can probably use this material in her future living. . . .

T-95:   . . . a child will lots of times define himself as a blackguard on his own. Because if he fails and does so lots of times—as he inevitably will—even if Mommy didn't call him a slob, he would probably tend to think he is worthless. It's sort of a normal, natural conclusion for a young child, who can't think straight because of his youth, to say, "Because I failed at A, B, C, and D, I'm bound to fail at X, Y, and Z; and therefore I'm thoroughly incompetent at everything." That's what we call overgeneralization; and human beings, especially young children, tend to overgeneralize. Now, unfortunately, we also help them to do this, in our society—in fact, in most societies. But they might well do it without social help, though probably to a lesser degree. Anyway, it behooves us to help them to think in a less overgeneralized manner. We'd better take the child who tends to overgeneralize and calmly show him, a thousand times if necessary, "Look, dear, because you did A, B, C, and D mistakenly, that doesn't mean—"

C-96:   "—that you're going to do X, Y, and Z wrongly."

T-97:   That's right! "And even if you do A, B, C, and D badly, and also do X, Y, and Z wrongly, that doesn't mean that you're a louse. It means, objectively, that you have deficiencies. So you're not Leonardo da Vinci. Tough!" But we don't teach them anything of the kind.

C-98:   No. "You have to excel in everything. If you don't, that's bad!"

T-99:   "That's terrible!" We don't even say it's bad. Because it is, of course, objectively bad; it's inconvenient; it's a nuisance when you fail; and you will get certain poor results if you keep failing. But it doesn't say anything about you personally, as a *human being,* except that you're the kind of a creature who often fails. It doesn't say that you're a worm—unless you define it so.

C-100: Well, I think I'll know what to look for.

T-101: Yes. It will take a little practice. It won't take very long, I'm sure, in your case, because you see the outlines, and I think you're very able to do this kind of thinking, which is highly important. Many people deliberately shy away from doing it, so they never see it. They're hopeless because, in a sense, they don't *want* to see it; they want the world to change, or others to change, rather than wanting to change themselves. But you want to see it, and you have seen a large hunk of it already, in dealing recently with your parents. Considering the short length of time that I saw you and that you've been working on it, you've done remarkably well. Now there's no reason why you can't see the bigger hunk of it—which applies to you much more than to your relations with your father and mother.

So you go off and look for these things we've been talking about. As I said, make a list, if you're not going to remember the things that come up during the week that you bother yourself about. Make a list of the major times when you feel upset, or when you believe you acted defensively instead of feeling overtly upset. Look for these things; come in, and we'll talk about them. I'll check what you find, just as I'd check your lessons if I were teaching you how to play the piano. You'll then be able to see your own blockings more clearly. There's no reason why not.

I continue to be encouraging to show Martha that she has been able to make good progress so far and that she should be able to continue to do so. But I stress that she well may not be able to do this entirely on her own at the present time and that therefore it would be best if she kept coming in to see me, to check her own impressions of what is bothering her and to make sure that she works concertedly against her internalized philosophies that lead her astray.

C-102: Because I know I need this right now. I mean I can feel the need for it. Logically, I know that my hang-up with relating to males is a big stumbling block; and this is something I have to overcome.

T-103: Yes. What I would advise you to do is to see me every week or so for therapy, or every other week or so; and also, if possible, join one of my therapy groups for awhile, where you'll see and relate to others who have similar problems to yours. You may get some insight into some of the things you're doing by watching them and showing them how to solve some of their difficulties. That's another helpful way, because we're often just too close to ourselves. But if we see the same kind of behavior in someone else, we say, "Ah, I do that, too!"

C-104: When do the groups meet? . . .

The client came for one more individual session and several group sessions of therapy, and then felt that she was doing very well and that she could manage things on her own. She returned, over the years, for other sessions from time to time, mainly to discuss the problems of her parents, her husband, her children, or other close associates. She continues to get along remarkably well. She is still in touch with me at intervals, largely to refer her friends and relatives for therapy sessions. She has reality (rather than emotional) problems with her parents; she is happily married and has two lively and seemingly little-disturbed children; she gets along well with her husband, in spite of his personal hang-ups; and she keeps writing successful books and taking great satisfaction in her work. She is hardly free from all disturbances, since she still has a tendency to become overwrought about people treating her unfairly. But she seems almost fully to accept herself, and most of her original problems are solved or managed. She still marvels at, and keeps telling her new acquaintances about, the relatively few sessions of REBT that helped her to look at, understand, and change her basic anxiety-creating and hostility-inciting philosophy of life.

Editors' Introduction

This case illustrates an important behavioral technique, covert sensitization, applied to a serious clinical problem, pedophilia. There is widespread pessimism among clinicians regarding the treatment of pedophilia, and this makes the success of this case all the more remarkable.

We selected the case because it illustrates how behavior therapists have embraced the use of cognitions as therapeutic tools. In addition, the case was written by Dr. David Barlow, arguably the most important figure in contemporary behavior therapy. Dr. Barlow has been an outspoken and eloquent advocate for the use of empirically supported treatments (ESTs).

Careful reading of this case will dispel the myth that behavior therapists are indifferent to relationship variables and the false belief that behavioral methods are applied in a lockstep manner without consideration for personality factors and family dynamics. We quickly see that Dr. Barlow is a sensitive therapist who tailors his treatment to the unique needs of his patient, and the case provides a glimpse of the genuine concern this therapist has for this very troubled patient.

It will be useful for students to think about how practitioners of the other therapeutic approaches represented in Case Studies in Psychotherapy *would have conceptualized the etiology and maintenance of this particular problem, and to speculate about how treatment—and outcome—might have differed. How would you have approached the case? Can a therapist's revulsion about a behavior like pedophilia influence his or her ability to help a client? How can a therapist put aside intense personal feelings in the interest of his or her clients?*

5 | COVERT SENSITIZATION FOR PARAPHILIA

David H. Barlow

CASE BACKGROUND

At the time of presentation, Reverend X was a 51-year-old married minister from the Midwest. He had three grown children, two females and a male, the youngest of whom was his 19-year-old daughter. He was tall and quite serious and although cooperative, did not volunteer a great deal of information at the initial interview. He came to my office after referral by a prominent psychiatrist in another state for assessment and possible treatment of heterosexual pedophilic behavior.

Reverend X reported that he had been touching and caressing girls between the ages of 10 and 16 for more than 20 years. He estimated at this time that there were probably more than 50 girls with whom he had had some interaction. Most typically this interaction was restricted to hugging or caressing their breasts. On occasion, he would also touch their genitals. He did not expose himself to girls nor did he ask them to touch him in any way. Generally, he reported achieving a partial erection during this type of contact but never ejaculated during one of these encounters. He did not report this to be primarily an erotic experience but rather continued to suggest that the emphasis was on an exchange of affection. In fact, during the initial interview he reported feeling little remorse about his activities for this reason, although he was deeply concerned over the effect of being "found out" on his family and his career.

Some 12 years before he presented for treatment, his activities were discovered for the first time and he was forced to leave his church in another state in the Midwest, but the matter was kept relatively quiet and he was able to take up a new position in a different state, a position he retained until just prior to treatment. Although he sought treatment and agreed to refrain from any physical interaction with young girls in his new church, he was soon as active as ever. This behavior continued on until several months before presenting for treatment.

According to Reverend X, in most of the cases the young girls responded positively to his advances and did not seem offended or frightened. In several instances this type of activity would continue with the girl for several months and it was with these girls that genital touching occurred.

During these years, although responsible administratively and spiritually for the entire parish, he took particular interest in activities involving young adolescent girls, such as the local Girl Scout troop. In addition to this activity, Reverend X, who was particularly attracted to the small breasts characteristic of young adolescent girls, would masturbate once or twice a week to pictures of girls with these features, which he found in what he referred to as "nudist magazines." In fact, he subscribed to a rather extensive series of pedophilic pornographic magazines, which, much to the embarrassment of himself and his family, continued to arrive at his old rectory for months after his discovery only to be received by the new occupants.

Several months before presenting for treatment he was confronted by the parents of an 11-year-old Girl Scout who were hearing "strange stories" about physical touching from their daughter and wanted to discuss them. His behavior was presented as a misunderstanding and the incident died down until the parents of another young girl with similar experiences mentioned them to the parents of the first girl. The story spread like wildfire and quickly led to outrage and dismissal from the parish by the bishop and suspension as a minister with strong recommendations to seek treatment.

Reverend X grew up a rather inhibited teenager with few lasting social contacts with girls. When he married at age 26, he engaged in sexual intercourse for the first time. He had begun dating at approximately age 22 and on only one occasion before marriage had he engaged in even light petting. Masturbatory fantasies in high school were centered on developing breasts.

After discovery 12 years ago at his previous parish, he was the client in a number of long-term psychotherapeutic relationships. He reported that none of these had had the slightest effect whatsoever on his sexual arousal patterns. At least one of his previous therapists had taken the approach that there must be something wrong within his marital relationship. This only angered him and was disconfirmed by his wife, who reported a normal and satisfying sexual and marital relationship.

Despite the incident, his relationship with his family remained excellent and his wife was extremely supportive, determined to stick by him through "thick and thin." His children were also quite supportive but seemed to largely dismiss the incidents or deny that they were anything but exaggerations and innuendos. He had never approached any of his children sexually.

ASSESSMENT AND BEHAVIOR ANALYSIS

The most striking aspect of the presentation of Reverend X alluded to previously and also mentioned by his referring psychiatrist was the absence of any remorse. Reverend X himself also commented on his relative absence of remorse and seemed puzzled by it since he had at least an intellectual appreciation of the seriousness of his acts. It became clear that before attempting formal intervention with covert sensitization it would be necessary to deal with his motivation to change, which would be likely to affect his compliance with covert sensitization procedures. Thus it became necessary to strip away some of the rationalizations that were interfering with his motivation for treatment.

The primary rationalization commonly found in pedophiles is the notion that they are somehow providing love and affection to children that is beneficial to them and that this affection may be restricted or absent from other sources. Indeed, this rationalization was clearly present in Reverend X, who considered his behavior to be primarily affectionate despite the occasional genital contact and masturbatory activity to "nudist magazines." The client was instructed to make a list of various specific rationalizations. He began working on these rationalizations at home. He was also asked to contemplate how his contacts were received by the girls and whether or not he was oblivious to any negative cues. It became apparent that he had established a strong "boundary" between "proper and improper" pedophilic behavior. For example, intercourse with a child or coercion was as repugnant to him as it would be to the average person. But fondling breasts and genitals was affectionate. Evidence for rationalization was present in the following reports or observations: (1) he reported that most children were very responsive to his advances; (2) his description of many of his episodes was objectified by his use of third person speech; (3) he was very indignant over the angry manner with which most of his congregation responded to him after discovery, thinking they were somehow ungrateful for all of his years of service to the parish (this included his bishop, whom he accused of not providing appropriate support); and (4) he had established boundaries between "good and bad" pedophilic behavior, as mentioned earlier.

In an attempt to break down some of these barriers, two scenarios were presented to him for consideration. First, he was asked how he would react if he discovered that one of his daughters had been fondled or molested by a strange adult male. Initially he digressed into problems of hypothetical questions but then replied that he had never considered that possibility and had probably blocked it out. In fact, in the remainder of the session he refused to consider the topic despite subsequent attempts to introduce it. In regard to the reaction of his parishioners, he was asked what his reaction would be if it was discovered that his bishop had been raping women in the back alleys of the city for several years on Saturday night. He was able to admit that his behavior was at least as repugnant as the hypothetical behavior of his bishop and that it would seem quite shocking indeed.

Thinking about these issues in and between the first several sessions sensitized Reverend X to several facets of his problem, and he was able to recognize, at least at a rational level, the horror that his behavior evoked in others and by inference, the repugnant nature of the behavior itself. Nevertheless, he was now requested in sessions to imagine that his daughter was being molested and to picture it as vividly as possible. He was instructed to feel it emotionally and then report his reactions. Second, he was asked to imagine a similar situation in which he was engaging in genital contact with his most recent victim with all of the parishioners watching.

During this time he was also given materials to read on the consequences of sexual abuse of children. In fact, he reported that he had been familiar with some of these materials before but had read them in a more abstract intellectual manner. During the next several weeks he reported that his masturbatory fantasies began to incorporate images of nameless, faceless people watching him and that his fantasies became a bit fuzzy, much like static on a television set.

By approximately the fourth session the patient clearly began to experience some of the horror and aversiveness of his behavior and actually demonstrated some negative affect and a few tears. This was a marked change from previous sessions characterized by little or no affect of any kind while discussing his behavior. Masturbation of any kind stopped. At this point steps preliminary to implementing covert sensitization were begun.

Detailed descriptions of his behavior and preliminary explorations of the most aversive consequences he could imagine allowed a behavior analysis prior to implementing formal covert sensitization. Self-monitoring revealed infrequent pedophilic fantasies at this time. The decreased frequency of his fantasies most likely related to the punishing effect of his recent discovery. Nevertheless, his pattern of pedophilic behavior was fairly consistent. Typically he would playfully approach a young girl who happened to be alone in a room at the church recreation center or perhaps in his car if he were driving her somewhere. He would then put his arms on her or around her and gradually move his hands to the breast area or, on occasion, the genital area. He would be very careful to ascertain if the girl would be likely to be responsive beforehand and if she remained responsive during the encounter. If there was any sign of resisting or lack of responsiveness he would quickly desist or revert to a wrestling or playing type of activity that did not involve breast or genital contact. On rare occasions the same behavior might occur during the summer while swimming in a nearby lake.

In addition to these rather restricted behavioral patterns, the client would experience a number of urges upon seeing young girls in various locations. These urges would range from a full-blown sexual thought sequence while watching a young girl to what he would call a "glimpse." During a glimpse he would not be aware of any frank sexual thoughts but would notice himself glancing at a young girl who was not directly in his line of sight and therefore represented someone who probably would not attract his attention if she were not the appropriate age and sex.

Since no behavior was occurring at this time and since fantasies (sexual thoughts in the absence of young girls) were also absent, self-monitoring was restricted to "urges" such as those described above. This "urge" once again was defined as a sexual thought, image, or impulse upon seeing a young adolescent girl. The client recorded all sexual urges on a self-monitoring record that he carried with him at all times. The record was divided into daily segments in which the patient could total the number of occurrences of full-blown urges or "glimpses" each day. The patient was instructed to record these urges or glimpses as soon as possible after their occurrence. Physiological assessment of sexual arousal patterns was also conducted using penile strain gauge measures. This assessment revealed continued marked responsiveness to pedophilic stimuli.

One further assessment procedure necessary before beginning covert sensitization is a determination of the worst possible consequences of the behavior in the patient's own mind. Reverend X reported, consistent with his reaction during the first several sessions of treatment, that being observed engaging in this behavior provoked a particularly strong negative emotional reaction in him. He also displayed some sensitivity to images of nausea and vomiting, which comprise a common set of aversive scenes in covert sensitization. In cases where nausea and vomiting are not particularly aversive, scenes of blood and injury or scenes of snakes or spiders crawling on one's skin can be very effective. With this information the patient was ready to begin covert sensitization trials.

TREATMENT PROGRAM

Prior to my initiating covert sensitization, I presented Reverend X with the following therapeutic rationale:

We will now initiate a procedure with the purpose of directly reducing remaining arousal to young girls using a technique called covert sensitization. This procedure involves having you imagine sexual scenes with young girls similar to those interactions you have actually experienced or masturbate to, and to pair an aversive image with that scene. This procedure has been successfully employed with individuals with similar problems in the past and we have every reason to believe that it will be very helpful in your case.

The purpose of covert sensitization is to neutralize what has become a very automatic uncontrollable sexual arousal to young girls. This will be accomplished by repeatedly imagining a very unpleasant scene in association with your typically sexually arousing scenes. It is very important that you imagine, as vividly as possible, all of the scenes that I present. In addition, this procedure is very useful because you will be learning a skill that you can apply to situations where in the past you would have become aroused. That is, if you find yourself becoming aroused by young girls you can utilize your aversive images in a self-control fashion and very quickly eliminate the arousal. Since this is basically a skill that you are learning, it is also very important that you do a fair amount of homework between sessions.

Initially, I will be presenting vivid descriptions of sexually arousing scenes based on everything we have talked about thus far. I want you to make yourself comfortable, close your eyes, and imagine the scene as if you are actually there. It is very important that you "live" the scene. You should feel, hear, and sense every part of the image. You should not see yourself in the scene but should actually be there. We will also develop some aversive scenes along the lines we have already discussed to be associated with the arousing scenes.

As noted, Reverend X had identified being caught in the act and observed by his family and close friends as perhaps the most aversive naturally occurring event he could think of. In addition, some preliminary exploration revealed a sensitivity to nausea and vomiting. Therefore, these two aversive scenes were used throughout covert sensitization trials.

> Sit back in the chair and get as relaxed as possible. Close your eyes and concentrate on what I'm saying. Imagine yourself in the recreation room of the church. Notice the furniture . . . the walls . . . and the feelings of being in the room. Standing to one side is Joan, a 13-year-old girl. As she comes toward you, you notice the color of her hair . . . the clothes she is wearing . . . and the way she is walking. She comes over and sits by you. She is being flirtatious and very cute. You touch her playfully and begin to get aroused. She is asking you questions about sex education and you begin to touch her. You can feel your hands on her smooth skin . . . on her dress . . . and on her breasts under her shirt.
>
> As you become more and more aroused, you begin taking off her clothes. You can feel your fingers on her dress as you slip it off. You begin touching arms . . . her back and her breasts . . . Now your hands are on her thighs and her buttocks. As you get more excited, you put your hand between her legs. She begins rubbing your penis. You're noticing how good it feels. You are stroking her thighs and genitals and getting very aroused.
>
> You hear a scream! As you turn around you see your two daughters and your wife. They see you there—naked and molesting that little girl. They begin to cry. They are sobbing hysterically. Your wife falls to her knees and holds her head in her hands. She is saying "I hate you, I hate you!" You start to go over to hold her, but she is afraid of you and runs away. You start to panic and lose control. You want to kill yourself and end it all. You can see what you have done to yourself.

The aversive scenes were presented in great detail in order to elicit arousal and to facilitate the imagery process. Initially, they were presented late in the chain of behavior. As treatment progressed, the aversive scenes were introduced earlier in the arousing sequence.

In addition to these scenes where Reverend X was caught by his family, other images involving nausea and vomiting were used. In these images as he would begin genital contact with young girls he would feel himself becoming more and more nauseous . . . feel the vomit working its way up into his throat and begin swallowing hard to attempt to keep it down. At that point he would start gagging uncontrollably until vomit and mucus began spilling out of his mouth and nose all over his clothes and the clothes of the young girl. In this particular case I embellished the scene by having him continue to vomit all over the lap of the young girl until the girl's flesh would actually begin to rot before his eyes and worms and maggots would begin crawling around in it. These embellishments are not effective with everyone but were very effective with Reverend X. During the scenes he would become visibly tense, rise in his chair, and be quite drained by the end of the session. During vomiting scenes patients on occasion will bring in a fresh shirt for fear that they might actually vomit during the sessions. This illustrates once again that there is no limit to the vividness of the scenes, and some dramatic presentations on the part of the therapist, at least initially, can be very helpful if the patient is able to process them in such a way that they are effective.

In the example presented earlier, the patient progressed rather far in the chain of sexual behaviors before the aversive scene was introduced. In general, as treatment progresses, the aversive scenes are introduced earlier in the arousing sequence. In this fashion, aversive scenes are paired with the very early parts of the chain, often the first glimpse, by the end of treatment. It is this early pairing that is rehearsed in a self-control fashion.

In this particular case these scenes were presented in two different formats. In the first format, referred to as "punishment," the sexually arousing scene was presented and resulted in the aversive scenes mentioned earlier. In the second format, described as "escape," the patient would begin the sexually arousing scene, contemplate briefly the aversive consequences, and then turn and flee the situation as quickly as possible, feeling greatly relieved and relaxed as he got farther away from the situation.

For Reverend X a typical session involved presenting five of the scenes, either three punishment and two escape or vice versa. The location of the scenes would be varied to conform to the typical locations that were relevant for this particular patient. The two aversive scenes would also be alternated in a random fashion or sometimes integrated or combined.

When it was clear that the patient could imagine these images vividly and was fully processing the information, he was asked to go through the trial himself in the presence of the therapist. Methods for overcoming difficulties in achieving clear images were discussed and practiced. The self-administered practices within sessions were interspersed with therapist-conducted trials. After several sessions, when it was clear that the patient could self-administer the procedure as effectively as the therapist, homework assignments were prescribed. The patient monitored the intensity of his self-administered sessions on a scale of 0 to 100, where 0 equaled no intensity whatsoever and 100 represented an intensity as vivid as real life. Initially, his practice sessions were rated in the 10% to 50% range. As time went on the practice sessions were more consistently rated in the 50% to 70% range, which was judged to be sufficiently intense to produce the desired effects. Initially sessions were prescribed once a day in which he would be asked to conduct three trials (imagine three scenes). After several weeks this was cut back to two practices a week to maximize the intensity. Scenes were varied slightly by the patient to prevent habituation.

During this time self-monitoring revealed occasional urges and glimpses but still no fantasies or masturbatory activity. In fact, the patient had cut back on masturbatory activity shortly after his apprehension and ceased altogether just before treatment began, as noted earlier. Nevertheless, occasional interviews with his wife, who remained extremely supportive, revealed some increase in sexual activity in their relationship, averaging two to three times per week. This relationship was described by both as improved and entirely satisfactory.

At this time the final phase of covert sensitization was introduced. In this phase the patient used the aversive images in vivo in a self-control fashion whenever an urge or even a glimpse occurred. This information was also noted on self-monitoring forms such that any urge or glimpse would be immediately consequated by an aversive image. While he found this somewhat difficult at first, Reverend X reported increasing facility in carrying out his part of the treatment and noted a gradually decreasing number of urges and glimpses.

RESULTS

Rather early in the course of treatment a reaction to Reverend X's behavior on the part of his community threatened to disrupt progress. Although he had moved out of the rectory and away from the church, some of his family remained in his hometown. On occasion he would return to town from his temporary residence, which was convenient to my office, to assist with some practical matters concerning an upcoming move that he and his wife were planning. He would also see a few old friends. During this period a very ugly reaction to his earlier apprehension occurred in the community. Rumors circulated describing very exaggerated accounts of his behavior as well as the fact that he was living in another state simply to wait out the statute of limitations and avoid criminal charges. It was also rumored that he had stopped seeking treatment and had a cavalier attitude toward his problem. This community reaction, which also affected his family, had a serious impact on therapy. A brief but deep state of depression retarded progress and forced a temporary cessation of covert sensitization sessions while the implications of the community reaction were discussed. In fact, Reverend X was deeply distressed by the incident, not only because of the vicious allegations, but also because it became clear that he still harbored some illusions that the community, which had showed deep support and respect for him during his years of service, would somehow welcome him back with open arms once his treatment was completed. Only when he fully appreciated that this was not going to happen and began to make realistic plans about permanently relocating was he able to continue on with therapy.

Four months after treatment began, pedophilic urges had dropped to zero and remained there. At this time Reverend X and his wife permanently relocated to another state, where he obtained work in a local hardware store. He would continue to commute approximately five hours each way for remaining treatment sessions such that he would have one long session every two weeks. Six months after treatment began, a full assessment revealed an excellent response. Treatment was terminated with plans for the first follow-up session to occur one month later and then at decreasing intervals after that as indicated.

Periodic follow-ups were conducted during the ensuing 18 months. A full evaluation at that time, including penile plethysmography, revealed no return of pedophilic arousal patterns. This pattern of results was supported by lengthy interviews with Reverend X as well as independent and separate interviews with his wife. Both individuals reported a satisfactory adaptation to their new location, where Reverend X had worked steadily and productively for the same employer and had been asked to take on additional supervisory responsibilities. The marital relationship, if anything, had continued to improve during the past year. He had begun to engage in extensive volunteer activity in his community.

DISCUSSION

Covert sensitization has proven very effective for paraphilic patterns of arousal, as noted earlier. Nevertheless, there were several aspects of this case that undoubtedly facilitated treatment. Reverend X received deep and sustaining support from his family not only during the initial crisis but also throughout treatment. This support extended to at least some of his old friends in his community who were aware of his problem and, increasingly, friends that he met in his new community, who, of course, were not aware of his problem. In view of the stigma so often attached to sexual offenders and the outright desertion by even close family and friends that often occurs, this support was undoubtedly very valuable to Reverend X.

In addition, throughout this period he maintained his deeply religious attitude and convictions. He attended service regularly and continued to express a desire to resume the provision of some service to the church, even if not on a full-time basis. Nevertheless, despite several inquiries to the church hierarchy, he received no response to his request and began to give up hope of resuming any vestiges of a career that had been at the very center of his existence and had provided deep meaning to his life for some 25 years.

More than two years following this contact and nearly four years after beginning treatment, another follow-up visit confirmed no return of pedophilic arousal patterns whatsoever. Reverend X continued to do extremely well in his new job and was now second-in-command of a small chain of hardware stores. He continued to be active in his community. The church continued to ignore his occasional letters asking for clarification of his status, and he had given up all hope of any return to even part-time duties. Nevertheless, he still hoped against hope that some day the church that he had served for so long might at least lift the suspension and allow him to occasionally conduct religious services for his immediate family. Beyond that his thoughts centered on his day-to-day life in his new community and the distant plan of retirement with his wife somewhere in the South in another 10 or 15 years.

Editors' Introduction

Aaron Beck, the leading figure in cognitive therapy, is an authority on suicide and depression. In the case that follows, the reader has an opportunity to see how Beck works with a depressed professional woman.

The cognitive approach to therapy is precise, straightforward, and methodological. Beck lays out a road map for therapy in the introduction to the case and then illustrates how the actual therapy sessions link to the therapy plan. Like Ellis, he challenges his patient's irrational beliefs, but he does so in a more probing, Socratic manner consistent with the philosophy of collaborative empiricism that is the foundation of cognitive therapy. This case is especially interesting because the depressed individual being treated is a clinical psychologist.

We believe this case nicely illustrates the sometimes subtle differences between cognitive therapy and two related approaches to therapy: rational emotive behavior therapy and cognitive behavior therapy. Once again, the student is given an opportunity to observe a master therapist at work, listening to the actual language used in the therapy sessions.

Aaron Beck has earned the admiration and respect of almost everyone in the world of psychotherapy, and he is the individual most responsible for the inclusion of at least some cognitive therapy techniques in the practice of almost all psychotherapists.

Every therapist and counselor will at some point treat suicidal clients, and most experienced therapists have lost patients to suicide. What feelings do you experience reading about this woman's suicidal ideation? How do you evaluate lethality in patients with suicidal thoughts? Will you feel comfortable working with seriously depressed individuals?

6

AN INTERVIEW
WITH A DEPRESSED
AND SUICIDAL PATIENT

Aaron T. Beck

Perhaps the most critical challenge to the adequacy of cognitive therapy is its efficacy in dealing with the acutely suicidal patient. In such cases the therapist often has to shift gears and assume a very active role in attempting to penetrate the barrier of hopelessness and resignation. Since intervention may be decisive in saving the patient's life, the therapist has to attempt to accomplish a number of immediate goals either concurrently or in rapid sequence: establish a working relationship with the patient, assess the severity of the depression and suicidal wish, obtain an overview of the patient's life situation, pinpoint the patient's "reasons" for wanting to commit suicide, determine the patient's capacity for self-objectivity, and ferret out some entry point for stepping into the patient's phenomenological world to introduce elements of reality.

Such a venture, as illustrated in the following interview, is taxing and demands all the qualities of a "good therapist"—genuine warmth, acceptance, and empathetic understanding—as well as the application of the appropriate strategies drawn from the system of cognitive therapy.

The patient was a 40-year-old clinical psychologist who had recently been left by her boyfriend. She had a history of intermittent depressions since the age of 12 years, and had received many courses of psychotherapy, antidepressant drugs, electroconvulsive therapy, and hospitalizations. The patient had been seen by the author five times over a period of 7 or 8 months. At the time of this interview, it was obvious that she was depressed and, as indicated by her previous episodes, probably suicidal.

In the first part of the interview, the main thrust was to *ask appropriate questions* in order to make a clinical assessment and also to try to elucidate the major psychological problems. The therapist, first of all, had to make an assessment as to how depressed and how suicidal the patient was. He also had to assess her expectations regarding being helped by the interview (T-1; T-8) in order to determine how much leverage he had. During this period of time, in order to keep the dialogue going, he also had to repeat the patient's statements.

It was apparent from the emergence of suicidal wishes that this was the salient clinical problem and that her hopelessness (T-7) would be the most appropriate point for intervention.

Several points could be made regarding the first part of the interview. The therapist accepted the seriousness of the patient's desire to die but treated it as a topic for further examination, a problem to be discussed. "We can discuss the advantages and disadvantages" (T-11). She responded to this statement with some amusement (a favorable sign). The therapist also tried to test the patient's ability to look at herself and her problems

Excerpt from Aaron T. Beck et al., *Cognitive Therapy of Depression* (pp. 225–243). Published in 1979 by Guilford Publications, Inc. Reprinted by permission of the publisher.

with objectivity. He also attempted to test the rigidity of her irrational ideas and her acceptance of his wish to help her (T-13–T-20).

In the first part of the interview the therapist was not able to make much headway because of the patient's strongly held belief that things could not possibly work out well for her. She had decided that suicide was the only solution, and she resented attempts to "get her to change her mind."

In the next part of the interview, the therapist attempted to isolate the participating factor in her present depression and suicidal ideation, namely, the breakup with her boyfriend. It becomes clear as the therapist tries to explore the significance of the breakup that the meaning to the patient is, "I have nothing" (P-23). The therapist then selects, "*I have nothing*" as a target and attempts to elicit from the patient information contradictory to this conclusion. He probes for a previous period of time when she did *not* believe "I have nothing" and also was not having a relationship with a man. He then proceeds (T-26) to probe for other goals and objects that are important to her; he seeks concrete sources of satisfaction (T-24–T-33). The therapist's attempt to establish that the patient does, indeed, "have something" is parried by the patient's tendency to discount any positive features in her life (P-32).

Finally, the patient does join forces with the therapist, and it is apparent in the latter part of the interview that she is willing to separate herself from her problems and consider ways of solving them. The therapist then moves to a consideration of the basic assumption underlying her hopelessness, namely, "I cannot be happy without a man." By pointing out disconfirming past experiences, he tries to demonstrate the error of this assumption. He also attempts to explain the value of shifting to the assumption, "I can make myself happy." He points out that it is more realistic for her to regard herself as the active agent in seeking out sources of satisfaction than as an inert receptacle dependent for nourishment on the whims of others.

The taped interview, which was edited down from 60 minutes to 35 minutes for practical reasons, is presented verbatim. (The only changes made were to protect the identity of the patient.) The interview is divided into five parts.

PART 1
QUESTIONING TO ELICIT VITAL INFORMATION

1. How depressed is the patient? How suicidal?
2. Attitude about coming to appointment (expectancy about therapy).
3. Emergence of suicidal wishes: immediate critical problem.
4. Attempt to find the best point for therapeutic intervention: hopelessness—negative attitude toward future (P-7).
5. Accept seriousness of patient's desire to die but treat it as a topic for further examination—"Discuss advantages and disadvantages" (T-11).
6. Test ability to look at herself—objectivity; test rigidity of her irrational ideas; test responsiveness to therapist (T-13–T-20).

PART 2
BROADENING PATIENT'S PERSPECTIVE

1. Isolate the precipitating factor—breakup with boyfriend; reduce use of questioning.
2. Determine meaning to patient of the breakup.
3. Immediate psychological problem: "I have nothing."

4. Question the conclusion, "I have nothing."

5. Probe for other objects that are important to her: concrete sources of satisfaction (T-24–T-33).

6. Shore up reality-testing and positive self-concept (T-35–T-37).

PART 3
"ALTERNATIVE THERAPY"

1. Therapist very active in order to engage patient's interest in understanding and dealing with her problem. Induce patient to examine options (T-38). "Eliminate" suicide as an option.

2. Undermine patient's all-or-nothing thinking by getting her to regard herself, her future, and her experiences in quantitative probabilities (T-45).

3. Feedback: important information as to success of interview. Look for (a) affect shift, (b) positive statements about herself, (c) consensus with patient regarding solution of problem (P-47).

PART 4
OBTAINING MORE ACCURATE DATA

1. More therapeutic collaboration: discussion about therapeutic techniques and rationale.

2. Testing her conclusions about "no satisfaction," indirectly disproving her conclusion.

3. Patient's spontaneous statement, "Can I tell you something positive?"

4. Periodic attempts to evoke a mirth response.

PART 5
CLOSURE

Reinforce independence (T-106), self-help, optimism.

Therapist (T-1):   Well, how have you been feeling since I talked to you last? . . .
Patient (P-1):   Bad.
T-2:   You've been feeling bad . . . well, tell me about it?
P-2:   It started this weekend . . . I just feel like everything is an effort. There's just completely no point to do anything.
T-3:   So, there are two problems; everything is an effort, and you believe there's no point to doing anything.
P-3:   It's because there's no point to doing anything that makes everything too hard to do.
T-4:   (*Repeating her words to maintain interchange. Also to acknowledge her feelings.*) Because there's no point and everything feels like an effort . . . And when you were coming down here today, were you feeling the same way?
P-4:   Well, it doesn't seem as bad when I am working. It's bad on weekends and especially on holidays. I sort of expected that it would happen.
T-5:   (*Eliciting expectancy regarding session*) You expected to have a hard time on holidays . . . And when you left your office to come over here, how were you feeling then?

P-5:   Kind of the same way. I feel that I can do everything that I have to do, but I don't *want* to.

T-6:   You don't want to do the things you have to.

P-6:   I don't want to do anything.

T-7:   Right . . . and what kind of feeling did you have? Feel low?

P-7:   (*Hopelessness to be target*) I feel that there's no hope for me. I feel my future . . . that everything is futile, that there's no hope.

T-8:   And what idea did you have about today's interview?

P-8:   I thought that it would probably help as it has always happened in the past . . . that I would feel better—temporarily. But that makes it worse because then I know that I am going to feel bad again.

T-9:   That makes it worse in terms of how you feel?

P-9:   Yes.

T-10:   And the reason is that it builds you up and then you get let down again?

P-10:   (*Immediate problem—suicide risk*) I feel like it's interminable, it will just go this way forever, and I am not getting any better . . . I don't feel any less inclined to kill myself than I ever did in my life . . . In fact, if anything, *I feel like I'm coming closer to it.*

T-11:   Perhaps we should talk about that a little bit because we haven't talked about the advantages and disadvantages of killing yourself.

P-11:   (*Smiles*) You make everything so logical.

T-12:   (*Testing therapeutic alliance*) Is that bad? Remember you once wrote something . . . that reason is your greatest ally. Have you become allergic to reason?

P-12:   But I can't try anymore.

T-13:   Does it take an effort to be reasonable?

P-13:   (*Typical "automatic thoughts"*) I know I am being unreasonable; the thoughts seem so real to me . . . it does take an effort to try to change them.

T-14:   Now, if it came easy to you—to change the thoughts, do you think that they would last as long?

P-14:   No . . . see, I don't say that this wouldn't work with other people. I don't try to say that, but I don't feel that it can work with me.

T-15:   So, do you have any evidence that it did work with you?

P-15:   It works for specific periods of time, and that's like the Real Me comes through.

T-16:   Now, is there anything unusual that happened that might have upset the apple cart?

P-16:   You mean this weekend?

T-17:   Not necessarily this weekend. As you know, you felt you were making good progress in therapy and you decided that you were going to be like the Cowardly Lion Who Found His Heart. What happened after that?

P-17:   (*Agitated, bows head*) It's too hard . . . it would be easier to die.

T-18:   (*Attempts to restore objectivity. Injects perspective by recalling previous mastery experience.*) At the moment, it would be easier to die—as you say. But, let's go back to the history. You're losing sight and losing perspective. Remember when we talked and made a tape of that interview and you liked it. You wrote a letter the next day and you said that you felt you had your Heart and it wasn't any great effort to reach that particular point. Now, you went along reasonably well until you got involved. Correct? Then you got involved with Jim. Is that correct? And then very predictably when your relationship ended, you felt terribly let down. Now, what do you conclude from that?

P-18:   (*Anguish, rejects therapist's venture*) My conclusion is that I am always going to have to be alone because I can't stay in a relationship with a man.

T-19:   All right, that's one possible explanation. What other possible explanations are there?

P-19:   That's the only explanation.

T-20:   Is it possible you just weren't *ready* to get deeply involved and then let down?

P-20A: But, I feel like I'll never be ready. (*Weeps*)

P-20B: I have never given up on him, even when I couldn't see him for a year at a time. He was always in my mind, all the time. So how can I think now that I can just dismiss him.

T-21:   This was never final until now. There was always the hope that . . .

P-21:   There wasn't, and he told me very clearly that he could not get involved with me.

T-22:   Right, but before January, it was very quiescent. You weren't terribly involved with him. It started up in January again. He did show serious interest in you.

P-22:   For the first time in four years.

T-23:   (*Attempts to restore perspective*) All right, so that's when you got involved again. Prior to January, you weren't involved, weren't thinking of him every minute and you weren't in the situation you are in now, and you were happy at times. You wrote that letter to me that you were happy, right? Okay. So that was back in January, you were happy and you did not have Jim. Now comes May, and you're unhappy because you have just broken up with him. Now, why do you still have to be unhappy, say, in July, August, or September?

P-23:   (*Presents specific target belief*) I have nothing.

T-24:   You weren't unhappy in January, were you?

P-24:   At first I was, that's why I called.

T-25:   All right, how about December? December you weren't unhappy. What did you have in December? You had something that made you happy.

P-25:   I was seeing other men. That made me happy.

T-26:   There are other things in your life besides men that you said you liked very much.

P-26:   Yes and I . . .

T-27:   (*Aims at target beliefs. Shows she had and has something.*) Well, there were other things you say were important that are not important right now. Is that correct? What were the things that were important to you back in December, November, and October?

P-27:   Everything was important.

T-28:   Everything was important. And what were those things?

P-28:   It's hard to even think of anything that I cared about.

T-29:   Okay, now how about your job?

P-29:   My job.

T-30:   Your job was important. Did you feel that you were accomplishing something on the job?

P-30:   Most of the time I did.

T-31:   (*Still aiming*) Most of the time, you felt you were accomplishing something on the job. And what about now? Do you feel you are accomplishing on the *job now?*

P-31:   (*Discounts positive*) Not as much as I could.

T-32:   (*Reintroduces positive*) You're not accomplishing as much as you could but even when you are "off," I understand that you do as well [as] or better than many of the other workers. Is that not correct?

P-32:   (*Disqualifies positive statement*) I can't understand why you say that. How do you know that? Because I told you that. How do you know that's true?

T-33:   I'm willing to take your word for it.

P-33:   From somebody who is irrational.

T-34:   (*Presents positive evidence of satisfactions and achievements.*) Well, I think that somebody who is as irrationally down on herself as you, is very unlikely to say something positive *about herself* unless the positive thing is so strong that it is unmistakable to anybody . . . In any event, you do get some satisfaction out of the job right now and you do feel you are doing a reasonably good job, although you are not doing as well as you would like to, but as well as you are capable. You're still doing a reasonably good job. You can see for yourself. Your clients' plans are improving? Are they being helped? Does anyone say they are appreciative of your efforts?

P-34: Yes.

T-35: They do tell you? Yet you are saying you are so irrational that I can't believe anything you say. Do you say, "You're just a dumb client . . . no judgment at all," to your clients?

P-35: I wouldn't say that about somebody.

T-36: Well, do you think it about yourself?

P-36: Yes.

T-37: (*Points out inconsistency. Underscores her capacity for rationality. Fortifies her professional role.*) So, you trust the word of your clients, but you won't trust your own word. You won't think of your clients as being irrational, and yet, you think of you—when you are the client—as being irrational. How can you be rational when you are the therapist and irrational when you are the patient?

P-37A: I set different standards for myself than what I set for anybody else in the world.

P-37B: Suppose I'll never get over it?

T-38: (*Changes the options—consider nonsuicidal solutions. Sweat it out or fight to solve problem.*) Suppose you'll never get over it? Well, we don't know whether you'll never get over it or not . . . so there're two things you can do. One is, you can take it passively and see, and you might find that you will get over it, since almost everybody gets over grief reactions. Or, you can attack the problem aggressively and actively build up a solid basis for yourself. In other words, you can capitalize on the chance . . .

P-38: (*Thinks of finding another man.*) I feel desperate. I feel that I have to find somebody right now—right away.

T-39: All right, now if you found somebody right away, what would happen?

P-39: The same thing would happen again.

T-40: (*Omits suicide as one of the options.*) Now, remember when we talked about Jim and you said back in January you decided that you would take that chance and you'd chance being involved, with the possibility that something would come of it positively. Now, you have two choices at this time. You can either stick it out now and try to weather the storm with the idea that you are going to keep fighting it, or you can get involved with somebody else and not have the opportunity for this elegant solution. Now, which way do you want to go?

P-40: (*Compulsion to get involved with somebody.*) I don't want to, but I feel driven. I don't know why I keep fighting that, but I do. I'm not involved with anybody now and I don't want to be, but I feel a compulsion.

T-41: That's right, because you're hurting very badly. Isn't that correct? If you weren't hurting you wouldn't feel the compulsion.

P-41: But I haven't done anything yet.

T-42: (*Emphasizes ideal option. Also turning disadvantage into advantage.*) Well, you know it's your decision. If you do seek somebody else, nobody is going to fault you on it. But I'm trying to show that there's an opportunity here. There's an unusual opportunity that you may never have again—that is to go it alone . . . to work your way out of the depression.

P-42: That's what I'll be doing the rest of my life . . . that's what worries me.

T-43: You really just put yourself in a "no-win" situation. You just acknowledged that if you get involved with another man, probably you would feel better.

P-43: Temporarily, but then, I'd go through the same thing.

T-44: I understand that. So now, you have an opportunity to not have to be dependent on another guy, but you have to pay a price. There's pain now for gain later. Now are you willing to pay the price?

P-44: I'm afraid that if I don't involve myself with somebody right away . . . I know that's dichotomous thinking . . . I think if I don't get immediately involved, that I will never have anybody.

T-45: That's all-or-nothing thinking.

P-45: I know.

T-46: (*Seeking a consensus on nonsuicidal option.*) That's all-or-nothing thinking. Now, if you are going to do it on the basis of all-or-nothing thinking, that's not very sensible. If you are going to do it on the basis of, "The pain is so great that I just don't want to stick it out anymore," all right. Then you take your aspirin temporarily and you'll just have to work it out at a later date. The thing is—do you want to stick it out right now? Now, what's the point of sticking it out now?

P-46: I don't know.

T-47: *You* don't really believe this.

P-47: (*Reaching a consensus.*) Theoretically, I know I could prove to myself that I could, in fact, be happy without a man, so that if I were to have a relationship with a man in the future, I would go into it not feeling desperate, and I would probably eliminate a lot of anxiety and depression that have in the past been connected to this relationship.

T-48: So, at least you agree, theoretically, on a logical basis this could happen. If you try to stick it out . . . Now, what do you think is the probability that this could happen?

P-48: For me?

T-49: For you.

P-49: For another person I'd say the probability is excellent.

T-50: For one of your clients?

P-50: Yeah.

T-51: For the average depressed person that comes to the Mood Clinic . . . most of whom have been depressed 7 years or more. You would still give them a high probability.

P-51: Listen, I've been depressed all of my life. I thought of killing myself when I was 14 years old.

T-52: (*Undermining absolutistic thinking by suggesting probabilities.*) Well, many of the other people that have come here too have felt this way. Some of the people that have come here are quite young and so have not had time to be depressed very long . . . Okay, back to this. Hypothetically, this could happen. This could happen with almost anybody else, this could happen with anybody else. But you don't think it can happen to you. Right . . . It can't happen to you. But what is the possibility . . . (you know, when we talked about the possibility with Jim, we thought it was probably five in a hundred that a good thing could come from it) . . . that you could weather the storm and come out a stronger person and be less dependent on men than you had been before?

P-52: I'd say that the possibility was minimal.

T-53: All right, now is it minimal like one in a hundred, one in a million . . . ?

P-53: Well, maybe a 10% chance.

T-54: 10% chance. So, you have one chance in ten of emerging from this stronger.

P-54: (*More perspective; disqualifies evidence.*) Do you know why I say that . . . I say that on the basis of having gone through that whole summer without a man and being happy . . . and then getting to the point where I am now. That's not progress.

T-55: (*Using database.*) I'd say that is evidence. That summer is very powerful evidence.

P-55:   (*Discredits data.*) Well, look where I am right now.

T-56:   The thing is, you did very well that summer and proved as far as any scientist is concerned that you could function on your own. But you didn't prove it to your own self. You wiped out that experience as soon as you got involved with a man. That experience of independence became a nullity in your mind after that summer.

P-56:   (*Mood shift. A good sign.*) Is that what happened?

T-57:   Of course. When I talked to you the first time I saw you, you said "I cannot be happy without a man." We went over that for about 35 or 40 minutes until I finally said, "Has there ever been a time when you didn't have a man?" And you said, "My God, that time when I went to graduate school." You know, suddenly a beam of light comes in. You almost sold me on the idea that you couldn't function without a man. But that's *evidence.* I mean, if I told you I couldn't walk across the room, and you were able to demonstrate to me that I could walk across the room, would you buy my notion that I could not walk across the room? You know, there is an objective reality here. I'm not giving you information that isn't valid. There are people . . .

P-57:   I would say, how could you negate that if it didn't happen?

T-58:   What?

P-58:   (*Asks for explanation. A good sign.*) I'd say what's wrong with my mind, having once happened, how can I negate it?

T-59:   (*Alliance with patient's rationality.*) Because it's human nature, unfortunately, to negate experiences that are not consistent with the prevailing attitude. And that is what attitude therapy is all about. You have a very strong attitude, and anything that is inconsistent with that attitude stirs up cognitive dissonance. I'm sure you have heard of that, and people don't like to have cognitive dissonance. So, they throw out anything that's not consistent with their prevailing belief.

P-59:   (*Consensus gels.*) I understand that.

T-60:   (*Optimistic sally.*) You have a prevailing belief. It just happens, fortunately, that that prevailing belief is wrong. Isn't that marvelous? To have a prevailing belief that makes you unhappy, and it happens to be wrong! But it's going to take a lot of effort and demonstration to indicate to you, to convince you that it is wrong. And why is that?

P-60:   I don't know.

T-61:   (*Since patient is now collaborating, he shifts to didactic strategy. Purpose is to strengthen patient's rationality.*) Do you want to know now why? Because you've always had it. Why? First of all, this belief came on at a very early age. We're not going into your childhood, but obviously, you made a suicide attempt or thought about it when you were young. It's a belief that was in there at a very young age. It was very deeply implanted at a very young age, because you were so vulnerable then. And it's been repeated how many times since then in your own head?

P-61:   A million times.

T-62:   A million times. So do you expect that five hours of talking with me is going to reverse in itself something that has been going a million times in the past?

P-62:   Like I said, and you agreed, my reason was my ally. Doesn't my intelligence enter into it? Why can't I make my intelligence help?

T-63:   Yeah, that's the reason intelligence comes into it, but that's exactly what I'm trying to get you to do. To use your intelligence.

P-63:   There's nothing wrong with my intelligence. I know that.

T-64:   I understand that. Intelligence is fine, but intelligence has to have tools, just as you may have the physical strength to lift up a chair, but if you don't believe at the time that you have the strength to do it, you're not going to try. You're going to say, "It's pointless." On the other hand, to give you a stronger example, you may have the physical strength to lift a heavy boulder, but in order to really lift it, you might have to use a crowbar. So, it's a matter of having the correct tool. It isn't simply a matter of having naked, raw intelligence, it's a matter of using the right tools. A person who has intelligence cannot solve a problem in calculus, can he?

P-64:   If she knows how to. (*Smiles.*)

T-65:   (*Reinforces confidence in maturity.*) All right. Okay. You need to have the formulas, that's what you're coming in here for. If you weren't intelligent, you wouldn't be able to understand the formulas, and you know very well you understand the formulas. Not only that, but you use them on your own clients with much more confidence than you use them on yourself.

P-65:   (*Self-praise, confirms therapist's statement.*) You wouldn't believe me if you heard me tell things to people. You'd think I was a different person. Because I can be so optimistic about other people. I was encouraging a therapist yesterday who was about to give up on a client. I said, "You can't do that." I said, "You haven't tried everything yet," and I wouldn't let her give up.

T-66:   All right, so you didn't even have a chance to use the tools this weekend because you had the structure set in your mind, and then due to some accidental factor you were unable to do it. But you concluded on the weekend that the tools don't work since "I am so incapable that I can't use the tools." It wasn't even a test was it? Now for the next weekend . . .

P-66:   (*Agrees.*) . . . It wasn't a true test . . .

T-67:   No, it wasn't even a fair test of what you could do or what the tools could do. Now for weekends, what you want to do is prepare yourself for the Fourth of July. You prepare for the weekends by having the structure written down, and you have to have some backup plans in case it gets loused up. You know you really do have a number of things in your network that can bring you satisfaction. *What are some of the things you have gotten satisfaction from last week?*

P-67:   I took Margaret to the movies.

T-68:   What did you see?

P-68:   It was a comedy.

T-69:   What?

P-69:   A comedy.

T-70:   That's a good idea. What did you see?

P-70:   (*Smiles*) It was called *Mother, Jugs and Speed.*

T-71:   Yeah, I saw that.

P-71:   Did you see that?

T-72:   Yeah, I saw that on Friday.

P-72:   (*Smiles*) I liked it.

T-73:   It was pretty good. A lot of action in that. So you enjoyed that. Do you think you could still enjoy a good movie?

P-73:   I can. If I get distracted, I'm all right.

T-74:   So what's wrong with that?

P-74:   Because then what happens . . . while I'm distracted the pain is building up and then the impact is greater when it hits me. Like last night I had two friends over for dinner. That was fine. While they're there . . . I'm deliberately planning all these activities to keep myself busy . . . and while they were there I was fine. But when they left . . .

T-75:   That's beautiful.

P-75:   The result was that the impact was greater because all this pain had accumulated . . .

T-76:   We don't know because you didn't run a control, but there is no doubt there is a letdown after you've had [a] satisfactory experience . . . so that what you have to do is set up a mechanism for handling the letdown. See what you did is you downed yourself, you knocked yourself and said, "Well . . . it's worse now than if I hadn't had them at all." Rather than just taking it phenomenologically: "They were here and I felt good when they were here, then I felt let down afterward." So then obviously the thing to pinpoint is what? The letdown afterward. So what time did they leave?

P-76: About 9.

T-77: And what time do you ordinarily go to bed?

P-77: About 10.

T-78: So you just had one hour to plan on.

P-78: To feel bad . . .

T-79: All right, one hour to feel bad. That's one way to look at it. That's not so bad, is it? It's only one hour.

P-79: But then I feel so bad during the hour. That's when I think that I want to die.

T-80: All right, what's so bad about feeling bad? You know what we've done with some of the people? And it's really worked. We've assigned them. We've said, "Now we want to give you one hour a day in which to feel bad." Have I told you about that? "I want you to feel just as bad as you can," and in fact sometimes we even rehearse it in the session. I don't have time today but maybe another time.

P-80: It's time-limited.

T-81: (*Alliance with patient as a fellow therapist.*) Yeah, and we have the people—I'd say, "Why don't you feel as bad as you can—just think of a situation, the most horribly devastating, emotionally depleting situation you can. Why don't you feel as bad as you possibly can?" And they really can do it during a session. They go out and after that they can't feel bad again even though they may even want to. It's as though they've depleted themselves of the thing and they also get a certain degree of objectivity toward it.

P-81: (*Helping out.*) It has to be done in a controlled . . .

T-82: It has to be done in a structured situation.

P-82: It has to be controlled.

T-83: That's true. It has to—that's why I say, "Do it in here, first."

P-83: Yes.

T-84: Then, I can pull them out of it . . . You need to have a safety valve.

P-84: If you do it at home . . . you might . . .

T-85: Right, the therapist has to structure it in a particular way. I'm just saying that one hour of badness a day is not necessarily antitherapeutic. And so it doesn't mean you have to kill yourself because you have one bad hour. What you want to do is to think of this as "my one bad hour for today." That's one way of looking at it. And then you go to sleep at 10 o'clock and it's over. You've had one bad hour out of 12. That's not so terrible. Well, you told yourself during that time something like this. "See, I've had a pretty good day and now I've had this bad hour and it means I'm sick, I'm full of holes, my ego is . . ."

P-85: See I'm thinking, "It never ends."

T-86: For one hour, but yeah, but that's not even true because you thought that you couldn't have any good times in the past, and yet as recently as yesterday you had a good day.

P-86: But what gives it momentum is that thought that it's not going to end.

T-87: Maybe the thought's incorrect. How do you know the thought is incorrect?

P-87: I don't know.

T-88: (*Retrospective hypothesis-testing.*) Well, let's operationalize it. What does it mean, "It's not going to end?" Does that mean that you're never going to feel good again in your whole life? Or does that mean that you're going to have an unremitting, unrelenting, inexorable sadness day in, day out, hour after hour, minute after minute. I understand that is your belief. That's a hypothesis for the moment.

Well, let's test the hypothesis retrospectively. Now you have that thought: "This is never going to end." You had that thought when? Yesterday at 9 a.m.

P-88:   Yes.

T-89:   Now that means that if that hypothesis is correct, every minute since you awoke this morning, you should have had unending, unrelenting, unremitting, inevitable, inexorable sadness and unhappiness.

P-89:   (Refutes hypothesis.) That's not true.

T-90:   It's incorrect.

P-90:   Well, you see, when I wake up in the morning, even before I'm fully awake the first thing that comes to my mind inevitably is that I don't want to get up. That I have nothing that I want to live for. And that's no way to start the day.

T-91:   That's the way a person who has a depression starts the day. That's the perfectly appropriate way to start the day if you're feeling depressed.

P-91:   Even before you're awake?

T-92:   Of course. When people are asleep they even have bad dreams. You've read the article on dreams. Even their dreams are bad. So how do you expect them to wake up feeling good after they have had a whole night of bad dreams? And what happens in depression as the day goes on? They tend to get better. You know why? Because they get a better feel of reality—reality starts getting into their beliefs.

P-92:   Is that what it is?

T-93:   Of course.

P-93:   I always thought it was because the day was getting over and I could go to sleep again.

T-94:   Go to sleep to have more bad dreams? The reality encroaches and it disproves this negative belief.

P-94:   That's why it's diurnal.

T-95:   Of course, and we have already disproven the negative belief, haven't we? You had that very strong belief last night—strong enough to make you want to commit suicide—that this would be unremitting, unrelenting, inevitable, and inexorable.

P-95:   (Cheerful) Can I tell you something very positive I did this morning?

T-96:   (Kidding) No, I hate to hear positive things. I'm allergic. Okay. I'll tolerate it. (Laughs.)

P-96:   (Recalls rational self instruction.) I got that thought before I was even awake, and I said, "Will you stop it, just give yourself a chance and stop telling yourself things like that."

T-97:   So what's wrong with saying that?

P-97:   I know. I thought that was a very positive thing to do. (Laughs.)

T-98:   (Underscores statement.) That's terrific. Well, say it again so I can remember.

P-98:   I said, "Stop it and give yourself a chance."

T-99:   (More hopeful prediction. Self-sufficiency.) When you had your friends over, you found intrinsic meaning there. This was in the context of no man . . . Now when the pain of the breakup has washed off completely, do you think you're going to be capable of finding all these goodies, yourself, under your own power, and attaching the true meaning to them?

P-99:   I suppose if the pain is less . . .

T-100: Well, the pain's less right now.

P-100: Does it matter?

T-101: Yeah.

P-101: But that doesn't mean it won't continue.

T-102: Well, in the course of time, you know, it's human nature that people get over painful episodes. You've been over painful episodes in the past.

P-102: Suppose I keep on missing him forever.

T-103: What?

P-103: Suppose I keep on missing him forever?

T-104: There's no reason to expect you to miss him forever. That isn't the way people are constructed. People are constructed to forget after a while and then get involved in other things. You had them before.

P-104: You spoke of a man who missed a mother for 25 years.

T-105: (*Emphasizes self-sufficiency.*) Well, I don't know . . . this may have been one little hang-up he had, but, I don't know that case . . . In general, that isn't the way people function. They get over lost love. All right? And one of the ways we can speed the process is by you, yourself, attaching meaning to things that are in your environment that you are capable of responding to . . . You demonstrated that . . .

P-105: Not by trying to replace a lost love right away?

T-106: (*Reinforcing independence.*) Replace it? What you're trying to do is find another instrument to happiness. He's become your mechanism for reaching happiness. That's what's bad about the whole man hang-up. It is that you are interposing some other unreliable entity between you and happiness. And all you have to do is to move this entity out of the way, and there's nothing to prevent you from getting happiness. But you want to keep pulling it back in. I say, leave it out there for a while, and then you'll see. Just in the past week you found that when you didn't have a man, you were able to find happiness without a man. And if you leave the man out of the picture for a long enough period of time, you'll see that you don't need him. Then if you want to bring him in as one of the many things that can bring satisfaction, that's fine, you can do that. But if you see him as the *only* conduit between you and happiness, then you are right back to where you were before.

P-106: Is it an erroneous thing to think that if I get to the point where I really believe that I don't need him, that I won't want him?

T-107: Oh, you're talking about him. I think it will just . . .

P-107: Any man . . . any man?

T-108: (*Undermines regressive dependency.*) . . . Well, you might still want him, like you might like to go to a movie, or read a good book, or have your friends over for dinner. You know, you still have to have relationships with your friends. But if they didn't come over for dinner last night it wouldn't plunge you into a deep despondency. I'm not underestimating the satisfaction that one gets from other people . . . but it's not a necessity . . . It's something that you, yourself, can relate to on a one-to-one basis . . . but one does, as one individual to another. You're relating to a man the way a child does to a parent, or the way a drug addict does to his drugs. He sees the drug as the mechanism for achieving happiness. And you know you can't achieve happiness artificially. And you have been using men in an artificial way. As though they are going to bring you happiness . . . rather than they are simply one of the things external to yourself by which you, yourself, can bring yourself happiness. *You* must bring *you* happiness.

P-108: I can . . . I've been focusing on dependency.

T-109: (*Emphasizing available pleasures.*) Well, you've done it. You've brought yourself happiness by going to the movies, by working with your clients, by having friends over for dinner, by getting up in the morning and doing things with your daughter. You have brought you happiness . . . but you can't depend on somebody else to bring you happiness the way a little girl depends on a parent. It doesn't work. I'm not opposed to it . . . I have no religious objection to it . . . It just doesn't work. Pragmatically, it is a very unwise way to conduct one's life. And in some utopian society after this, children will be trained not to depend on others as the mechanism for happiness. In fact, you can even demonstrate that to your daughter . . . through your own behavior, she can find that out.

P-109:   She's a very independent child.

T-110:   (*Probing for adverse reaction to interview.*) Well, she's already found that out. Okay, now do you have any questions? Anything that we discussed today? Is there anything that I said today that rubbed you the wrong way?

P-110:   You said it would be damaging . . . not damaging . . . but you think it would deprive me of more opportunity to test this out if I were to go to another man.

T-111:   Well, it's an unusual opportunity . . .

P-111:   It's not so unusual, because I might get involved with somebody else.

T-112:   (*Turning disadvantage into advantage.*) Well, yes, but this is like the worst—you said this is the worst—depression you felt for a long time. It's a very *unusual* opportunity to be able to demonstrate how you were able to pull yourself from the very deepest depths of depression onto a very solid independent position. You may not have that opportunity again, really, and it would be such a very sharp contrast. Now, you don't have to do it, but I'm saying it's really a very rich chance, and it does mean possibly a lot of gain. I don't want to make any self-fulfilling hypotheses, but you've got to expect the pain and not get discouraged by it. What are you going to say to yourself . . . if you feel the pain tonight? Suppose you feel pain after you leave the interview today, what are you going to say to yourself?

P-112:   "Present pain for future gain."

T-113:   Now where are you now on the hopelessness scale?

P-113:   Down to 15%.

T-114:   It's down to 15% from 95%, but you have to remember that the pain is handled in a structured way, the way I told you about the people who make themselves feel sad during that one period. It has to be structured. If you can structure your pain, this pain is something that's going to build you up in the future, and, indeed, it will. But if you see yourself as just being victimized by these forces you have no control over, . . . you're just helpless in terms of the internal things and external things . . . then you are going to feel terrible . . . And what you have to do is convert yourself from somebody who feels helpless, right? . . . And you are the only person who can do it . . . I can't make you strong and independent . . . I can show you the way, but if you do it, you haven't done it by taking anything from me; you've done it by drawing on resources within yourself.

P-114:   How does it follow then that I feel stronger when I have a man? If things are going . . .

T-115:   (*Counteracts assumption about getting strength from another person. Empirical test.*) You mean you make yourself feel strong because you yourself think, "Well, I've got this man that's a pillar of strength, and since I have him to lean on, therefore, I feel strong." But, actually, nobody else can give you strength. That's a fallacy that you feel stronger having a man, but you can't trust your feelings. What you're doing is just probably drawing on your own strength. You have the definition in your mind. "I'm stronger if I have a man." But the converse of that is very dangerous . . . which is, "I am weak if I don't have a man . . ." What you have to do, if you want to get over this is to disprove the converse, "I am weak if I don't have a man." Now, are you willing to subject that to the acid test? Then you will know. Okay, well suppose you give me a call tomorrow and let me know how you're going and then we can go over some of the other assignments.

It was apparent by the end of the interview that the acute suicidal crisis had passed. The patient felt substantially better, was more optimistic, and had decided to confront and solve her problems. She subsequently became involved in cognitive therapy on a more regular basis and worked with one of the junior staff in identifying and coping with her intrapersonal and interpersonal problems.

This interview is typical of our crisis intervention strategies but is a departure from the more systematic approach used during the less dramatic phases of the patient's depression. We generally attempt to adhere to the principle of collaborative empiricism in our routine interviews and deviate from standard procedures for a limited period of time only. Once the crisis is over, the therapist returns to a less intrusive and less active role and structures the interview in such a way that the patient assumes a greater responsibility for clarifying and devising possible solutions to problems.

Editors' Introduction

Irvin Yalom is the world's leading proponent of existential psychotherapy, and arguably the world's foremost authority on group therapy—his book on the topic remains one of the best selling books in the history of psychology. This particular case was selected by Yalom to illustrate his chapter with Ruthellen Josselson in Current Psychotherapies; *it is especially valuable because it shows existential therapy being applied in the context of group psychotherapy. Yalom has a lively expository style, and he is probably the best writer in psychotherapy, with the possible exception of Jay Haley.*

This case illustrates the way Yalom approaches dream analysis, and it shows how he deals with denial during therapy. It also raises the interesting—and difficult—question about the allocation of scarce resources (like psychotherapy) on a patient who is dying and will only live a few weeks more. Is therapy less—or more—justified in cases like this?

How would you have responded with a client like Carlos who minimizes the psychological effects of rape and the trauma that results from the experience? How will you respond when you find a client's values, beliefs, and behaviors repugnant? Does the fact that Carlos is dying from cancer affect the way you feel about him?

You have now had an opportunity to read sequential cases that demonstrate the approaches, methods, and styles of four of the world's leading therapists: Albert Ellis, David Barlow, Aaron Beck, and Irvin Yalom. Do these four case studies help you understand the sometimes subtle differences in the approaches they take? Do any of these approaches to therapy seem to resonate with your own values and style? Do you feel a personal affinity or identify with any of these four therapists?

7 | "IF RAPE WERE LEGAL ..."

Irvin Yalom

"Your patient is a dumb shit and I told him so in the group last night—in just those words." Sarah, a young psychiatric resident, paused here and glared, daring me to criticize her.

Obviously something extraordinary had occurred. Not every day does a student charge into my office and, with no trace of chagrin—indeed, she seemed proud and defiant—tell me she has verbally assaulted one of my patients. Especially a patient with advanced cancer.

"Sarah, would you sit down and tell me about it? I've got a few minutes before my next patient arrives."

Struggling to keep her composure, Sarah began, "Carlos is the grossest, most despicable human being I have ever met!"

"Well, you know, he's not my favorite person either. I told you that before I referred him to you." I had been seeing Carlos in individual treatment for about six months and, a few weeks ago, referred him to Sarah for inclusion in her therapy group. "But go on. Sorry for stopping you."

"Well, as you know, he's been generally obnoxious—sniffing the women as though he were a dog and they [were] bitches in heat, and ignoring everything else that goes on in the group. Last night, Martha—she's a really fragile borderline young woman, who has been almost mute in the group—started to talk about having been raped last year. I don't think she's ever shared that before—certainly not with a group. She was so scared, sobbing so hard, having so much trouble saying it, that it was incredibly painful. Everyone was trying to help her talk and, rightly or wrongly, I decided it would help Martha if I shared with the group that I had been raped three years ago—"

"I didn't know that, Sarah."

"No one else has known either!"

Sarah stopped here and dabbed her eyes. I could see it was hard for her to tell me this—but at this point I couldn't be sure what hurt worse: telling me about her rape, or how she had excessively revealed herself to her group. (That I was the group therapy instructor in the program must have complicated things for her.) Or was she most upset by what she had still to tell me? I decided to remain matter-of-fact about it.

"And then?"

"Well, that's when your Carlos went into action."

My Carlos? Ridiculous! I thought. As though he's my child and I have to answer for him. (Yet it was true that I had urged Sarah to take him on: she had been reluctant to introduce a patient with cancer into her group. But it was also true that her group was down to five, and she needed new members.) I had never seen her so irrational—and so challenging. I was afraid she'd be very embarrassed about this later, and I didn't want to make it worse by [offering] any hint of criticism.

"What did he do?"

"He asked Martha a lot of factual questions—when, where, what, who. At first that helped her talk, but as soon as I talked about my attack, he ignored Martha and started doing the same thing with me. Then he began asking us both for more intimate details. Did the rapist tear our clothing? Did he ejaculate inside of us? Was there any moment when we began to enjoy it? This all happened so insidiously that there was a time lag before the group began to catch on that he was getting off on it. He didn't give a damn about Martha and me, he was just getting his sexual kicks. I know I should feel more compassion for him—but he is such a creep!"

"How did it end up?"

"Well, the group finally wised up and began to confront him [about] his insensitivity, but he showed no remorse whatsoever. In fact, he became more offensive and accused Martha and me (and all rape victims) of making too much of it. 'What's the big deal?' he asked, and then claimed he personally wouldn't mind being raped by an attractive woman. His parting shot to the group was to say that he would welcome a rape attempt by any woman in the group. That's when I said, 'If you believe that, you're fucking ignorant!'"

"I thought your therapy intervention was calling him a dumb shit?"

That reduced Sarah's tension, and we both smiled.

"That, too! I really lost my cool."

I stretched for supportive and constructive words, but they came out more pedantic than I'd intended. "Remember, Sarah, often extreme situations like this can end up being important turning points *if* they're worked through carefully. Everything that happens is grist for the mill in therapy. Let's try to turn this into a learning experience for him. I'm meeting with him tomorrow, and I'll work on it hard. But I want you to be sure to take care of yourself. I'm available if you want someone to talk to—later today or anytime this week."

Sarah thanked me and said she needed time to think about it. As she left my office, I thought that even if she decided to talk about her own issues with someone else, I would still try to meet with her later when she settled down to see if we could make this a learning experience for *her* as well. That was a hell of a thing for her to have gone through, and I felt for her, but it seemed to me that she had erred by trying to bootleg therapy for herself in the group. Better, I thought, for her to have worked on this first in her personal therapy and then, even if she still chose to talk about it in the group—and that was problematic—she would have handled it better for all parties concerned.

Then my next patient entered, and I turned my attention to her. But I could not prevent myself from thinking about Carlos and wondering how I should handle the next hour with him. It was not unusual for him to stray into my mind. He was an extraordinary patient; and ever since I had started seeing him a few months earlier, I thought about him far more than the one or two hours a week I spent in his presence.

"Carlos is a cat with nine lives, but now it looks as if he's coming to the end of his ninth life." That was the first thing said to me by the oncologist who had referred him for psychiatric treatment. He went on to explain that Carlos had a rare, slow-growing lymphoma which caused problems more because of its sheer bulk than its malignancy. For ten years the tumor had responded well to treatment but now had invaded his lungs and was encroaching upon his heart. His doctors were running out of options: they had given him maximum radiation exposure and had exhausted their pharmacopoeia of chemotherapy agents. How honest should they be? they asked me. Carlos didn't seem to listen. They weren't certain how honest he was willing to be with himself. They did know that he was growing deeply depressed and seemed to have no one to whom he could turn for support.

Carlos was indeed isolated. Aside from a seventeen-year-old son and daughter—dizygotic twins, who lived with his ex-wife in South America —Carlos, at the age of thirty-nine, found himself virtually alone in the world. He had grown up, an only child, in Argentina. His mother had died in childbirth, and twenty years ago his father succumbed to the same type of lymphoma now killing Carlos. He had never had a male friend. "Who needs them?" he once said to me. "I've never met anyone who wouldn't cut you dead for a dollar, a job, or a cunt." He had been married only briefly and had had no other significant relationships with women. "You have to be crazy to fuck any woman more than once!" His aim in life, he told me without a trace of shame or self-consciousness, was to screw as many different women as he could.

No, at my first meeting I could find little endearing about Carlos's character—or about his physical appearance. He was emaciated, knobby (with swollen, highly visible lymph nodes at elbows, neck, [and] behind his ears) and, as a result of the chemotherapy, entirely hairless. His pathetic cosmetic efforts—a wide-brimmed Panama hat, painted-on eyebrows, and a scarf to conceal the swellings in his neck—succeeded only in calling additional unwanted attention to his appearance.

He was obviously depressed—with good reason—and spoke bitterly and wearily of his ten-year ordeal with cancer. His lymphoma, he said, was killing him in stages. It had already killed most of him—his energy, his strength, and his freedom (he had to live near Stanford Hospital, in permanent exile from his own culture).

Most important, it had killed his social life, by which he meant his sexual life: when he was on chemotherapy, he was impotent; when he finished a course of chemotherapy, and his sexual juices started to flow, he could not make it with a woman because of his baldness. Even when his hair grew back, a few weeks after chemotherapy, he said he still couldn't score: no prostitute would have him because they thought his enlarged lymph nodes signified AIDS. His sex life now was confined entirely to masturbating while watching rented sadomasochistic videotapes.

It was true—he said, only when I prompted him—that he was isolated and, yes, that did constitute a problem, but only because there were times when he was too weak to care for his own physical needs. The idea of pleasure deriving from close human (nonsexual) contact seemed alien to him. There was one exception—his children—and when Carlos spoke of them, real emotion, emotion that I could join with, broke through. I was moved by the sight of his frail body heaving with sobs as he described his fear that they, too, would abandon him: that their mother would finally succeed in poisoning them against him, or that they would become repelled by his cancer and turn away from him.

"What can I do to help, Carlos?"

"If you want to help me—then teach me how to hate armadillos!"

For a moment Carlos enjoyed my perplexity, and then proceeded to explain that he had been working with visual imaging—a form of self-healing many cancer patients attempt. His visual metaphors for his new chemotherapy (referred to by his oncologists as BP) were giant B's and P's—Bears and Pigs; his metaphor for his hard, cancerous lymph nodes was a bony-plated armadillo. Thus, in his meditation sessions, he visualized bears and pigs attacking the armadillos. The problem was that he couldn't make his bears and pigs be vicious enough to tear open and destroy the armadillos.

Despite the horror of his cancer and his narrowness of spirit, I was drawn to Carlos. Perhaps it was generosity welling out of my relief that it was he, and not I, who was dying. Perhaps it was his love for his children or the plaintive way he grasped my hand with both of his when he was leaving my office. Perhaps it was the whimsy in his request: "Teach me to hate armadillos."

Therefore, as I considered whether I could treat him, I minimized potential obstacles to treatment and persuaded myself that he was more *un*socialized than malignantly antisocial, and that many of his noxious traits and beliefs were soft and open to being modified. I did not think through my decision clearly and, even after I decided to accept him in therapy, remained unsure about appropriate and realistic treatment goals. Was I simply to escort him through this course of chemotherapy? (Like many patients, Carlos became deathly ill and despondent during chemotherapy.) Or, if he were entering a terminal phase, was I to commit myself to stay with him until death? Was I to be satisfied with offering sheer presence and support? (Maybe that would be sufficient. God knows he had no one else to talk to!) Of course, his isolation was his own doing, but was I going to help him to recognize or to change that? Now? In the face of death, these considerations seemed immaterial. Or did they? Was it possible that Carlos could accomplish something more "ambitious" in therapy? No, no, no! *What sense does it make to talk about "ambitious" treatment with someone whose anticipated life span may be, at best, a matter of months?* Does anyone, do I, want to invest time and energy in a project of such evanescence?

Carlos readily agreed to meet with me. In his typical cynical mode, he said that his insurance policy would pay ninety percent of my fee, and that he wouldn't turn down a bargain like that. Besides, he was a person who wanted to try everything once, and he had never before spoken to a psychiatrist. I left our treatment contract unclear, aside from saying that having someone with whom to share painful feelings and thoughts always helped. I suggested that we meet six times and then evaluate whether treatment seemed worthwhile.

To my great surprise, Carlos made excellent use of therapy; and after six sessions, we agreed to meet in ongoing treatment. He came to every hour with a list of issues he wanted to discuss—dreams, work problems (a successful financial analyst, he had continued to work throughout his illness). Sometimes he talked about his physical discomfort and his loathing of chemotherapy, but most of all he talked about women and sex. Each session he described all of his encounters with women that week (often they consisted of nothing more than catching a woman's eye in the grocery store) and obsessing about what he might have done in each instance to have consummated a relationship. He was so preoccupied with women that he seemed to forget that he had a cancer that was actively infiltrating all the crawl spaces of his body. Most likely that was the point of his preoccupation—that he might forget his infestation.

But his fixation on women had long predated his cancer. He had always prowled for women and regarded them in highly sexualized and demeaning terms. So Sarah's account of Carlos in the group, shocking as it was, did not astonish me. I knew he was entirely capable of such gross behavior—and worse.

But how should I handle the situation with him in the next hour? Above all, I wished to protect and maintain our relationship. We were making progress, and right now I was his primary human connection. But it was also important that he continue attending his therapy group. I had placed him in a group six weeks ago to provide him with a community that would both help to penetrate his isolation and also, by identifying and urging him to alter some of his most socially objectionable behavior, help him to create connections in his social life. For the first five weeks, he had made excellent use of the group but, unless he changed his behavior dramatically, he would, I was certain, irreversibly alienate all the group members—if he hadn't done so already!

Our next session started uneventfully. Carlos didn't even mention the group but, instead, wanted to talk about Ruth, an attractive woman he had just met at a church social. (He was a member of a half-dozen churches because he believed they provided him with ideal pickup opportunities.) He had talked briefly to Ruth, who then excused herself because she had to go home. Carlos said goodbye but later grew convinced that he had missed a golden opportunity by not offering to escort her to her car; in fact, he had persuaded himself that there was a fair chance, perhaps a ten- to fifteen-percent chance, he might have married her. His self-recriminations for not having acted with greater dispatch continued all week and included verbal self-assaults and physical abuse—pinching himself and pounding his head against the wall.

I didn't pursue his feelings about Ruth (although they were so patently irrational that I decided to return to her at some point) because I thought it was urgent that we discuss the group. I told him that I had spoken to Sarah about the meeting. "Were you," I asked, "going to talk about the group today?"

"Not particularly, it's not important. Anyway, I'm going to stop that group. I'm too advanced for it."

"What do you mean?"

"Everyone is dishonest and playing games there. I'm the only person there with enough guts to tell the truth. The men are all losers—they wouldn't be there otherwise. They're jerks with no *cojones,* they sit around whimpering and saying nothing."

"Tell me what happened in the meeting from your perspective."

"Sarah talked about her rape, she tell you that?"

I nodded.

"Ariel Martha did, too. That Martha. God, that's one for you. She's a mess, a real sickie, she is. She's a mental case, on tranquilizers. What the hell am I doing in a group with people like her anyway? But listen to me. The important point is that they talked about their rapes, both of them, and everyone just sat there silently with their mouths hanging open. At least I responded. I asked them questions."

"Sarah suggested that some of your questions were not of the helpful variety."

"Someone had to get them talking. Besides, I've always been curious about rape. Aren't you? Aren't all men? About how it's done, about the rape victim's experience?"

"Oh, come on, Carlos, if that's what you were after, you could have read about it in a book. These were real people there—not sources of information. There was something else going on."

"Maybe so, I'll admit that. When I started the group, your instructions were that I should be honest in expressing my feelings in the group. Believe me, I swear it, in the last meeting I was the only honest person in the group. I got turned on, I admit it. It's a fantastic turn-on to think of Sarah getting screwed. I'd love to join in and get my hands on those boobs of hers. I haven't forgiven you for preventing me from dating her." When he had first started the group six weeks ago, he talked at great length about his infatuation with Sarah—or rather with her breasts—and was convinced she would be willing to go out with him. To help Carlos become assimilated in the group, I had, in the first few meetings, coached him on appropriate social behavior. I had persuaded him, with difficulty, that a sexual approach to Sarah would be both futile and unseemly.

"Besides, it's no secret that men get turned on by rape. I saw the other men in the group smiling at me. Look at the porno business! Have you ever taken a good look at the books and videotapes about rape or bondage? Do it! Go visit the porno shops in the Tenderloin—it'd be good for your education. They're printing those things for somebody—there's gotta be a market out there. I'll tell you the truth, *if rape were legal, I'd do it*—once in a while."

Carlos stopped there and gave me a smug grin—or was it a poke-in-the-arm leer, an invitation to take my place beside him in the brotherhood of rapists?

I sat silently for several minutes trying to identify my options. It was easy to agree with Sarah: he *did* sound depraved. Yet I was convinced part of it was bluster, and that there was a way to reach something better, something higher in him. I was interested in, grateful for, his last few words: the "once in a while." Those words, added almost as an afterthought, seemed to suggest some scrap of self-consciousness or shame.

"Carlos, you take pride in your honesty in the group—but were you really being honest? Or only part honest, or easy honest? It's true, you were more open than the other men in the group. You did express some of your real sexual feelings. And you do have a point about how widespread these feelings are: the porno business must be offering something which appeals to impulses all men have.

"But are you being completely honest? What about all the other feelings going on inside you that you *haven't* expressed? Let me take a guess about something: when you said 'big deal' to Sarah and Martha about their rapes, is it possible you were thinking about your cancer and what you have to face all the time? It's a hell of a lot tougher facing something that threatens your life *right now* than something that happened a year or two ago.

"Maybe you'd like to get some caring from the group, but how can you get it when you come on so tough? You haven't yet talked about having cancer." (I had been urging Carlos to reveal to the group that he had cancer, but he was procrastinating: he said he was afraid he'd be pitied, and didn't want to sabotage his sexual chances with the women members.)

Carlos grinned at me. "Good try, Doc! It makes a lot of sense. You've got a good head. But I'll be honest—the thought of my cancer never entered my mind. Since we stopped chemotherapy two months ago, I go days at a time without thinking of the cancer. That's goddamn good, isn't it—to forget it, to be free of it, to be able to live a normal life for a while?"

Good question! I thought. Was it good to forget? I wasn't so sure. Over the months I had been seeing Carlos, I had discovered that I could chart, with astonishing accuracy, the course of his cancer by noting the things he thought about. Whenever his cancer worsened and he was actively facing death, he rearranged his life priorities and became more thoughtful, compassionate, wiser. When, on the other hand, he was in remission, he was guided, as he put it, by his pecker and grew noticeably more coarse and shallow.

I once saw a newspaper cartoon of a pudgy lost little man saying, "Suddenly, one day in your forties or fifties, everything becomes clear. . . . And then it goes away again!" That cartoon was apt for Carlos, except that he had not one, but *repeated* episodes of clarity—and they always went away again. I often thought that if I could find a way to keep him continually aware of his death and the "clearing" that death effects, I could help him make some major changes in the way he related to life and to other people.

It was evident from the specious way he was speaking today, and a couple of days ago in the group, that his cancer was quiescent again, and that death, with its attendant wisdom, was far out of mind.

I tried another tack. "Carlos, before you started the group I tried to explain to you the basic rationale behind group therapy. Remember how I emphasized that whatever happens in the group can be used to help us work in therapy?" He nodded.

I continued, "And that one of the most important principles of groups is that the group is a miniature world—whatever environment we create in the group reflects the way we have chosen to live? Remember that I said that each of us establishes *in* the group the *same kind of social world we have in our real life?*"

He nodded again. He was listening.

"Now, look what's happened to you in the group! You started with a number of people with whom you might have developed close relationships. And when you began, the two of us were in agreement that you needed to work on ways of developing relationships. That was why you began the group, remember? But now, after only six weeks, all the members and at least one of the co-therapists are thoroughly pissed at you. And it's your own doing. You've done *in* the group what you do *outside* of the group! I want you to answer me honestly: Are you satisfied? Is this what you want from your relationships with others?"

"Doc, I understand completely what you're saying, but there's a bug in your argument. I don't give a shit, not one shit, about the people in the group. They're not real people. I'm never going to associate with losers like that. Their opinion doesn't mean anything to me. I don't *want* to get closer to them."

I had known Carlos to close up completely like this on other occasions. He would, I suspected, be more reasonable in a week or two, and under ordinary circumstances I would simply have been patient. But unless something changed quickly, he would either drop out of the group or would, by next week, have ruptured beyond repair his relationships with the other members. Since I doubted very much, after this charming incident, whether I'd ever be able to persuade another group therapist to accept him, I persevered.

"I hear those angry and judgmental feelings, and I know you really feel them. But, Carlos, try to put brackets around them for a moment and see if you can get in touch with anything else. Both Sarah and Martha were in a great deal of pain. What other feelings did you have about them? I'm not talking about major or predominant feelings, but about any other flashes you had."

"I know what you're after. You're doing your best for me. I want to help you, but I'd be making up stuff. You're putting feelings into my mouth. Right here, this office, is the one place I can tell the truth, and the truth is that, more than anything else, what I want to do with those two cunts in the group is to fuck them! I meant it when I said that if rape were legal, I'd do it! And I know just where I'd start!"

Most likely he was referring to Sarah, but I did not ask. The last thing I wanted to do was enter into that discourse with him. Probably there was some important Oedipal competition going on between the two of us which was making communication more difficult. He never missed an opportunity to describe to me in graphic terms what he would like to do to Sarah, as though he considered that we were rivals for her. I know he believed that the reason I had earlier dissuaded him from inviting Sarah out was that I wanted to keep her to myself. But this type of interpretation would be totally useless now: he was far too closed and defensive. If I were going to get through, I would have to use something more compelling.

The only remaining approach I could think of involved that one burst of emotion I had seen in our first session—the tactic seemed so contrived and so simplistic that I could not possibly have predicted the astonishing result it would produce.

"All right, Carlos, let's consider this ideal society you're imagining and advocating—this society of legalized rape. Think now, for a few minutes, about your daughter. How would it be for her living in the community—being available for legal rape, a piece of ass for whoever happens to be horny and gets off on force and seventeen-year-old girls?"

Suddenly Carlos stopped grinning. He winced visibly and said simply, "I wouldn't like that for her."

"But where would she fit, then, in this world you're building? Locked up in a convent? You've got to make a place where she can live: that's what fathers do—they build a world for their children. I've never asked you before—what do you really want for her?"

"I want her to have a loving relationship with a man and have a loving family."

"But how can that happen if her father is advocating a world of rape? If you want her to live in a loving world, then it's up to you to construct that world—and you have to start with your own behavior. You can't be outside your own law—that's at the base of every ethical system."

The tone of the session had changed. No more jousting or crudity. We had grown deadly serious. I felt more like a philosophy or religious teacher than a therapist, but I knew that this was the proper trail. And these were things I should have said before. He had often joked about his own inconsistency. I remember [him] describing with glee a dinner-table conversation with his children (they visited him two or three times a year) when he informed his daughter that he wanted to meet and approve any boy she went out with. "As for you," pointing to his son, *"you* get all the ass you can!"

There was no question now that I had his attention. I decided to increase my leverage by triangulation, and I approached the same issue from another direction:

"And, Carlos, something else comes to my mind right now. Remember your dream of the green Honda two weeks ago? Let's go back over it."

He enjoyed working on dreams and was only too glad to apply himself to this one and, in so doing, to leave the painful discussion about his daughter.

Carlos had dreamed that he went to a rental agency to rent a car, but the only ones available were Honda Civics—his least favorite car. Of several colors available, he selected red. But when he got out to the lot, the only car available was green—his least favorite color! The most important fact about a dream is its emotion, and this dream, despite its benign content, was full of terror: it had awakened him and flooded him with anxiety for hours.

Two weeks ago we had not been able to get far with the dream. Carlos, as I recall, went off on a tangent of associations about the identity of the female auto rental clerk. But today I saw the dream in a different light. Many years ago he had developed a strong belief in reincarnation, a belief that offered him blessed relief from fears about dying. The metaphor he had used in one of our first meetings was that dying is simply trading in your body for another one—like trading in an old car. I reminded him now of that metaphor.

"Let's suppose, Carlos, that the dream is more than a dream about cars. Obviously renting a car is not a frightening activity, not something that would become a nightmare and keep you up all night. I think the dream is about death and future life, and it uses your symbol of comparing death and rebirth to a trade of cars. If we look at it that way, we can make more sense of the powerful fear the dream carried. What do you make of the fact that the only kind of car you could get was a green Honda Civic?"

"I hate green and I hate Honda Civics. My next car is going to be a Maserati."

"But if cars are dream symbols of bodies, why would you, in your next life, get the body, or the life, that you hate above all others?"

Carlos had no option but to respond. "You get what you deserve, depending on what you've done or the way you've lived your present life. You can either move up or down."

Now he realized where this discussion was leading, and began to perspire. The dense forest of crassness and cynicism surrounding him had always shocked and dissuaded visitors. But now it was his turn to be shocked. I had invaded his two innermost temples: his love for his children and his reincarnation beliefs.

"Go on, Carlos, this is important—apply that to yourself and to your life."

He bit off each word slowly. "The dream is saying that I'm not living right."

"I agree, I think that *is* what the dream is saying. Say some more on your thoughts about living right."

I was going to pontificate about what constitutes a good life in any religious system—love, generosity, care, noble thoughts, pursuit of the good, charity—but none of that was necessary. Carlos let me know I had made my point: he said that he was getting dizzy, and that this was a lot to deal with in one day. He wanted time to think about it during the week. Noting that we still had fifteen minutes left, I decided to do some work on another front.

I went back to the first issue he had raised in the hour: his belief that he had missed a golden opportunity with Ruth, the woman he had met briefly at a church social, and his subsequent head pounding and self-recrimination for not having walked her to her car. The function that this irrational belief served was patent. As long as he continued to believe that he was tantalizingly close to being desired and loved by an attractive woman, he could buttress his belief that he was no different from anyone else, that there was nothing seriously wrong with him, that he was not disfigured, not mortally ill.

In the past I hadn't tampered with his denial. In general, it's best not to undermine a defense unless it is creating more problems than solutions, and unless one has something better to offer in its stead. Reincarnation is a case in point: though I personally consider it a form of death denial, the belief served Carlos (as it does much of the world's population) very well; in fact, rather than undermine it, I had always supported it and in this session buttressed it by urging that he be consistent in heeding all the implications of reincarnation.

But the time had come to challenge some of the less helpful parts of his denial system.

"Carlos, do you really believe that if you had walked Ruth to her car you'd have a ten-to-fifteen-percent chance of marrying her?"

"One thing could lead to another. There was something going on between the two of us. I felt it. I know what I know!"

"But you say that every week—the lady in the supermarket, the receptionist in the dentist's office, the ticket seller at the movie. You even felt that with Sarah. Look, how many times have you, or any man, walked a woman to her car and *not* married her?"

"O.K., O.K., maybe it's closer, to a one-percent or half-percent chance, but there was still a chance—if I hadn't been such a jerk. I didn't even *think* of asking to walk her to the car!"

"The things you pick to beat yourself up about! Carlos, I'm going to be blunt. What you're saying doesn't make any sense at all. All you've told me about Ruth—you only talked to her for five minutes—is that she's twenty-three with two small kids and is recently divorced. Let's be very realistic—as you say, this is the place to be honest. What are you going to tell her about your health?"

"When I get to know her better, I'll tell her the truth—that I've got cancer, that it's under control now, that the doctors can treat it."

"And—?"

"That the doctors aren't sure what's going to happen, that there are new treatments discovered every day, that I may have recurrences in the future."

"What did the doctors say to you? Did they say *may* have recurrences?"

"You're right—*will* have recurrences in the future, unless a cure is found."

"Carlos, I don't want to be cruel, but be objective. Put yourself in Ruth's place—twenty-three years old, two small children, been through a hard time, presumably looking for some strong support for herself and her kids, having only a layman's knowledge and fear of cancer—do you represent the kind of security and support she's looking for? Is she going to be willing to accept the uncertainty surrounding your health? To risk placing herself in the situation where she might be obligated to nurse you? What really are the chances she would allow herself to know you in the way you want, to become involved with you?"

"Probably not one in a million," Carlos said in a sad and weary voice.

I was being cruel, yet the option of *not* being cruel, of simply humoring him, of tacitly acknowledging that he was incapable of seeing reality, was crueler yet. His fantasy about Ruth allowed him to feel that he could still be touched and cared for by another human. I hoped that he would understand that my willingness to engage him, rather than wink behind his back, was my way of touching and caring.

All the bluster was gone. In a soft voice Carlos asked, "So where does that leave me?"

"If what you really want now is closeness, then it's time to take all this heat off yourself about finding a wife. I've been watching you beat yourself up for months about this. I think it's time to let up on yourself. You've just finished a difficult course of chemotherapy. Four weeks ago you couldn't eat or get out of bed or stop vomiting. You've lost a lot of weight, you're regaining your strength. Stop expecting to find a wife right now, it's too much to ask of yourself. Set a reasonable goal—you can do this as well as I. Concentrate on having a good conversation. Try deepening a friendship with the people you already know."

I saw a smile begin to form on Carlos's lips. He saw my next sentence coming: "And *what better place to start than in the group?*"

Carlos was never the same person after that session. Our next appointment was the day following the next group meeting. The first thing he said was that I would not believe how good he had been in the group. He bragged that he was now the most supportive and sensitive member. He had wisely decided to bail himself out of trouble by telling the group about his cancer. He claimed—and, weeks later, Sarah was to corroborate this—that his behavior had changed so dramatically that the members now looked to him for support.

He praised our previous session. "The last session was our best one so far. I wish we could have sessions like that every time. I don't remember exactly what we talked about, but it helped me change a lot."

I found one of his comments particularly droll.

"I don't know why, but I'm even relating differently to the men in the group. They are all older than me but, it's funny, I have a sense of treating them as though they were my own sons!"

His having forgotten the content of our last session troubled me little. Far better that he forget what we talked about than the opposite possibility (a more popular choice for patients)—to remember precisely what was talked about but to remain unchanged.

Carlos's improvement increased exponentially. Two weeks later, he began our session by announcing that he had had, during that week, two major insights. He was so proud of the insights that he had christened them. The first, he called (glancing at his notes) "Everybody has got a heart." The second was "I am not my shoes."

First, he explained "Everybody has got a heart." "During the group meeting last week, all three women were sharing a lot of their feelings, about how hard it was being single, about loneliness, about grieving for their parents, about nightmares. I don't know why, but I suddenly saw them in a different way! They were like me! They were having the same problems in living that I was. I had always before imagined women sitting on Mount Olympus with a line of men before them and sorting them out—this one to my bedroom, this one not!"

"But that moment," Carlos continued, "I had a vision of their naked hearts. Their chest wall vanished, just melted away leaving a square blue-red cavity with rib-bar walls and, in the center, a liver-colored glistening heart thumping away. All week long I've been seeing everyone's heart beating, and I've been saying to myself, 'Everybody has got a heart, everybody has got a heart.' I've been seeing the heart in everyone—a misshapen hunchback who works in reception, an old lady who does the floors, even the men I work with!"

Carlos's comment gave me so much joy that tears came to my eyes. I think he saw them but, to spare me embarrassment, made no comment and hurried along to the next insight: "I am not my shoes."

He reminded me that in our last session we had discussed his great anxiety about an upcoming presentation at work. He had always had great difficulty speaking in public: excruciatingly sensitive to any criticism, he had often, he said, made a spectacle of himself by viciously counterattacking anyone who questioned any aspect of his presentation. I had helped him understand that he had lost sight of his personal boundaries. It is natural, I had told him, that one should respond adversely to an attack on one's central core—after all, in that situation one's very survival is at stake. But I had pointed out that Carlos had stretched his personal boundaries to encompass his work and, consequently, he responded to a mild criticism of any aspect of his work as though it were a mortal attack on his central being, a threat to his very survival.

I had urged Carlos to differentiate between his core self and other, peripheral attributes or activities. Then he had to "disidentify" with the non-core parts: they might represent what he liked, or did, or valued—but they were not *him,* not his central being.

Carlos had been intrigued by this construct. Not only did it explain his defensiveness at work, but also he could extend this "disidentification" model to pertain to his body. In other words, even though his body was imperiled, he himself, his vital essence, was intact.

This interpretation allayed much of his anxiety, and his work presentation last week had been wonderfully lucid and nondefensive. Never had he done a better job. Throughout his presentation, a small mantra wheel in his mind had hummed, "I am not my work." When he finished and sat down next to his boss, the mantra continued, "I am not my work. Not my talk. Not my clothes. None of these things." He crossed his legs and noted his scuffed and battered shoes: "And I'm not my shoes either." He began to wiggle his toes and his feet hoping to attract his boss's attention so as to proclaim to him, "I am not my shoes!"

Carlos's two insights—the first of many to come—were a gift to me and to my students. These two insights, each generated by a different form of therapy, illustrated, in quintessential form, the difference between what one can derive from group therapy, with its focus on communion *between,* and individual therapy, with its focus on communion *within.* I still use many of his graphic insights to illustrate my teaching.

In the few months of life remaining to him, Carlos chose to continue to give. He organized a cancer self-help group (not without some humorous crack about this being the "last stop" pickup joint) and also was the group leader for some interpersonal skills groups at one of his churches. Sarah, by now one of his greatest boosters, was invited as a guest speaker to one of his groups and attested to his responsible and competent leadership.

But, most of all, he gave to his children, who noted the change in him and elected to live with him while enrolling for a semester at a nearby college. He was a marvelously generous and supportive father. I have always felt that the way one faces death is greatly determined by the model one's parents set. The last gift a parent can give to children is to teach them, through example, how to face death with equanimity—and Carlos gave an extraordinary lesson in grace. His death was not one of the dark, muffled, conspiratorial passings. Until the very end of his life, he and his children were honest with one another about his illness and giggled together at the way he snorted, crossed his eyes, and puckered his lips when he referred to his "lymphooooooooooooomma."

But he gave no greater gift than the one he offered me shortly before he died, and it was a gift that answers for all time the question of whether it is rational or appropriate to strive for "ambitious" therapy in those who are terminally ill. When I visited him in the hospital he was so weak he could barely move, but he raised his head, squeezed my hand, and whispered, "Thank you. Thank you for saving my life."

In this interesting case reprinted from The International Gestalt Journal, *a highly respected and experienced therapist shares a verbatim segment of her time with a patient and then allows four colleagues to critique her work. One of those four colleagues is Lynne Jacobs, coauthor of the Gestalt therapy chapter in* Current Psychotherapies. *Sally Denham-Vaughan then responds to the four critiques of her work. The case permits the reader to see firsthand the many different ways in which the therapist could have directed the therapy session.*

The therapists reviewing the case were blind to the identity of the therapist providing services, and the therapist whose work was reviewed did not know the identities of the four reviewers. This is why the reviewers sometimes use male pronouns when referring to the female therapist.

Although only representing about 15 minutes of a therapy session, the case illustrates the commitment of the therapist and the isolation and loneliness of the patient, as well as some core Gestalt principles such as field theory, the importance of presence, contact and awareness, contact boundaries, retroflection, and the conceptual limits imposed by diagnostic labels.

How would you have handled this case? What would you have done differently? Read the case a second time to see if you can identify choice points where you might have made different choices from those made by the therapist. What are your reasons for preferring different interventions?

8 | FIRST OR NOWHERE?

Sally Denham–Vaughan

To avoid criticism, do nothing, say nothing, be nothing.
—Elbert Hubbard

What follows is a transcript of part of a session (approximately 15 minutes) that took place in the summer of 2002.

BACKGROUND

Briefly, Louisa has been in therapy with me for some 3½ years now, and we have had 143 weekly sessions. I first met her following admission to a psychiatric hospital, where she had been sectioned (an involuntary patient) for treatment of her mental health problems and especially suicidal behavior. She had been in the hospital for some 3 months, and upon being discharged, it was agreed that she should be referred for psychotherapy. Her formal diagnosis is of borderline personality disorder (BPD), with comorbid Axis 1 disorders, including severe bulimia and severe depressive disorder. In terms of her personality disorder, she fulfils all the *DSM IV* features for a diagnosis of BPD, and I have assessed her using the SIDP IV. Within this classificatory system, she can also be described as having avoidant and dependent traits.

In terms of personal history, Louisa is the second born of twins conceived on a honeymoon night. She believes that the pregnancy was unplanned, that her parents were ill prepared for children, and especially that her mother and father had a preference for boys.

The first-born twin, Michael, she describes as having always been "first, quicker, louder, more positive, and more creative." She has great difficulty owning and accepting her identity, feeling that neither her birthday nor even her name truly belonged to her. (If she had been a boy, she would have been called Louis.)

Over time in therapy, we have covered a wide range of areas, including attempting to manage her active suicidal behaviors, which include serious self-harm and severe bulimic difficulties. Both of these problems have been formulated as reflecting a fundamental feeling that she should not exist, but that if she is on this planet, then she should make only a positive contribution to others and have no needs of her own. Just being aware of her wants and desires triggers tremendous self-criticism.

Louisa is single and lives near her parents. She is 35 years of age, does not have a partner, and has never been married. She has very few friends, or indeed even acquaintances,

From *International Gestalt Journal* 2003, 26/1, p. 14–20. Reprinted with permission.

and does describe herself as being profoundly lonely. She lives in a small house with a range of animals, which are her "substitute family," including two dogs, two cats, and a range of hens and geese. She also has two horses.

This transcript comes after approximately 20 minutes of the session. Louisa has come into the session extremely upset having had the experience of reversing her car, hitting an object, and getting out only to discover that she had run over her new kitten. The kitten was killed by this incident and Louisa has been blaming and berating herself for the animal's death. I have been trying to facilitate her staying in contact with herself and me without dissociating or having a "panic attack." (Both these phenomena have occurred in previous sessions.) The main themes so far have been repetitive statements to the effect that this whole incident is certainly her fault and proof that she shouldn't exist.

TRANSCRIPT

Every act of creation is first of all an act of destruction.

—Pablo Picasso

Client (00:00):   It just feels that I shouldn't be here . . . and that I shouldn't even bring that up.

Therapist (00:12): Do you believe that I think you shouldn't bring that up?

C (00:21): I don't know, I feel so awful, always harping back to the past. Why was I born? I just feel so awful. You'll think I'm so awful, bringing it all up again.

T (00:39): Sounds like the past has spontaneously arrived here, rather than you having gone looking for it.

C (00:43): No.

T (00:46): It's rather that it's come and found you.

C (00:49): It feels like it's a "come-back" you see that I can't just forget it. It's like it keeps on repeating itself, and it's just going to keep on repeating itself. The memories keep coming back, and it keeps on happening. Something will happen, sooner or later, and the pattern is there . . . all the same.

T (01:21): What is the pattern? What does it look like?

C (01:29): (angrily, hopelessly) I don't know.

T (01:43): I'm wondering then . . . what's the connection? What is repeating? (Pause)

C (02:08): That I should just keep out . . . that there is nothing I can create or get right.

T (02:21): So that's what's being repeated? That's the connection. That's what it means to you.

C (02:27): Well, everything I try to do, I get it wrong. Not just get it wrong . . . I kill things. I do it . . . (Pause)

T (02:53): So there is the connection . . . then this is the pattern you come down to.

C (02:55): Oh God; it's so awful. (Pause)

T (03:15): (reflectively) I imagine a spiral, a vortex; I wonder how it seems to you.

C (03:20): It's all down to me being here.

T (03:25): What's the feeling that goes with that . . . that it's all down to you being here?

C (03:31): Horrible, hateful; . . . that it's all down to me . . . my mistakes. What is the point of me being here? I've always said that I haven't got a function in life; but at least if I haven't got a function, if I don't get things wrong . . . no one gets hurt.

T (03:50): Sounds like you've got back to that very early decision that "I shouldn't be here"; and if I am here, I should have no needs, make no waves, and definitely get nothing wrong.

C (04:06): Well at least then I'm not doing any harm by being here. But as soon as I start taking part . . . Oh.

T (04:20): You look in such pain, physical pain when you say that.

C (04:30): Well, I just can't bear me. I've just had all these things happen to me . . . it's just like something's trying to get rid of me; but it doesn't quite happen.

T (05:05): (*beginning to feel anxious that she is dissociating*) Can you try and make a bit of contact with me?

C (05:15): Sorry, sorry.

T (05:17): I wasn't meaning to criticize you . . . I was just concerned you were disappearing, hating, and punishing yourself.

C (05:28): Self-pity.

T (05:30): No . . . not self-pity . . . self-hatred, that's what I see.

C (05:35): Mmmmmm.

T (05:41): Do you remember when we talked about the early decision; that "I just shouldn't be here"?

C (05:52): Well, it feels like it keeps coming back. It's here right now . . . I shouldn't be here. That's true.

T (06:01): So you think that's the truth . . . and that the pattern you are seeing reflects the truth, which is at the heart of that decision.

C (06:13): Are you saying that I'm wrong?

T (06:18): What I'm trying to say is that this decision is your interpretation of a set of events, but I think you know that I believe something different . . . that your existence is important.

C (06:31): (*slowly and with emphasis*) Maybe I'd believe that if I'd been born a single person. But it's like, when there's twins, it's like a repeat one has been made. Like an afterthought; so in effect, my brother's the one that was meant to be born. You know, he's the one who can create, and I'm the . . . oh . . . I can't explain it . . . a by-product. . . . A repeat, with nothing to make me separate, important. He's the one who was meant to be born. He's the one who is making a contribution, being useful to life, making a difference to life, and it's like I'm looking on.

T (07:56): I notice I feel really sad when you say that.

C (08:01): Well, what is the point to my life? I've just always been there to create problems, to be surplus.

T (08:23): I'm wondering what it's like for you to say that here, with me . . . to say that to me.

C (08:31): Well, I think it's your experience. That I'm just one more . . . there are plenty of clients, I'm just one more, a problem. Not even getting better, just killing things.

T (08:50): Do you know; that is absolutely not my experience of being here with you . . . now . . . or over time. (*Pause*) But I feel very sad when I hear you say that; and I understand and feel . . . I feel it here in my body as well as in my emotions; . . . that that's what you believe. I notice I have a sort of choking; almost like I shouldn't be even breathing . . . and I'm wondering if that is telling me something about how strongly you believe you shouldn't exist.

C (09:14): Well, when you've always been with someone who's so . . . oh, . . . everything that you're not; but he even looks the same; . . . well there comes a time when you just think . . . it's not even that I'm second; I just shouldn't be at all. It's a feeling that just comes up. You know, something happens and it'll bring me back to it. (*Pause*)

T (09:50): So, what is it like for you, that I'm here with you now . . . different from you . . . and with such a different belief about you, and a different experience of you too? I'm just wondering if that makes you feel apart from me.

C (10:23): No, . . . I really want to believe you, to be *with* you.

T (10:30): I feel really moved and pleased when you say that. I'm glad you *want* to believe me. So let's start with that. I'm wondering if you think I'm being genuine, real with you now. If I'm saying my truth or if I'm just trying to reassure you.

C (10:53): I know you wouldn't lie to me; but I know you couldn't agree with me; that's not your role, to agree with me about that.

T (11:09): Well, I neither agree nor disagree. I have a response, a reaction; I have a truth that is based on my own understandings, and my experience of being with you.

C (11:20): (*looking confused*) What?

T (11:27): For example, if I think of being with you, I can recall many times and memories of both good and bad times: successes and failures. So there is contrast and difference. It is not all the same . . . all problems . . . all sad. My view of the pattern does not lead me to your conclusion; I do see and believe there is purpose in your life. I just believe that life, including your life, is purposeful. There are not "mistakes" or afterthoughts. (*Pause*)

C (12:21): I'm just thinking of one of my little dogs. He was born last and almost died. But you know, I really really wanted him to live . . . almost more than the others. And when they got old enough to go to homes, he was the one I kept.

T (12:36): So you chose him.

C (12:41): Oh yes . . . (*Pause*) I suppose I identified with him. Coming last; being a nuisance . . . he wouldn't eat or feed properly so I bottle-fed him for a while.

T (12:58): So why did you choose him if he was such a nuisance?

C (13:07): Well, I loved him: I know he reminded me of me; but I just thought it wasn't his fault, being small. And do you know, he really fought for life . . . and he's grown up; and he's a lovely little dog.

T (13:25): So, is he really a nuisance?

C (13:31): No; not now; and not then really; he just needed a lot . . . well; a bit more than the others; but he was worth it. I mean he had the chance to go either way didn't he? He could easily have died either before he was born, or at birth, or even later . . . but he didn't.

T (14:02): So he really fought for life?

C (14:10): Oh yes.

T (14:15): With a purpose . . . a sense of purpose.

C (14:17): (*smiles*) Well he's a real fighter, even now. (*Pause*)

T (14:31): (*feeling moved*) I'm not surprised you identify with this little dog. So much in common. I'm thinking that even while part of you has found it so hard to take your life; and accept you are alive and have needs; part of you has really fought to stay alive. (*Pause*) I was just really appreciating the fighter in you. Thinking about the struggles you've had . . . the struggles we've had; and I just had a really warm, pleased sense of your aliveness. (*Pause*)

C (15:15): It's still a struggle.

T (15:23): I do know that Louisa, I see that; I really see your struggle; and I've seen and felt it today especially with what happened to your kitten.

C (15:32): I don't know how to cope with that.

T (15:39): Of course not; how could you know . . . it's an awful experience. And: I see you struggling to cope; as I've seen you struggling with many things; and I trust that struggle will bring you through.

The session moves on to a new figure focusing on Louisa thinking about and considering things she might do to support herself at this time. I felt that we had touched a very dark place in her, and one that lies at the center of her issues. I felt relieved that we had come through with a strong contact that was maintained for most of the session. This felt different from previous sessions discussing difficult events.

COMMENT 1: AN INDIVIDUALISTIC OR FIELD-ORIENTED POINT OF VIEW?

Jacques Blaize

First, I would like to thank the unidentified therapist for taking such a risk in publishing this transcript and being willing to be criticized. So I am pleased to accept this opportunity to open some tracks of reflection and not to say what the therapist should have done or not, which would be too simplistic because of the context: a few minutes of therapy, isolated from the whole of the therapy.

POSSIBLE EFFECTS OF THE DIAGNOSIS

My first comment is about the influence of the diagnosis on the therapeutic situation: It seems to me that the therapist is sometimes very careful and, maybe, anxious. (He says himself that he feels "anxious that she is dissociating.") And I cannot help thinking that the diagnosis of "borderline personality disorder, with comorbid Axis 1 disorders" is a determinant factor in the therapist's field organization.

This question is, for me, more general than the present case. A plausible hypothesis would be that the knowledge of such a diagnosis itself contributed to the increase in the therapist's anxiety and that this anxiety itself raised the patient's feelings of insecurity. Also, it is possible to argue that the prior information about a risk of dissociation could increase the probability of such dissociation. This is not to say that the therapist was too careful! Nor do I say that it would have been better not to know the diagnosis. I only want to underline that knowing the diagnosis structures the field in a particular way; not knowing it would structure the field in another, different, particular way.

So the title "First or Nowhere?" could apply not only to the patient's problem but also to the ongoing therapeutic situation: Is it possible to work only with a pure "here and now," or as therapists, have we necessarily to cope with some "first," always present? Here, the "first," or better, the "before" would be the knowledge of the so-called diagnosis.

AN OSCILLATING ATTITUDE: SOMETIMES INDIVIDUALISTIC, SOMETIMES FIELD-ORIENTED

My second remark is about the therapist's attitude. It seems to me that he very often oscillates between a field attitude and an individualistic one.

Thus, at the very beginning of the transcript, when the patient says, "I shouldn't bring that up," the therapist answers: "Do you believe that I think you shouldn't bring that up?" (00:12) This is, for me, a field posture: The therapist here makes the hypothesis that the feeling of the patient belongs not to her as a separate person, but that this feeling is the result of the therapeutic field's organization, and therefore that he has, as therapist, contributed to it. But immediately after, and even though the patient continues addressing him directly ("You'll think I'm so awful . . ." [00:21]), the therapist seems to withdraw, sending back the patient to herself and to her past, contributing so to an individualistic position ("Sounds like the past has spontaneously arrived here . . ." [00:39]).

Another example can be found when the therapist asks the patient to try making a bit of contact with him (05:05). The patient says "sorry," and then the therapist answers that he was not meaning to criticize her. For me it is an individualistic position, referring to therapist and patient as isolated persons. A field position would be to look at the emergence of this theme of criticizing in the therapeutic situation.

For me these examples raise the question: What is the meaning of this oscillation between the individualistic and the field-oriented attitudes? Maybe, when the therapist leaves the field's posture, he is, out of awareness, avoiding the contact with his patient, protecting himself. Maybe also, he chooses this deliberately, considering for instance that continuing the contact would be too unbearable for the patient. Maybe, maybe . . . Here, only the wider context of the whole of the therapy, or the comments of the therapist himself could help us to opt for one or another of these hypotheses.

SUGGESTING POSSIBILITIES OR INTENDING TO CHANGE THE PATIENT?

My third question involves the nature of the therapeutic project: The therapist opens the possibility of different truths (06:18). And it seems to me that it is an important moment, creating a stronger contact between the therapist and the patient. My question is: Is the therapist's aim only to open the field of possibilities or also to lead the patient to change her negative image of herself, to try to convince her she is wrong?

Sometimes it seems clear that the therapist searches only to open the field of possibilities, for instance, when he says: "Well, I neither agree nor disagree. I have a response, a reaction. I have a truth that is based on my own understandings . . ." (11:09). But sometimes it also seems that the therapist tries to influence the patient, especially when he tells her his feelings. So when he says, "I notice I feel really sad when you say that" (07:56), or "but I feel very sad . . . almost like I shouldn't be even breathing" (08:50), it is as if he was asking her to change and to protect him. And a few minutes later, when the patient says, "I really want to believe you, to be *with* you" (10:23), the therapist answers, "I feel really moved and pleased when you say that. I'm glad you *want* to believe me" (10:30). Here also it is as if the aim of the therapist was to lead the patient to another, better, image of herself.

Of course, I am aware that my formulations are excessive, and I imagine that the intentions of the therapist were not so clear, not so obvious. But it is to open the significance of the therapist's self-disclosure. Telling his feelings is a possible way toward the exploration of the field; it can also be a means to influence the patient.

IMPLICIT RETROFLECTED DEMAND?

Another question is about the function of retroflection: If the therapist comes to develop many efforts and arguments to change the patient, it is probably because the patient, through retroflection, and quite massive retroflection, as seems to be the case here, is effectively asking him to try and convince her that she is not so awful! So the therapist has to choose: He can accept such an implicit demand, and it seems that this is the choice of the therapist in our present transcript; he could also work to bring to light the function of retroflection and how it strongly contributes to the field's organization. It is a matter of the therapist's strategies and beliefs.

SUPPORTING THE PATIENT OR THE ONGOING EXPERIENCE?

My last comment will be about the little dog the patient evokes, near the end of the transcript. She says: "He was born last and almost died. But you know, I really really wanted him to live . . . almost more than the others" (12:21). And a few minutes later: "Well he's a real fighter, even now" (14:17). Here, the therapist seems to refer the patient to her own struggle for life, saying, "I was just really appreciating the fighter in you. Thinking about the struggles you've had . . ." (14:31). It could be, once more, an individualistic position, the patient being invited to become conscious of her fighting capacities.

But the therapist adds, ". . . the struggles we've had!" Saying that, he includes himself in the process; he assumes with his patient the role that she has assumed with the little dog, the role of a desiring human being. If the dog has survived, it is not only because of her own efforts; it is above all because of the desire of the patient that this dog should live. And if the patient, sometimes, exhibited suicidal behaviors, I guess it may be connected to a lack of other people's desire for her to be alive, maybe especially from her parents.

So it's possible to imagine that the therapy session here related is, fundamentally, an attempt to supply an archaic loss of attention and desire, which could explain that most of the time the therapist seems concerned with giving support to his patient more than with giving support to the ongoing experience, including the exploration of the here and now process of organization/disorganization of the therapeutic field.

COMMENT 2: THE UNDOING OF A RETROFLECTION

Marie–Claude Denis

> The retroflector abandons any attempt to influence his environment by becoming a separate and self-sufficient unit, reinvesting his energy back into an exclusively intrapersonal system and severely restricting the traffic between himself and the environment.
>
> —Polster & Polster, 1974, p. 71

Louisa's therapy session "First or Nowhere?" relates what must have been a most significant moment in the client's life. A dramatic event, the client killing one of her pet kittens, turned out to be her entry into the "real" world, thanks to the patient and skilful facilitation of her therapist.

I think this excerpt can be considered as a beautiful example of the undoing of a retroflection where the client (a) emerges into the "real" world, out of her self-arranged, closed-in world, (b) gains access to a fuller range of experience, involving her whole person (including physical sensations and affects) instead of returning to her stereotyped cognitive beliefs, (c) contacts the other as a separate and differentiated person instead of falling back to her opinion of the other, and (d) recognizes her identity. This session is very rich and dense in reporting the process of moving from a defensive retroflective position to a contactful experience.

THE RETROFLECTING LOUISA AND HER "TRANSITIONAL" PETS

> In retroflection, the split often creates internal abrasion and considerable stress because it remains self-contained and does not move into the required action. Movement towards growth, therefore, would be to redirect energy so that the internal struggle is opened. Instead of operating only within the individual, energy becomes free to move towards a relationship with something outside oneself. The undoing of retroflection consists of the search for the appropriate other.
>
> —Polster & Polster, 1974, p. 85

While being avoidant, engaging into self-destructive behavior, and refraining from contactful action, Louisa can be said to be a retroflector. She cloisters herself in the belief that she shouldn't exist. She seems to have constructed a world for herself where her personal dilemma of being a twin is repeatedly reproduced with numerous pairs of pet animals. From the story reported, we understand these animals to be genuine transitional objects, as Winnicott and Winnicott (1982) conceived them, one of whom literally catapulted Louisa into "reality." Somehow petrified by the fear of "getting it wrong" if she did anything, she refrained from action. But that day, when she did happen to act inadvertently and commit her most dreaded deed, killing one of her cherished pets, she has been projected through the phobic layer, right into the impasse leading to face the real her.

What or whom did Louisa kill when she hit her kitten? Did the fact of being a twin have anything to do with Louisa's retroflective behavior? Did she unconsciously feel like killing her brother? When hurting herself, was she retroflecting a smoldering anger toward him? Did she need her brother to feel whole? Or on the contrary, did she feel he shouldn't exist in order for her to be?

LIVING IS ENGAGING INTO ACTION

Only hypothesis can be drawn to answer these questions. One can only guess that a link may exist somewhere along that line. But we can witness that, killing her kitten, she broke the walls between herself and the outside world: The catastrophic idea she had of herself has been made real. As awful as the experience could be, it opened the way to genuine feelings that she has been able to express and share with the therapist's help. It also led to recognize her right to exist, just like this little dog of hers who, like her, came last, had been a "nuisance," but whom she nurtured and loved.

This process of coming into the world couldn't have succeeded without the therapist's intervention. How did the therapist facilitate this happening?

THE "APPROPRIATE OTHER"

Though the goal is for the individual to seek contact with otherness, the work-through of the inner struggle must frequently come first. In retroflection, since the impulse to do or be done to in contact with others is severely overshadowed, the interaction within the divided self must be re-energized with awareness. Close attention to the physical behavior of the individual is one way to identify where the battle is taking place . . .

—Polster & Polster, 1974, p. 87

Louisa's therapist must have been good for her since the therapy has been lasting for more than 3 years. How has she been the "appropriate other" to help Louisa come out of her cognitive bound, closed in space? While Louisa was projected into reality by the accident of killing her kitten (one could say by this accidental loss of one of her transitional objects), how did she help Louisa come to acknowledge her feelings and open up to a caring and loving space?

Some indications come out clear in the excerpt showing how the therapist worked through Louisa's emergence into a shared ("real") world, helped her to access a fuller range of experience and gain a sense of her identity. Deeply rooted in an I-Thou dialogue, the therapist asked for projections ("Do you believe that I think . . ."; "I'm wondering if you think I'm genuine"), specifications ("What's the connection? What's being repeated?"), or feeling ("What's the feeling that goes with that?").

At all times, the therapist has been very present and empathic to the client ("You look in such pain"), pointing to retroflective behavior ("I was concerned you were disappearing, hating, and punishing yourself"), specifying feelings or emotions ("not self-pity . . . self-hatred"). She opposed the client's belief with her own ("I believe something different . . . your existence is important"; "it's not my experience of being here with you"). She expressed personal feelings and physical sensations as a reverberation of the client's experience ("I feel sad when you say that"; "I notice I have a sort of choking, almost like I shouldn't even be breathing"). She pointed to the present moment and to the relation between the two of them ("I'm wondering what it's like for you to say that here, with me"), confronting the client on the difference ("I'm here with you now . . . different from you . . . and with such a different belief about you"). She made room for polarities and opposing situations, making for complete and differentiated experience ("I have a truth based on my understanding, and my experience of being with you"; "I recall many memories of both good and bad times: successes and failures"). This altogether opened the way to the expression of love ("I loved him"), understanding ("he reminded me of me"), acceptance of needs ("he just needed a lot"), and recognition of worth ("he was worth it").

Underlying all of the techniques used, I trust that the therapist's capacity to be true and to share her thoughts and feelings have been critical in Louisa's therapeutic progress toward full and genuine contact.

REFERENCES

Polster, E., & Polster, M. (1974). *Gestalt therapy integrated.* New York: Vintage Books.

Winnicott, D. W., & Winnicott, C. (1982). *Playing and reality.* London: Routledge.

COMMENT 3: THE ECOLOGY OF PSYCHOTHERAPY

Joel Latner

Whenever I hear about a patient not my own, I look for something in the description, which brings the person and the situation alive to me. With my thus activated imagination, I can penetrate empathically into some part of their life and know who they are and what is important to them to find my own truth and my version of theirs. This is in principle not different from what I do with my own patients when they talk about their friends and families. If the descriptions have a kernel of the independent life of the person being talked about, the person comes alive and the descriptions can inform my judgment of what I am hearing. In this way, I hear about the person who is talking to me (my patient or, in this case, the therapist) and also the person who is being described.

So I notice the descriptions each person gives: the patient's characterization of his or her life and its distinctive features and the facts that they consider important. In this case, it includes what her therapist refers to as her "serious self-harm," her feeling that she should not exist, and her self-criticism. Similarly, the therapist's description of Louisa's diagnosis, her admission to a hospital, her suicidal behavior, her "avoidant" and "dependent" traits.

At the same time, I remain open to the possibilities that "coming alive" suggests: a unique life lived, distinct from the descriptions, not reported, not understood, not conceptualized.

I know that these stories of the therapist and the patient have their own descriptive and explanatory power, and I take note of the way these are used by each of them. Typically, I find such descriptions and self-definitions mildly oppressive because they are evidently restrictive and categorical, and at the same time ("Holding Both!"—see Latner, 2001) in my mind and my imagination, I take them seriously and also retain my own ability to make my own judgments. So I start out with this tension between what I am given and knowing that we all are desperate to construct a coherent picture of who we are and of what our lives consist. We do this the best way we can, with what we are given: what we are told, what categories of understanding our culture gives us, and what serves to stitch together and hold together a picture of ourselves.

COMING ALIVE

So I had my customary difficulty here until I found my footing in the actuality of the events reported in this transcript. The therapists says he has been "trying to facilitate her staying in contact with herself and me," and I wonder what she is doing to be out of contact (how she achieves this), what she is in contact with, and what contribution he makes to this situation. Asking myself these questions reminds me of my own perspective as I find what is transpiring in the session—in this case, how the therapist works — and also it helps make these two people alive for me.

But then I read further in the transcript, and I see how the therapist does what he says he does: He insists on his presence and his questions, taking her seriously and asking her to be clearer for him and to engage him. He says, "What is the pattern, what does it look like?" (01:21) He is saying, in effect, "What are you talking about? I don't follow you; tell me so that I can understand you." And she answers him, finally, "Oh God, it's so awful" (02:55). This sounds like it could be something uttered from her visceral connection with her life as she knows it. But it is followed by a pause and the therapist's "reflective" comment; he imagines a vortex. It strikes me that this image is perhaps designed to be a characterization of "Oh God, it's so awful," but he is too literal; he is trying to imagine what she means by "patterns," and it comes out too abstractly. Not as the vortex she *is*, or the vortex she is *in*. He offers something mental, too abstract. She can only respond in the same way, abstractly, and in terms of how she thinks, by saying how she thinks about this new incident—killing her kitten—is in the categorical realm of what she knows already, "down to me being here."

The therapist tries again. He asks for what is missing (for him, and for me too), something direct and emotional (03:25), which embodies the self-loathing in the words she uses, "horrible, hateful . . . my mistakes"; to my eyes (and heart), he doesn't get what he asks for. I am sympathetic to his efforts, but he is asking for something she cannot deliver—not the way he is asking it. She does not know how to feel what she is talking about. (And the therapy is not focused on this, on her meaning what she says and on learning how to do this. It is difficult, isn't it, to mean what you say?)

Though he keeps looking indirectly for this, saying that she looks to be in such pain (04:20) when she says ". . . as soon as I start taking part . . . Oh" (04:06). Then he says she makes him more anxious (05:05), saying, "I just can't bear me . . ." (04:30), and he reports that he believes she might be dissociating (05:05). I would agree with him that she is perhaps dissociating, but not more than before. Louisa seems persistently disconnected from what she is saying—though he acts as though she is making sense (!)—but at the same time, paradoxically, the power of what she is saying moves him, "you look in such pain . . ." (04:20).

The therapist then asks for what is lacking, "Can you try and make a bit of contact with me" (05:05). This is a key moment, a key intervention. He is aware of the gap between how stirred up she is and how disconnected she is from herself and also from him. He asks her to come forth. She catches a part of his meaning very well, distorting it through the prism of her self-hate. He is suggesting that she should do something she is not doing, and she apologizes and then asks if he is saying she is wrong (06:13).

Another way to think about what is occurring is that Louisa lives in a world of her ideas, disconnected from a good deal of the actuality of her life, including her therapist. He sees this and attempts to intervene, though there is not much in the transcript which indicates that this is—as it ought to be, for Louisa and for her therapist—the central focus of her therapy. She needs to learn to be contactful, by which I mean open to contacting the other as fully as she does herself and allowing the play of contact, within and without, to be free of her control. This is what we in Gestalt therapy call spontaneity. Instead, she tends toward being self-involved, contacting herself, imposing her preoccupations on her perceptions. How can she do what he is asking? It seems to me she does not know how.

She tries, doing it in her characteristic manner, turning it into what she knows, the ideas she characterizes as "self-pity," and her familiar thoughts about the patterns of her life mistakes. As I read the transcript, I think the therapist could perhaps have broken through her self-involved and self-defining awareness of him if he had said, instead, "When you look like you are in such pain, I feel so sad and worried about you. I don't mind feeling this way—please, I'm not blaming you for your reaction—but I want to help you, and I think if you saw my interest in you and my affection and concern for you, it would make a difference."

I know, of course, there is a potential in saying this that she will feel blamed by him—as she has already—but instead of asking her to do what she cannot do and to do it without specific instructions. (What does "make a bit of contact with me" mean to someone like Louisa? She thinks she is making contact!) Saying what I have suggested creates a new situation: an immediate and compelling reality in which the therapist acts more like a human being, undefined and unique, not a "therapist," the familiar (and classic) role of a passive person who reflects at a remove and does not engage or react.

This role is one of our legacies from our heritage in psychoanalysis, where the analyst wishes to disappear to allow the patient's projections to be played out in the room. But it is anachronistic. We have learned that patients will project, no matter what we do (as will we), and we cannot utilize the actuality of the here and now if we do not attend to it. I think it is also a legacy of our fear of our founder and his putative bad behavior in therapy. We will be beyond reproach (by whom?), but as we recede, we will also take no risks. This part of the transcript is an instance of the risk of taking no risks.

Sure enough, as the meeting continues (06:13–06:18), the therapist takes a more human stance in the therapy. He reflects her at 06:01, and she, asking for his engagement and reading him correctly says, "Are you saying I'm wrong?" (06:13). She says, in effect, where do you stand? And he says, in effect, without denying her beliefs, yes, I think you are not correct in how you see things; I see things from my perspective as well as yours, and "I believe something different."

This is contactful, and he engages her vividly. She reiterates her ideas (are they convictions or just repetitive ideas?), and he strides forth into the room at 07:56, saying, "I notice I feel really sad when you say that," only hedging his daring with "I notice." And he is bolder still at 08:50, "That is absolutely not my experience of being here with you . . . I notice I have a sort of choking . . . telling me how strongly you believe you shouldn't exist." This is the essential contact from the therapist, telling Louisa how it is for another human, the one who has devoted these 143 hours of his professional life to her care, to be with her. He has brilliantly abandoned the safety of his obscurity, his clinical distance, and instead of asking her to meet him, he does it himself. (Who knows? If he continues in this direction, soon he will tell her about himself, his life, his loves, his family, his dis-appointments, and she will find the actuality of this world unavoidable!)

She responds, arriving in the room with him. He says, directly and engagingly, "What is it like . . . I'm here with you . . . and a different experience of you . . . I'm just wondering if that makes you feel apart from me" (09:50). (Better: What is it like *for you?*) Louisa replies, obliquely, "I really want to believe you . . ." and then, striding forward, "to be *with* you" (10:23).

The next words from both of them circle around this meeting they have initiated. He backs off, "wondering"(10:30), consulting his thought processes, but trying also to find again the pulsing vein he had touched. She tells him something important about the man she has known these 4 years, "I know you wouldn't lie to me" (10:53). He gets didactic—backing off—and she responds with apparent confusion (11:20). The therapist's sentences at this point, explaining his ideology ("So there is contrast and difference. . . . I just believe that life, including your life, is purposeful" [11:27]), show him stepping back from the vitality of their meeting—what is he afraid of?—into ideas and beliefs, reasserting the morass she and he were struggling in previously.

This is a critical moment, where it is clear that he can control the tone of the therapy and the "disease" of his patient. In fact, the form of his statements is not different from the ones he was hearing from her earlier. He says what he believes about life in general, and therefore her life; earlier in the transcript, she was telling him how she sees her life in general. Here he is encouraging a generalized present. At this point, it seems as though he has lost touch with what was important and lively about this encounter and how he can make this occur. He is either not aware of the way he controls the extent of their intimacy, or he is afraid of it. He is again taking the distant and parental benign-teacher–therapist position and telling her his good ideas, in contrast to her bad ones about patterns and self-hate.

But Louisa is a straightforward person (and she seems healthier than we have been led to believe), and her response is refreshingly concrete: "I'm just thinking of one of my little dogs" (12:21). The topics she touches on as she continues, reminiscing about her dog are—not coincidentally—love, acceptance, and the struggle to grow (13:07). But the therapist insists on his teacherly posture with her ("So, is he really a nuisance?" [13:25]). The therapist realizes he is moving in the wrong direction and tosses away this unconstructive stance and says he is moved. "I just had a really warm, pleased sense of your aliveness" (14:31).

Louisa steps back a moment (What's with this guy? He's here and then he's gone!? And then he's back!?!) and takes her familiar infirm position, saying, "It's still a struggle" (15:15). And so the therapist too returns to his kindly role, full of hope and encouragement (15:23 and 15:39), "I see you struggling to cope . . . and I trust that struggle will bring you through." I read into his words his feeling of joy at her spontaneous emergence and his pleasure at his knowledge of his part in it, but this is not the best way to say it.

CONCLUSION

In his summary paragraph, the therapist says they had touched a dark place in her, and they had also maintained a strong contact for most of the rest of the session. I wished he had considered himself more in the course of the therapy and in his final comment, which is misleading. It directs our attention to the wrong place and suggests that this disturbed woman has dark places in her. This term expresses his overly intrapsychic perspective. It is not necessary to ignore the inner world, but he looks too insistently away from himself and to Louisa. Properly, he should embrace them both.

I would say that the place they had touched was the result of the efforts of two people who fail to touch each other because of the ways they encapsulate themselves and blunt their contacting. He does this by his impersonal methods, his intellectualizing interventions, and the way he hides what is distinctive about him. Louisa encapsulates herself by organizing her awareness and her social milieu (her therapist, in this case) to focus on her mental constructions—without regard for the rest of her awareness or her qualities: her capacity for engagement, her emotions, her feelings, her liveliness, her creative resources. But each of them persevered and, because of the daring of the therapist and Louisa's responsiveness—they both have good instincts, a taste for life!—they made something important.

I don't see any sign that he has yet recognized what they did, unfortunately, or how they can repeat it, but I am optimistic that they can again create a life between them that is vital and engaging and that they will each grow in it.

REFERENCE

Latner, J. (2001). Alles einbeziehen—Gedanken über Ganzheitlichkeit [Holism—Holding all]. In F.-M. Staemmler (Ed.), *Gestalttherapie im Umbruch—Von alten Begriffen zu neuen Ideen* [Gestalt therapy in upheaval—From old terms to new ideas] (pp. 117–141). Köln, Germany: Edition Humanistische Psychologie. Also in *British Gestalt Journal 2001, 10/2*, 106–113, as "The sense of gestalt therapy: Holism, reality and explanation"; as "Lo Holistico: Abarcandolo Todo" in *Figura/Fondo, 11*, 2002. The article was accepted for publication in *Cahiers de Gestalt-thérapie* in 2002.

COMMENT 4: BEING A REPEAT, REPEATING BEING

Lynne Jacobs

So much of the therapeutic process is circular. There are the repetitive loops, and then there are the recursive loops, and loops that have aspects of both repetition and recursiveness.

REPETITIVE AND RECURSIVE LOOPS OF EXPERIENCING

The repetitive loops reflect imprisonment in, and also investment in, a closed system of negative expectation, dread, and despair. In general, I believe the imprisonment in dread and negativity is an outgrowth of trauma. On the other hand, the investment in the closed system is a creative adjustment (the creative nature of which has been long forgotten, needing reawakening in therapy), one whereby the negativity, dread, and despair that characterized one's reactions to trauma are used in the service of maintaining a sense of security. One's conviction that the next moment of existence offers no possibility for richness, but only pain and misery, offers a sure and secure guideline about life. Such a conviction removes uncertainty, and uncertainty is messy. Uncertainty leaves one open to rising hopes and crashing disappointments, to loves and losses, to enthusiasms and embarrassments. Uncertainty draws us toward the world and all its vagaries, whereas a firm conviction about the hopelessness of life draws us away from the roller coaster that living inevitably is.

Recursive loops, on the other hand, are the manifestations of the fluidity and movement of present-centeredness, in which one's history and one's future are intermixed oscillating grounds for each other. In other words, a recursive loop is an inevitable outgrowth of contacting. In a recursive loop, one may touch upon very familiar themes and yet do so in a way that casts new light upon the theme, reshuffles the images of one's history into a different Gestalt, or opens a surprising new pathway into the next moment. Every so-called "new" experience, contact with novelty, is only *relatively* new; it is emergent from the ground of our history. "New" experience reorganizes our history as it also becomes our history, the ground for the next moment and so on.

Therapist and patient each bring repetitive loops to their relationship. They also both bring recursive loops or at least an aptitude for their development. And over the course of therapy, they will develop some dance steps together. The ritualized dance steps will draw on the repetitive tendencies of both and will become a unique but still relatively closed system. Both will have to work together to "open up" the dance to greater degrees of improvisation if their relationship is to develop. The development of the patient is an emergent phenomenon of a "recursive loop dance" that draws on the shift, in both partners, from relating in a repetitive loop to relating in recursive loops.

ATTUNEMENT TO REPETITION

Louisa and her therapist[1] have lived through many a repetition. Louisa, with her pronounced tendency to dissociate, probably knows from direct experience what trauma is. This anguished woman who describes beautifully and compellingly the annihilation of being a pointless repetition herself ("Maybe I'd believe that [my existence is important] if I'd been born a single person. But it's like, when there's twins, it's like a repeat one has been made. Like an afterthought; so in effect, my brother's the one that was meant to be born. . . . [I am] surplus." [06:31–08:01]) lives in a very familiar loop that she and her therapist have traveled many times, illustrated by the following exchange:

C (03:31): Horrible, hateful; . . . that it's all down to me . . . my mistakes. What is the point of me being here? I've always said that I haven't got a function in life; but at least if I haven't got a function, if I don't get things wrong . . . no one gets hurt.

T (03:50): Sounds like you've got back to that very early decision that "I shouldn't be here;" and if I am here, I should have no needs, make no waves, and definitely get nothing wrong.

C (04:06): Well at least then I'm not doing any harm by being here. But as soon as I start taking part . . . Oh.

T (04:20): You look in such pain, physical pain when you say that.

The theme of utter negation has had many repetitions in the history of this therapeutic relationship. This theme of repetitive loops is not often addressed in Gestalt therapy literature, with its emphasis on fresh, new experiences, and yet I hazard a guess that we are all familiar with the enervating and demoralizing influence of such repetition.

My belief is that part of the transformative power of the relatively newer moments of contact derives from the shared history of having lived together in the repetitive loop. Further, I believe that the recursive evolution of this therapy session, which moved from heartbreak (of killing her cat), into familiar repeat ("It feels like it's a 'come-back' you

[1]For simplicity's sake, I will write as if the therapist is male.

see that I can't just forget it. It's like it keeps on repeating itself, and its just going to keep on repeating itself. The memories keep coming back, and it keeps on happening. Something will happen, sooner or later, and the pattern is there . . . all the same" [00:49]), into heartfelt shared engagement with Louisa's darkest thoughts and feelings (the later two-thirds of the transcript), into a newer perspective (reflected in her loving/ self-loving discussion of her puppy), derived in large part from the therapist's openness to the repetitive loop. I cannot emphasize this enough: *The therapist's willingness to really know the patient from within her repetitive experiential world was fundamental to making it possible for the patient to emerge, even if momentarily, from that world.*

Our paradoxical theory of change emphasizes the importance for the patient of identifying with his or her immediate, ongoing, moment-by-moment experience. The same is required of the therapist, I believe, although with a twist. The therapist needs to be able to identify with his or her own experiencing and also to attempt to stay in contact with the patient's experiencing at the same time. This is often done through practicing "inclusion" (Buber, 1967, p. 173). One means whereby one might practice inclusion is through emotional attunement. By attunement I mean attempting to find an emotional resonance with the patient's emotional state and perspective.[2] I contrast this notion with the emphasis some other therapists place on focusing on the quality of patients' contacting. Obviously, at various points in our therapeutic work, we will want to experiment with various modes of contacting. But there is a big difference between an exploratory atmosphere that has been built on being well met and respected for your current solutions and one that is built on an atmosphere that suggests there is a right way to contact and a wrong way.

The transcript provides a lucid example of how repetitive loops begin to break out into recursive loops through an ongoing process in which the therapist attempts to really know the patient's experience. There are plenty of examples of the therapist attempting to feel his way into the patient's perspective. Here are some from the first third of the transcript:

T (03:15): (reflectively) I imagine a spiral, a vortex; I wonder how it seems to you.
T (03:25): What's the feeling that goes with that . . . that it's all down to you being here?
T (04:20): You look in such pain, physical pain when you say that.

An important point here is that the therapist's efforts to formulate an attuned understanding of the patient's struggles did not result, as some people fear, in an entrenchment of the patient in her repetitive loop. Rather, his attunement, his emotional resonance, seemed to provide a platform that deepened the conversation, made it more emotional, *and* ultimately more exploratory.

In particular, the therapist also attempts to track the patient's experience of the therapist's impact. This is a special case of attunement, and an interesting effect of his questions about his potentially difficult affect on Louisa is that Louisa's conversation often began to open into the recursive looping following his queries about her experience of being with him.

The patient began by saying she shouldn't even bring up her repetitive pessimistic version of herself. The therapist asks, "Do you believe that I think you shouldn't bring that up?" (00:12). At this point, she does not really explore his question but begins her descent into what the therapist called a downward spiral (might that have been his experience?). At another point, he asks her, "I'm wondering what it's like for you to say that

[2]There is some confusion among Gestalt therapists about the concept of "attunement," a concept that first gained wide currency in contemporary psychoanalysis (Stolorow et al., 1987) and in child development studies (Stern, 1985). I think that Gestalt therapists who criticize attunement as a surrender or diminishment of the therapist's phenomenology are mistaken (see, e.g., Philippson, 2001; Resnick, 1995). The practice of attunement in fact requires *exquisite* ongoing awareness of one's own phenomenology. That is why actually practicing inclusion or attunement is so difficult to do!

here, with me . . . to say that to me" (08:23). In response, the patient voiced her *ideas* about the therapist's feelings, which opened the door for them to have a long conversation about their differing *experiences* of being with her. Their conversation about differing experiences of being with her vacillated back and forth between familiar and new and ran through the rest of the session. We can see here the interweaving of repetition and recursiveness that runs through many a therapy session.

The therapist also listened, throughout the session, both with an ear for the emotional tone of her misery but [also] for something that might reach past the immediate moment, something that might provide some perspective. Hence, the references earlier to "patterns," which he elaborates as: "Sounds like you've got back to that very early decision that 'I shouldn't be here,' and if I am here, I should have no needs, make no waves, and definitely get nothing wrong" (03:50).

I think most of us look for such fundamental themes, patterns, and repetitions, and we look to put them into words, in part in the hope that the words will create a slight shift in perspective. Instead of just living from the negative theme, our hope is that labeling the theme might allow for exploration of the theme.

Another important contribution from the therapist is that he offered his own experience as part of the evolution of a recursive dialogue in which they were both implicated. Some of the therapist's statements seem to be an attuned responsiveness to the patient's interest in conversation that is outside the repetitive loop. Other statements seem more reactive to the therapist's distress (as when the therapist was worried about another dissociative episode), and yet they all emerge from the ground of genuine interest in the patient's experiential world (which is the therapist's contribution to living through the paradoxical theory of change). When the therapist reacted to his own anxiety, the exchange did not go well, although they both were able to recover quickly. When he spoke from a more centered state, the patient appeared genuinely interested, engaging in conversation with him.

RECURSIVE DANCE

By the time they were engaged in Louisa's moving story about her puppy, with its obvious parallels to her own story, they were dancing together smoothly, daring to try a few new moves, building the moves out from their original choreography. They were in a recursive loop, still addressing her fundamental themes, but in creative new ways. They weren't throwing away the old steps; they were adding new ones that emerged from their way of dancing the older steps together while being open to experimenting with new steps. The experiments were built upon skill with the old steps, but having new steps puts the old steps into a different context now. The old steps are not the only steps they know.

My guess is that Louisa is just beginning to dance new steps. She is at the edge of her imprisonment, the new steps a beginning of breakout. I said at the beginning of my remarks that I thought repetitive loops were both a reaction to trauma and also reflected a self-protective investment in sameness and security. The figure at this moment seems to be her imprisonment. At another moment, it may be her investment. Ultimately, unless her investment is also explored, the new dance steps will be small gains and in fact may be assimilated back into a repetitive loop.

However, at this point, such a focus would seem to me to be ill-timed and might well reimprison Louisa in her sense of worthlessness. There may be moments that emerge later; for instance, she may become aware that she is anxious when she dares to believe her therapist truly does value her, when the investment side of the polarity can become a momentary focus. When that begins to happen, there may be stretches of time when the therapist and patient will go back and forth (in recursive loops!) between imprisonment and investment. Then still newer dance steps will develop again, some uncoordinated, with "who is leading here?" being fought out, and others thrillingly mutually coordinated. But for now, we have all born witness to the tiny but awesome beginnings of a new dance.

What a privilege to have been allowed a glimpse of an intense, moving, therapeutic encounter. I am grateful to the therapist and to the client for letting all of us walk along the way for a bit with them. I was moved deeply by both of you, your courage, and honest dialogue with each other. I wish you both all the best.

REFERENCES

Buber, M. (1967). *A believing humanism: Gleanings* (M. S. Friedman, Trans.). New York: Simon & Schuster.

Philippson, P. (2001). *Self in relation*. Highland, NY: Gestalt Journal Press.

Resnick, R. (1995). Gestalt therapy: Principles, prisms and perspectives. *British Gestalt Journal, 4/1,* 3–13.

Stern, D. (1985). *The interpersonal world of the infant.* New York: Basic Books.

Stolorow, R., Brandchaft, B., & Atwood, G. (1987). *Psychoanalytic treatment: An intersubjective approach.* Hillsdale, NJ: Analytic Press.

FIRST OR NOWHERE?
A QUEST FOR EXISTENCE:
RESPONSE TO THE COMMENTS

Sally Denham-Vaughan

In my response to the comments, I wish to take the opportunity to explore a number of themes. First, I want to write briefly about my process of offering the transcript and then receiving feedback. This is something that was, somewhat to my surprise, remarked upon by a number of the commentators. Second, I shall attempt to explain my process regarding some of the interventions made (or indeed not made) in the transcript. Finally, I wish to highlight one or two key themes that this exercise raises.

MY BASIC ATTITUDE

With regard to my process of offering and receiving, I was particularly struck by the supportive nature of the feedback I have received. I heard the commentators highlighting the risks involved in offering the transcript, their general support and curiosity for the work, and also their appreciation of the opportunity to glimpse an intimate moment in an ongoing therapy. I was struck by the "reaching out" I felt from these unidentified watchers and began to reflect with interest upon aspects in myself that had enabled me to undertake my role in this joint venture.

It was, unsurprisingly perhaps, a risky and scary business for me to reveal my therapeutic work. I had what I imagined to be fairly usual fears of being criticized, shown to be theoretically lacking or methodologically clumsy, and was particularly anxious that the comments were made by "unknown strangers" rather than within the context of a dialogue.

I wondered then in more detail what had impelled me forward! I kept coming up with the phrase "I trusted I would not be annihilated."

I felt moved by these words. I also reflected on the fact that perhaps it is this aspect of my character that is supporting me in working with Louisa, who both fears annihilation and, in this transcript, finds herself to be the cause of it in a very literal sense. I was therefore struck by how central this, possibly naive, trusting in my ability to survive, and indeed finding support for myself in that process, had been in the exercise and also in the therapy.

I wondered if this possibly reflected a basic attitude that underpins my work, which I think is central to many of us within the Gestalt community. It is the belief that growth and change are possible and that the organism orientates itself naturally toward these ends.

I now wish to deal with some of the individual comments.

RESPONSE TO COMMENT I

I consider myself a fairly classic Gestalt therapist in that I work with elements of field theory, dialogue, and phenomenology. I was delighted that this first commentator picked up on possible tensions between these maps, which I think are often glossed over.

I now wish to talk about this with specific reference to the issue of diagnosis, which is also noted in comment three.

As stated in my introduction, I work in the British National Health Service, where Gestalt therapy is, unfortunately, rapidly disappearing. One of the reasons for this, I believe, has been our ongoing ambivalence regarding the issue of diagnosis and pre-configuration of the field with reference to specific client groups. In particular, Gestalt psychotherapy has little to say about "evidence-based" work with the Axis 1 disorders named in *DSM-IV* and lacks a coherent model of brief therapy that can be reliably agreed upon.

Thus, there are times when I find myself balancing an internal tension between the need to work in a way that recognizes the system within which I work—that is, "field congruence,"—without losing my identity as a Gestalt therapist. Specifically, I experience a "pull" to engage in an "I-it" mode of relating that challenges my commitment to both dialogue and the phenomenological principle of horizontality.

I *am* constantly aware of the potential abuses that can result from rote labeling and psychopathologizing of people. As a trainee (when I was already a practicing clinical psychologist), I was struck by Clarkson's statement, "to label people can be to strip them of the unique way in which they have chosen to give meaning to their existence and their historical context" (1989, p. 23). Within my environment, this process does occur.

Regrettably, however, I have witnessed this same process at work within a range of Gestalt settings. Therefore, I would ask that we attempt to own our shadow rather than comfortably project it onto the mental health system. Any semantic form can be misused if misapplied, including Gestalt psychotherapy language.

I believe I share with Louisa a dialectic tension in experiencing the environment as *both* potentially destructive *and* potentially lifesaving, at times even life enhancing. Perhaps it is no surprise that these themes are also paralleled within Louisa's therapeutic journey and in the brief vignette of our work together that the transcript describes.

Second, I was somewhat confused by some of the examples that this commentator described as expressing an "individualistic" stance. My experience is of oscillating, intentionally, around four key aspects in the current phenomenal field. These include myself as an individual, the client as an individual (both of us with unique intrapsychic structures), the "between" of our relationship, and the environment that frames and configures our meeting. For me, these elements comprise the "total situation" that a field perspective demands we examine (Lewin, 1951, p. 288).

In addition, Parlett (1991) states that therapy "may include the past-as-remembered-now or the future-as-anticipated-now, which will form part of the person's experiential field in the present" (p. 71). Thus, the temporal focus is the present as it combines past and the anticipated future.

I thereby recognize that I may have a different "take" with regard to a field theoretical mode of working from this writer, as mine *includes* attention to individual intrapsychic experience as it emerges in the context of specific field conditions. For example, one aspect that I am alert to with regard to Louisa's process is her tendency to constellate herself as a burden in relationship. My experience is that too intense, prolonged, or intimate contact between us triggers her into initial confluence, followed by intense shame and isolation. I therefore attempt to keep the contact available, but "calibrate" it in line with my previous experiences of her responding with either feelings of abandonment or shame if the contact is either underplayed or overmade.

I judge this way of working as wholly consistent with a "field" paradigm, recognizing her process with me across time and emergent in the here-and-now relational frame. To me, this is not an "individualistic" way of formulating her case but recognition of the self as process model being meshed with a field theoretical stance. As such, both Louisa and I emerge as ourselves at the boundary formed by our meeting. The entire phenomenal field is present in this meeting, shaping and forming not just our relationship but also the selves who are available to the meeting.

I was interested in comments where again this commentator made for me a false dichotomy between my being open to either "the field of possibilities" or "leading the patient." This raises an interesting dialectic tension surrounding work with patients where their current experience of themselves is *truly* unbearable and overwhelming. When I contact Louisa in that place, I wish to validate not only where she is now but also her sense that this place is unbearable and she needs to get out of it as fast as possible!

At these moments, I am questioning the value of us as Gestalt therapists holding too tightly to the notion of the paradoxical theory of change and believing that it is always acceptable to stay with the client and his or her experience in any state that is expressed. My sense is that here we confront a real theoretical tension with very fragile clients, between the phenomenological method and the practice of the dialogic relationship. My reality is that I have now lived with Louisa's wish to kill herself for some 4 years. On the one hand, living with this for that length of time has reassured me that she is unlikely to kill herself. On the other hand, I have also validated her desire to kill herself so frequently and felt the intensity of her desire so strongly that I now hold this as part of my inclusive relational stance with Louisa. I thus have an emotional response to her self-destructive feelings and behaviors, which I see being authentically presented in this vignette. My experience is of attempting to be present with this while also demonstrating my respect for her ultimate decision regarding whether to end her life.

Finally, I was struck by this commentator's last paragraph, where she or he imagines that the therapy session is fundamentally an attempt to supply an archaic loss of attention and desire. It is indeed within my awareness that Louisa carries archaic longings for specific types of contact, commonly known as self-object needs, which were unmet in her childhood (see Kohut, 1971). I would say that my experience is of wishing to give support to these longings, as well as to the ongoing experience of exploring the here and now. I do not see these as an "either–or" that we can follow in therapy. Indeed, Yontef's and Jacobs's "relational Gestalt therapy" (see Jacobs, 1992, 1995; Yontef, 1993, 2002), which combines elements of self-psychology with Gestalt therapy theory, emphasizes the importance of both these activities occurring simultaneously within the therapeutic encounter.

RESPONSE TO COMMENT 2

I appreciated this commentator looking at the work through the lens of moderations to contact. In particular, I resonated with the idea of "creative adjustments" that have been used to survive traumatic field conditions in the past, becoming embedded as "fixed Gestalt" (see Perls, Hefferline, & Goodman, 1951).

With Louisa, I am frequently reminded of how her original needs were often denied or distorted, and continue to be so, due to a danger being perceived in pursuing their satisfaction. Currently, the whole of Louisa's being—physical, emotional, and cognitive—frequently moderates contact in these fixed ways.

I felt especially pleased that this commentator seemed to have so accurately picked up the fears of annihilation/annihilating that emerge from Louisa's work. She does indeed admit to historical feelings of wishing to kill her twin so that she could have been "the only one." In many ways, the dreadful experience of killing her kitten is an incarnation of this most terrible (to her) aspect of her personality. Interestingly, however, this theme manifests itself within the therapy as ongoing dreams consisting of her twin killing her. It is indeed the case that the twins did frequently compete for a range of situations, including both being attracted to a young man who eventually had a relationship with both twins but chose to stay with Louisa's brother! She experienced this loss of an early lover as an "annihilation" of her sexuality and has since been abused and raped twice in other relationships.

I felt very met by this commentator in the work and, although the particular map of moderations to contact is not one that I commonly use, I would agree that retroflection is a key contact style for Louisa and add that it is also key for myself. Thus, my ability to cognitively attune, possibly project, and occasionally miss her through retroflecting my more spontaneous, contactful aspects are all part of our therapeutic journey together.

This has perhaps been most powerfully described when Louisa has equated her fear of people with my current fear of riding horses (an activity which she is a master at). She has on more than one occasion said that if I were willing to get back on a horse under her instruction, she would be willing to attend a social group. These moments provide us with very powerful contact when we can both connect with what feels to be an irrational, but overriding, fear that prevents action. At the current time in therapy, we are using the metaphor of me getting on a horse (and I am experimenting with the notion of this as a reality) as an active way of exploring and supporting her overcoming her fear of relationships and contact.

RESPONSE TO COMMENT 3

I was struck by this therapist's attention to the detail in the work. In particular, I found the section on "coming alive" full of momentum and had a sense of this writer feeling into the "sequential imperative" of the work. The detail of the analysis reminded me of Erv Polster's (1991) notion of "tight therapeutic sequences," where each individual intervention is viewed as either sharpening or diffusing the figure.

I was particularly interested in comments regarding my perception, and anxiety, around Louisa's dissociation. The phrase "Louisa seems persistently disconnected from what she is saying—though he [the therapist] acts as though she is making sense (!) . . ." was fascinating to me because Louisa does indeed make sense to me. Whether this is because as individuals we have similar processes regarding contact style, or whether this is simply because I know sufficient ground of her story to have a sense of coherent narrative, one cannot be sure.

I do believe that here this commentator is highlighting a critical choice point of mine regarding how to "be" in the therapeutic relationship. My dilemmas lie in the realm of how to respond, without, as Beaumont (1993) describes, causing a breakdown of contact by either too much intimacy or too much stress.

In some ways, it is true that as an individual I tend toward retroflection and as a therapist can stay within my comfort zone by making insufficient contact. I can only say that this does not seem to be the reality of the ongoing nature of this particular therapy. Rather, my sense is that I have become more delicate and sparing with contact as I have gotten to know Louisa better. It is easy for her to be overwhelmed by contact, descend into dissociation and then shame, with a clear sense of being a failure at not being able to "handle" relationships. It is true that there are moments of excellent contact between us; however, I do configure her dissociation as a creative adaptation to trauma, and my sense is that Louisa and I carefully calibrate our contact.

My main dilemma is therefore around how *much* contact to offer, given her beliefs that only a "twin" who is with her 24 hours a day will be able to provide enough, that I am paid to do the work, and that any needs for contact on her part are burdensome to the other! She thus experiences a tremendously conflictual situation of feeling insatiably needy and dreadfully ashamed of her needy part.

I am curious that this commentator states that "we cannot utilize the actuality of the here and now . . ." if we do not attend to clients' projections. My way of working with projections, I would argue, is more, rather than less, contactful. I favor the method of initially looking for the "perception" that may be concealed within the projected material but out of my awareness. At these points, therefore, I will tend to examine my own behavior/self-configuration to see what has triggered a particular comment from the client. This work is largely informed by that of Stolorow, Brandchaft, and Atwood (1987, pp. 38ff.) in describing their rupture and repair cycle. This seems to be a path that Louisa and I frequently travel together, with her seeming to find my willingness to take responsibility for my side of the relationship very freeing and supportive of her moving forward into more contact. I have a clear sense of being in the immediate actuality of the present while working in this way.

I found this commentator's curiosity regarding my potential fears of Louisa's neediness in the relationship very interesting. I am sure it will not wholly surprise some readers to hear that I am a child of a twin, who had the experience of a twin dying in childhood. My own childhood thus frequently involved being invited to provide a lost twin relationship.

Through my own therapy, I am well aware of how demanding I found this. While it gives me a fairly unique insight into Louisa's neediness, it also gives me a great wariness of ongoing confluence, or being seen to promise to deliver something that I personally and professionally am unable to provide. I am aware that through Louisa's therapy I stand to learn, grow, explore, and examine this issue again and again. This truly is a case where both of us gain from the meeting, and I am grateful to Louisa for this opportunity.

In retrospect, I can imagine that this piece of information would have enabled the commentators to go far deeper into the relational process between Louisa and myself. I can only say that, having met the commentators through their writing, I now feel able to move forward into more contact regarding my own process. Such is the nature of dialogue and retroflection as a contact style!

RESPONSE TO COMMENT 4

I felt very in tune with this writer's comments regarding trauma, creative adjustment, and security, although the notion of repetitive and recursive loops of experience is not a language that I would use, favoring instead notions of creative adjustment, fixed Gestalts, and needed/repeated relational themes.

There were a number of occasions when I found myself so attuned to this writer's formulation of the case that it left relatively little to write and respond to. This left me musing about the notion of confluence and the basic biological necessity that we ground ourselves in as Gestalt therapists. That is, human neural networks are excited by novelty and change. I agreed with this writer that, historically, the stance of Gestalt therapy theory has been to build upon this fact (perhaps due to the effect of Fritz Perls's personality), and we tend to favor action, differentiation, and newness over repetition, calmness, and stillness. We are traditionally a "libidinous" brand of therapy, tending to suit resilient, explorative clients rather than fragile individuals seeking to enact old patterns and have the therapist fulfill additional ego-functions.

I was reminded of Stratford and Brallier's (1979) classic paper describing Gestalt psychotherapy with "profoundly disturbed" people. These writers employ the metaphors of "solvent" and "glue," suggesting the latter as being more helpful with more fragile clients. With Louisa, I seem to shuttle between the gluepot and the solvent spray, attempting to release old stuck patterns as far as we are able, without destabilizing and dissolving her to an intolerable degree. I found this writer's notion of recursive and repetitive loops forming at the contact boundary provided an elegant form for describing this process, and one which I can imagine incorporating into my work with other clients. I also found myself having a sense of confirmation in my work with Louisa; a notion that although we seem to recycle old patterns for much of our time together, fresh, new, and potentially transformative moments arise spontaneously from the ground of our meeting. Indeed, it is the sense of this possibility that supports me in holding the pole of "life" in our work together, especially in those dark moments when Louisa's hold on this seems very fragile.

Interestingly, as I write this some 12 months after the session described in the transcript, I am impacted by a moment that happened today. It has been a beautiful spring day, and Louisa left a message on my voice-mail. Usually, these signal moments of distress and requests for contact and support. Today, however, the content was different. "Sally, I am just ringing to let you know that I've been out with the dogs and I noticed the colors everywhere. I couldn't believe how vivid everything looked and the strange thing was that as I noticed this, I had a sense of aliveness everywhere around me. I remembered you saying that therapy was one way of discovering a capacity for joy in living and I wanted to tell you that I'd had a brief sense of what that might be like today."

I'm sure it will not surprise readers to know that I have been powerfully affected by that call; I looked up from my writing, glanced out the window, and thought, "It *is* gorgeous out there; she's right." In that instant, I realized that not only had Louisa described a potentially transformative moment for her, but she had also improved the quality of my life in that moment. In doing this, she also powerfully reinforced my ability to hold the "libidinous" pole of the therapy for her. I wondered if this moment was an example of a recursive loop, having the potential to grow, change, and heal both the individuals who are present. It certainly felt like it!

I was particularly pleased that the theme of Louisa being a twin was given a central position in how this writer viewed the relational dance. In addition, I was struck by the attention to the process of attunement, which I regard as an essential part of my practice of inclusion. As I said earlier, my aim here is to be fully present in my own experience while attempting to see the situation as the client has constructed it. I would agree that this practice does require an oscillation between the intrapsychic worlds of two individuals who are together working at an emergent relational boundary.

Finally, I appreciated how this commentator also gave a very elegant description of my tracking of the impact of my presence upon Louisa. This was framed within the notion of the recursive loop of being a burden, but it very accurately attuned to my own struggles to calibrate my contact in a way that Louisa found growthful.

SUMMARY

Having read the four comments on the transcript, I am left with a sense of range and variety between the writers. In many ways, for me this is part of the excitement, creativity, and vitality of Gestalt psychotherapy.

On a more somber note, however, I can feel myself left with some lingering discomfort at quite how much variation there is in the maps and models that have been used to discuss the work. I am reminded of some hot debates that have taken place in various Gestalt conferences regarding "What is and is not Gestalt therapy?" This question has traditionally caused me to bridle, feeling a sense of stultification, control, and judgment being potentially used to erode the spontaneous and vital aspect that is at the heart of our work. I believe that Gestalt psychotherapy is unique in its ability to orientate to growth, health, and change as well as distress, despair, and pain, and I am committed to bringing this work to my more fragile clients within the healthcare system.

I now find myself, however, reflecting again upon what are the essential qualities of Gestalt therapy and Gestalt therapy theory. What precisely is it that enables us to describe a case as one that employs "a Gestalt therapy frame" as opposed to say an integrationist perspective or an intersubjective one?

This process of defining Gestalt therapy is not just of theoretical interest but also of intense pragmatic value. My fear is that if we cannot agree on ways of describing and formulating cases, then we cannot fulfill the fundamental requirements needed to research the validity and efficacy of our approach. Namely, the work should be able to be described and replicated in method if not in practice.

Maybe it is this issue at the heart of our approach that explains why we have failed to respond to the challenge of providing adequate research into the outcome of Gestalt psychotherapy. This lack of validation and empirical support is now proving a serious difficulty for those of us wishing to work in environments where an "evidence-based approach" is called for. I firmly believe that if we are to respond to this challenge, it is only by describing cases and beginning to agree on ways of discussing our approach that we will begin to put forward some key signposts and milestones that we might all be able to converge around.

REFERENCES

Beaumont, H. (1993). Martin Buber's 'I-Thou' and fragile self-organisation: Gestalt couples therapy. *British Gestalt Journal, 2/2,* 85–95.

Clarkson, P. (1989). *Gestalt counseling in action*. London: Sage.

Jacobs, L. (1992). Insights from psychoanalytic self-psychology and intersubjectivity theory for Gestalt therapists. *The Gestalt Journal, 15/2,* 25–60.

Jacobs, L. (1995). Self psychology, intersubjectivity theory, and Gestalt therapy: A dialogic perspective. In R. Hycner & L. Jacobs (Eds.), *The healing relationship in Gestalt therapy: A dialogic/self psychology approach* (pp. 129–158). Highland, NY: Gestalt Journal Press.

Kohut, H. (1971). *The analysis of the self*. New York: International Universities Press.

Lewin, K. (1951). *Field theory in social science: Selected theoretical papers* (D. Cartwright, Ed.). New York: Harper & Brothers.

Parlett, M. (1991). Reflections on field theory. *British Gestalt Journal, 1/2,* 69–81.

Perls, F. S., Hefferline, R. F., & Goodman, P. (1951). *Gestalt therapy: Excitement and growth in the human personality*. New York: Julian Press.

Polster, E. (1991). Tight therapeutic sequences. *British Gestalt Journal, 1/2,* 63–68.

Stolorow, R. D., Brandchaft, B., & Atwood, G. E. (1987). *Psychoanalytic treatment: An intersubjective approach*. Hillsdale, NJ: Analytic Press.

Stratford, C. D., & Brallier, L. W. (1979). Gestalt therapy with profoundly disturbed persons. *The Gestalt Journal, 2/1,* 90–103.

Yontef, G. M. (1993). *Awareness, dialogue, and process: Essays on Gestalt therapy*. Highland, NY: Gestalt Journal Press.

Yontef, G. M. (2002). The relational attitude in Gestalt therapy theory and practice. *International Gestalt Journal, 25/1,* 15–35.

Editors' Introduction

This case study was specifically selected by Myrna Weissman and Lena Verdeli to illustrate the principles of interpersonal psychotherapy (IPT) they describe in their chapter in Current Psychotherapies. *Although this approach is used in the treatment of a wide variety of disorders, it was initially developed as a treatment for depression, and most of the research done with IPT has looked at the therapy as an intervention used with depressed clients. This case illustrates the use of IPT to treat a depressed woman who is romantically involved with a married man.*

The patient is a part of a randomized clinical trial, and treatment is specific, detailed, and manualized. The treatment focuses on interpersonal disputes, and the therapist (a) seeks information; (b) explores parallels in various relationships; (c) explores relationship patterns; and (d) explores the client's communication patterns. In addition, the therapist signals what is likely to be significant; provides supports; explores affect; explores options; helps with problem solving; draws analogies; and challenges the client when necessary. The therapist also attempts to identify, describe, and classify the most salient themes that emerge during the course of therapy.

Do you think you will find comfort in an approach to therapy that is detailed, exacting, and specific—or is it likely that you will be more comfortable with an approach in which the therapist has wider latitude in determining "what do I do next?" Are manualized treatments best for inexperienced therapists? How much latitude can a therapist take with a manualized approach while still maintaining fidelity to the basic principles promulgated by the manual?

9 | A CASE STUDY FOR THE NEW IPT THERAPIST

Marie Crowe and Sue Luty

Background. X was a 42-year-old divorced female with a son aged 25. She heard about the study from a friend and self referred, aware that she had depressive symptoms. The diagnosis of major depressive disorder of moderate severity was made on the initial assessment interview by an experienced psychiatrist.

X's depression had occurred in the context of her mother's death from cancer three years previously, followed by the death of her father one year later. Major family conflict had then developed as her three half-siblings from her father's first marriage contested the will with her and her other three biological siblings. The patient lived alone in her own home and found her supports came from younger adults, many of whom were her son's friends. She had an active sporting life and worked with elderly people which she enjoyed and regarded as low stress. However, the lack of a supportive partner/intimate relationship was difficult for her.

X had no previously diagnosed episodes of depression but had been "down" during her violent marital relationship which had ended 15 years previously. All her intimate relationships since the divorce from her husband were "difficult," and she described herself as a person who was well liked by friends but was "not good at choosing men." X was brought up in a blended family with constant conflict between the two sets of half-siblings. Her father was a heavy drinker, and she had only recently begun to have a positive relationship with him. At the age of 16, she became pregnant and left home to marry the father of her child. She had always been close to her mother.

Symptomatically at the commencement of psychotherapy, she described low mood, loss of enjoyment, insomnia, loss of appetite, and described life as being "crappy; what's the point of going on?"

The psychotherapist and patient identified interpersonal role disputes as a focus. This involved relating X's symptoms to the dispute, determining the stage of the dispute and how it was perpetuated, understanding how nonreciprocal role expectations related to the dispute and exploring parallels in other relations.

Psychotherapeutic Interventions

From the transcripts of the sessions, there was an analysis of the psychotherapeutic interventions utilized by the psychotherapist which involved identifying and tracking the nature of the interventions used, when they were used, and their effect on the patient.

Excerpt from Crowe, M., & Luty, S. (2005). The process of change in interpersonal psychotherapy (IPT) for depression: A case study for the new IPT therapist. *Psychiatry, 68* (1), 43–54. Reprinted with permission.

This was then compared to Weissman's (2000, p. 25) description of the specific focus for interpersonal disputes:

- Seeking information on different levels
- Exploring parallels in other relationships
- Exploring relationship patterns
- Exploring the communication patterns that [the] patient draws on

Weissman has identified that although the techniques used in IPT are common to other psychodynamic psychotherapies, there are differences in how they are used. In IPT the techniques are used to treat a depressive episode rather than to increase insight. "Each technique is used in a specific sequence and with varying frequency, depending on the characteristics of the patient and the particular interpersonal problem the patient describes." The following are the psychotherapist's interventions that were identified by analyzing the transcripts of the sessions with X.

Seeking Information. During the beginning phase, the psychotherapist was setting the scene for the process of psychotherapy and conducting the interpersonal inventory.

- What is he like as a person?
- How often do you see him?
- What kind of things do you do together?
- Do you ever clash at all?
- Would you want the relationship to be different?

The information sought in this beginning phase enabled the therapist to formulate an interpersonal inventory that identified who was significant in the patient's life and any relationship issues that the patient found unsatisfactory.

Exploring Parallels in Other Relationships. The psychotherapist helped the patient to identify parallels between what she was currently experiencing and what had happened in past relationships:

- Has that happened to you in the past?
- Is that something you have done before?
- I guess you have learned this way of dealing with things.
- Your tendency has been to rush and fix things—"well, I will do it if no one else will."

The therapist also linked how the patient was currently responding to relationship issues and the way she had dealt with them in the past:

- Remember with your mom dying, things just took over and you didn't have time to really grieve.
- Did it bring up issues for you, about the losses before? Are there similarities to your mom?

The therapist explored what the patient had learned in past relationships that worked well for her and suggested that she identify the successful aspects so she could apply them to her current situation:

- You might be able to draw on things you have achieved in the past on what it was that worked.
- You have been able to see the elements that made it something you enjoyed and maybe you can create that again in a different way.

Most of these interventions occurred in the early middle sessions and appeared less often towards the end of the sessions.

Exploring Relationship Patterns. In the middle sessions, the therapist began to explore the patterns that the patient was describing in her relationships:

- It seems that there is a type of role that you have gotten yourself into.
- I guess that demonstrates that you chose a backward step because you knew there would be conflict.

The therapist moved from exploration to naming some of the patterns that were emerging:

- What do you think leads you to not being able to be assertive?
- Looking at different decisions, it might have been that you were trying to be all things to all people.
- It has been easier for you to sort of focus on other people rather than on yourself.

This shifted from exploration to suggesting how the patient might make some changes to the patterns:

- You have learned how not to compromise when probably what you need to do is practice compromise.
- We have already talked about you being in the caring role; maybe it is not what you want to do . . . you have overly stressed yourself and put yourself in situations of multi-tasking, but the future could be "let me do what I want to do," "let me do what I enjoy," or "I could be doing something that I feel much more motivated to do."

Another aspect of this phase involved the therapist suggesting how the patient might make changes:

- I guess this is a crucial thing about expectations in relationships, about being clear about what you want and what he wants.
- Perhaps you need to be clear about what you want for yourself, and that would make a difference.
- It is about looking after you, not other people, so that you can work through issues.

These interventions enabled both the therapist and the patient to identify repetitive experiences and patterns that were occurring in the patient's relationships.

Exploring Communication Patterns. This psychotherapeutic intervention involved clarifying how the patient communicated her feelings and wishes:

- How do you give him the message?
- Is that giving him the message that you don't actually want to see him?
- Is she [his wife] aware that you feel awful?

It also involved identifying problems in the patient's communication style:

- I guess sometimes you don't really talk about how badly you feel about yourself.
- What do you think leads you to not being able to be assertive?
- So that is a kind of giving excuses sort of thing.

The therapist encouraged the patient to try different ways of communicating by exploring it from the other person's perspective:

- What does she [his wife] need to be able to do to forgive you, do you think? What would you expect in that situation?

As the patient began to practice the changes in communication style, the therapist provided her with feedback:

- So you were direct with him, you were honest.
- So you stuck to your guns?
- Have you talked to her about it? What have you done about it?
- I guess you are still not saying I am not interested, I would like to be friends but that's all.

Other Interventions. Although the therapist utilized techniques specific to IPT, other techniques were also applied, but within an IPT context.

Signaling What Is Significant. One of the strategies that the therapist utilized in early sessions was to signal to the patient when she brought up an issue significant to the IPT process:

- That was an important thing to know about.
- It's good to voice that and just being aware of why.

Providing Support. Another strategy that was important in developing a therapeutic relationship involved providing the patient with acknowledgement of what she was experiencing and providing support for how she was managing:

- I see you have already made some fast steps . . . you have come to some decisions just by exploring them and thinking about them more in terms of "how helpful is this?"
- And you have been changing; you have been making some quite significant decisions which wouldn't have been easy.

Exploring Affect. Throughout the sessions the therapist drew connections between how the patient was feeling and how she expressed her feelings to others:

- What about the fact that you have been hurt; what about dealing with that a little bit; do you see what I mean?
- And how did you feel when that happened?

Exploring Options. The therapist encouraged the patient to explore the options she had in dealing with issues in her relationships:

- What were your choices; did you choose to retaliate or withdraw?
- It is a choice that you have got—you can either go and tolerate it or not go.
- What other choices do you have?

Problem-Solving. Throughout the middle phases in the IPT process, significant attention was given to approaching issues using problem-solving techniques:

- Let's look at what is going to be good for you and what is not, because that might help clarify the goal or what the need is.
- That's the same kind of thing with life decisions; you kind of narrow it down and start testing the waters, and if doesn't work, it doesn't work.

Drawing Analogy. A technique the therapist used which engaged the patient was that of making an analogy:

- When you say you are not sure [about what to do], it's like saying, I'm not sure about that color; what will I do? I will try that color, let's have a look, let's just see. Maybe I made the wrong decision or maybe I could go with that.

Challenging. The therapist also gently challenged some of the beliefs that underpinned the patient's decisions and challenged her to practice some new strategies:

- Is it really selfish? Following something you want to do, why should that be selfish just because other people say it is?

- I wonder if you can go away with a sense of testing the waters?

Weissman and colleagues suggest that the general goals of treatment in interpersonal role disputes are to help the patient first identify the dispute, then make choices about a plan of action, and finally modify maladaptive communication patterns or reassess expectations, or both, for a satisfactory resolution of the interpersonal dispute. Improvements may take the form of a change in the expectations and behavior of the patient and/or the other person; changed and more accepting patient attitudes with or without attempts to satisfy needs outside the relationship; or a satisfactory dissolution of the relationship.

The general IPT treatment strategy with interpersonal disputes is to help the patient understand how nonreciprocal role expectations relate to the dispute and begin steps that will bring about resolution of disputes and role negotiations. This involves movement from exploration to action.

The aim is to help patients recognize their complex, mixed feelings of anger, fear, and sadness, and devise strategies for managing them. Depressed patients typically have difficulty in asserting their needs and in appropriately expressing anger in interpersonal situations.

The Patient's Response to IPT

The following section presents the themes that emerged from the transcripts as the patient dealt with her mood and her relationships with others.

Struggling. The patient described her relationships with family members and friends and also identified a pattern of avoidance when faced with conflicts—"I do try to avoid as much as I can to do with them." She also expressed some uncertainty about relationship expectations—"I don't know what I expect from my friends; I don't know if what I expect is realistic." She described how she learned avoidance as a child:

> Most of our childhood was just spent trying to not be seen essentially, all we heard was a lot of yelling . . . all we heard was lots of yelling and screaming and the less you were noticed the better.

The patient also revealed a number of significant losses that she had experienced over the previous two years, including the death of both parents and of a close friend, and how she had not allowed herself to fully experience her grief.

> I tell you at that stage I still hadn't grieved for mum, death was fine, I don't know to be honest, I didn't really feel much, I wasn't feeling anything.

It also became apparent that she often took on most of the responsibilities in her relations with others and that she managed any interpersonal disputes either by avoidance or placating.

> At the time, I thought keeping everything smooth was fine, I mean not just for me but for everyone, doing what I thought was best for all of us.

However when she entered psychotherapy she was feeling overwhelmed by the responsibilities she had taken on.

> Before, I always managed to survive but just recently I stopped [being able to survive], it is such a struggle.

The patient had been able to identify that her struggle with depression was associated with her pattern of 1) avoiding conflict and a role where she became the pacifier, and 2) her feelings of grief that she suppressed rather than feel overwhelmed by.

Deconstructing. During this phase of the psychotherapy, the patient identified a theme of selflessness that influenced her decision-making in regard to relationships.

A lot of the things I have chosen to do is because I don't want to be selfish.

She identified a fear of being regarded as selfish underpinning many of her decisions and that many of her decisions were influenced by her attempt to not appear selfish.

I think a lot of things I do and why I make a lot of decisions is to oppose that I am just being selfish, but it doesn't make me any happier.

The patient made the connection that although she had strived not to be selfish, it had not made her happy. She was able to identify what had made her happy and the elements which were most satisfying.

I liked being free . . . it is a feeling where you have got to rely on yourself and it is just you against everything, just you with nature, and it is a great feeling. You have to rely on your own know-how, your own skill, strength.

The patient identified self-reliance as a significant experience that brought her happiness but which was currently absent in her life, a life that involved many relationships in which she felt responsible for others. She also accepted the therapist's challenge to think about selfishness differently.

I think maybe I have done my time and maybe I am allowed to . . . be selfish.

As a result of beginning to see some patterns in her relationships, the patient then expressed trepidation about becoming involved in a new relationship.

I am scared of the whole thing about relationships, because there seems to be a pattern, you have to do what other people want you to do, otherwise they don't work.

Her uncertainty about relationships related to the role of pacification she had adopted.

Make it smooth, try and smooth it over, be the mediator, make the peace, do what ever they want to keep it quiet.

She described the struggle she had been having as feeling overwhelmed and not in control of what had been happening to her.

Sometimes it is very hard to keep on that Pollyanna kind of thing when things are just constantly happening and to me it just sometimes you know, you are just starting to feel good and something else pops up, something else trips you up.

The patient had been able to deconstruct her experiences in relationships with others and identified the particular aspects that were causing her problems: her judgments about selfishness, her need to feel self-reliant, and a need to feel more in control of her life.

Connecting. This next phase in the improvement trajectory occurred as the patient began to make connections for herself between her mood and what had been happening in her relationships. The first connection she made was about her need to trust herself more.

Maybe if I can't trust myself I can't trust other people.

After exploring what had been happening she realized that not all aspects of her life were bad.

I say, look our lives aren't really that bad when you look at the good things.

She also realized that she had not always been as passive as she had perceived herself.

A lot of them have been kind of a non-decision, I have to admit, but that is a decision in itself.

The patient made some connections between the role she had been assuming in relationships and her mood.

I thought keeping everything smooth was fine, I mean not just for me but for everyone, doing what I thought was best for all of us . . . I was thinking what's the point and then I thought things have got to change, they've certainly got to change.

At this point in the psychotherapy, she began to realize that things were not as hopeless as she thought and that change was possible.

I guess it is actually determination; you have just got to keep plugging on and on and on and maybe have a bit of optimism.

She had made a connection between her mood and her role in relationships, which enabled her to consider other possibilities. She described the process of change as a process of remediation but recognized that it was not going to be easy.

This is like my remedial life lessons . . . but it is so hard, it's actually really hard to do.

She reminded herself of the importance of attending to her own needs which she had not considered important before.

The thing that keeps ringing through is unless you are true to yourself, you know, life ain't going to work. Now it is ringing through, it didn't ring through before; I didn't even hear anything before.

In response to the therapist's identification of the achievements she had made, the patient realized that she had made progress and that she wanted to make further progress.

Pat on the back, yeah, yeah, sometimes if I get time I can sit and think OK yeah little changes, not major ones, and I can see them, I mean other people might not but I can see them. Maybe just wanting a change is good . . . yeah I am getting it, I am sure I am getting there. I wasn't so certain this week, but I still want to get there which is good. I still take little steps, but it just means trusting myself which is the hard one.

The significant themes that emerged through this phase of the patient's improvement were related to the connections she made about the roles she had been assuming in relationships and how she could make changes.

Practicing. This next phase involved putting into action what she had learned from the connections she had made about her lack of assertiveness and her over-responsible role in relationships.

I actually just said no, look I can't cope, I can't do it, I have other things to do; she was really nice, so that was alright.

She began to set boundaries around her role.

It's their problem. It's not my problem.

She realized what she had been gaining from putting other's needs before her own.

I mean it is lovely that they all love you and want you there and need to see you but it is kind of like a bit here bit there, bit there—you are just pulled in millions of directions. But I survived that too.

With the realization of the trap she had set for herself in wanting to be wanted, by placing her own needs as subordinate, she was able to identify that she needed to communicate what she wanted in a more direct manner.

I am just going to have to be more honest with him and say definitely not. It is throwing me out; I really don't need to worry about having a relationship . . . I just didn't really know whether I wanted to be myself at that stage.

As she began to practice different roles and different methods of communicating, the patient became clearer about what it was that she needed.

I just want time to be me.

The positive experience of being more assertive and being more direct enabled the patient to make a clear statement about what it was she needed.

Reconstructing. The final phase of the improvement trajectory involved the patient being able to articulate a reconstructed sense of self. She gave herself permission to accept her feelings as important and described herself in a more positive manner.

Maybe it is just kind of a reaffirmation of the fact that it is OK to feel how I am feeling and um you know, I am not such a drop kick after all.

She realized that she needed to refocus her energy on herself and her own needs rather than expending it on meeting others' needs.

I was just thinking instead of giving all these other people my energy I could actually focus on myself.

She also described an occasion when she was tempted to revert to an old relationship pattern and how she resisted this because of the progress she had made.

At one stage I thought it would actually be nice to go and get a big hug from [male friend] and have sex and lie in his arms and just cuddle and I thought no, no, NO, NO . . . this is a nice temporary measure and I thought yeah this is OK.

Towards the final IPT sessions, the patient identified a significant improvement in mood and how this has not resulted in a major life reconstruction but rather a reconstruction in the way she perceived herself and the changes she had made.

I feel better, I was just thinking today, the situation hasn't changed, I just don't feel as bad about it . . . I know that I am just feeling OK, it is feeling good, I am feeling like a person, I mean there are still things I need to think about like work and how I feel about that . . . but basically as a human being I am feeling OK, and it doesn't mean my life has changed that much, I mean I am still in the same position but it feels OK.

The improvement in mood that was facilitated by the IPT process had enabled the patient to have a more hopeful view of her future.

Now that I am feeling better I might actually be able to see where the opportunities are, whereas I was just so wound up, I just couldn't see anything. I just couldn't see a damn thing, I needed a guide dog.

The patient employed the metaphor of a guide dog to describe how she had experienced the IPT sessions. It had enabled her to make sense of her mood, connect it to her pattern of interpersonal relationships, and change some of her roles and communication styles.

DISCUSSION

This case study of the patient's improvement can be validated by plotting her mood based on self-reported BDI-II scores. (See Figure 1.) From this figure, it can be seen that the patient was experiencing severe depressive symptoms at the commencement of IPT (BDI-II range: severe 29–63, moderate 20–28, mild 14–19, minimal 0–13). Her symptoms improved at a consistent rate until she rated them as mild at the end of her 12 sessions of IPT. During the 3-month follow-up, the symptoms were in the non-depressed range. This is consistent with the process of recovery in IPT observed by Weissman and colleagues. It is of interest that there was a marked improvement in mood during the second week of IPT and then the process of improvement was more gradual over the following weeks.

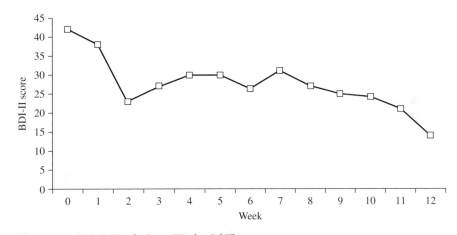

Figure 1.   BDI-II Totals Over Weeks Of Therapy

The Process of Change

At the commencement of IPT, this patient rated her depressive symptoms as severe. Her symptoms occurred in an interpersonal context; she was engaged in relationships that were both contributing to and being affected by her mood. The role she had adopted in her relationships, that of a pacifier, involved her taking responsibility for others. She described learning this behavior as a child as a way of protecting herself in family conflicts, and it could be regarded as a motivating influence for her to learn to suppress her feelings. A deconstruction of what it meant to be "selfish" enabled the patient to make connections between trusting herself and trusting others—and between her pacifier role and the need to be "true" to herself. After making these connections she was able to practice different communication strategies which enabled her to be more direct and assertive. In the final sessions, it was evident that she had developed confidence in these new practices and in herself.

The IPT enabled the patient to make a shift from regarding herself and her situation as hopeless to "feeling like a person" and seeing opportunities in her future. She described the content of her IPT sessions as "remedial life lessons" and the process like having "a guide dog," enabling her to make significant changes which she attributed to seeing things more clearly.

This case study provides details about the process of IPT which is helpful for therapists working with IPT or training to become an IPT therapist. Further in-depth validation or replication of the process of change in IPT will enable a more comprehensive understanding of the factors that influence a positive response to the psychotherapeutic process.

Editors' Introduction

With family therapy there is the same dilemma we faced with behavior therapy: Dozens of good teaching cases are available, but it is virtually impossible to select a single case that will adequately illustrate the multiple and variegated techniques used by most family therapists. Ultimately we elected to use a strategic therapy case to serve as an exemplar of family therapy.

We feel fortunate to have been able to locate the following case by Peggy Papp. It demonstrates the effective treatment of the family of a young anorectic woman and demonstrates the use of a "Greek Chorus"—a group of observing therapists who remain behind a one-way mirror. The Greek Chorus is always available to consult with the therapist, and the group will periodically make recommendations about treatment. Family therapists, more than any other group, have used such procedures to good advantage. Would you feel comfortable having your own work scrutinized this closely?

The case describes the treatment of a young woman with anorexia nervosa. The longer this life-threatening disorder remains untreated, the more intractable it becomes. How would this client have been treated differently if seen by a psychoanalyst, a behavior therapist, or someone practicing rational emotive behavior therapy? Would a person-centered therapist, committed to authenticity in the therapeutic relationship, feel comfortable with the manipulation inherent in the use of paradoxical intention? How do you feel about this therapeutic tactic? How do the values of a therapist affect decisions about which tools in the psychotherapist's armamentarium are appropriate in any given case?

10 | THE DAUGHTER WHO SAID NO

Peggy Papp

This case illustrates the step-by-step process of putting concepts into practice over time. It describes the treatment of a 23-year-old anorectic daughter and her family who present the classical pattern of an anorectic family: a high degree of enmeshment, covert alliances between the generations, subverted conflict, and power struggles fought with guilt and martyrdom.

The parents, in rigidly symmetrical positions, are in constant conflict and divert this conflict through Rachel, the anorectic daughter, hence isolating her from her siblings and the world of her peers. The therapeutic dilemma centers around what will happen to Rachel and the various members of her family if she gives up her symptom and becomes a full-blown woman. The consultation group is used to debate this dilemma, and the sibling subsystem is enlisted to free Rachel from her involvement in the parental generation.

Twenty sessions were held over the period of one year with a one-, two- and three-year follow-up. All sessions were videotaped and observed behind a one-way mirror.

For the purpose of clarity, the case is broken down into stages according to the following outline.

Stage I: *Forming a hypothesis*

    Step 1: Gathering information

    Step 2: Connecting the symptom with the family system

Stage II: *Setting the terms for therapy*

    Step 1: Defining the therapeutic dilemma

    Step 2: Setting the terms for change

Stage III: *Putting the therapeutic contract into operation*

    Step 1: Involving father in the therapeutic dilemma

    Step 2: Dramatizing the therapeutic dilemma

Stage IV: *Coping with the forces of change*

    Step 1: Defining change within the therapeutic contract

Stage V: *Coping with the fallout from change*

    Step 1: Defining resistance within the therapeutic framework

    Step 2: Shifting the definition of the problem

    Step 3: Prescribing enmeshment

Stage VI: *Enlisting the sibling subsystem*

    Step 1: Forming a coalition with the sisters

    Step 2: Differentiating from the sisters

Stage VII: *Saying no to therapy*

    Step 1: Pushing the prescription to the breaking point

    Step 2: Escalating the therapeutic triangle

    Step 3: Opposing the group

    Step 4: Supporting autonomy

Stage VIII: *Solidifying change*

    Step 1: Anticipating and rehearsing a regression

    Step 2: Redefining the marital relationship

Stage IX: *Prescribing a farewell ritual*

Follow-up

STAGE I
FORMING A HYPOTHESIS

Step 1: Gathering Information

The information I obtained from the first session is summarized here since information gathering tends to make tedious reading. Rachel, 23, requested therapy for herself, and her sisters, Clare, 31, and Sandy, 26; her mother agreed to participate in therapy, but her father emphatically refused. Having been pushed into various kinds of therapy by his wife for the last five years, he told Rachel in no uncertain terms she would have to solve her problem herself.

I agreed to see the family without him, believing I could involve him later. Some therapists will not see the family unless everyone is present for the first session. Since my way of dealing with resistance is indirect rather than direct, my decisions are based on an evaluation of each case. In this situation it seemed important to go along with father's resistance since it was obviously a reaction to his wife's pressure. Also, the intensity of his feelings was a good indication he could be involved at a later date.

Only mother and Rachel appeared for the first interview as Sandy was in the hospital having her first baby and Clare refused to come after a fight with Rachel.

Rachel appeared frail and flat-chested, but animated, with huge dark eyes and a thin face. She was exceptionally articulate, expressing herself in colorful language and sometimes adding a comic delivery. Her mother, a large, handsome, robust woman with short, white hair, stylishly cut, possessed the style and flair of a seasoned actress. With the exuberance of Lady Bountiful she embraced family therapy, saying she "believed" family members should help one another and she would do anything to help Rachel. She tempered each criticism of her with "there's really nothing wrong with you, you're a wonderful child, but—."

Rachel had begun dieting four years ago during her second year at college. Since that time she had slowly but steadily lost weight until she finally weighed 89 pounds. She had not menstruated for a year and a half. During the last three years she had made several attempts to leave home but failed, each time feeling depressed, isolated, lonely, and coming back home. She now had an interim job as a secretary but was dissatisfied with it. Although living at home, she was talking about moving into an apartment of her own.

The primary concern of Rachel and her mother was not her weight loss or her diet, but the psychological implications, which they saw in terms of Rachel's intrapsychic problems. Rachel's previous individual therapy of one year had focused on the classical individual symptoms of anorexia—high expectations, overachievement, perfectionistic attitudes, obsessions, and control over the body—but had not connected these in any way with the family system.

The mother was interested in our helping Rachel with her high expectations of herself, describing her as being "obsessively and rigidly perfectionistic." She also stated Rachel had been a rebellious child all her life. "I have been worried about Rachel since she learned to say no. It has been no and no and no and no and no and no and no ever since then. She has not wanted to adopt any of our standards, and I question her judgment." She gave as an example of this Rachel's not wanting to join B'nai B'rith or date Jewish boys, and her tendency to pick a boy up off the street and make a date with him. Rachel accused her mother of matchmaking. "I feel like it's mating season. I'm in heat and it's time to find a male for me quick before I'm not eligible anymore. I don't enjoy that." Mother then mentioned drugs, and Rachel admitted she had experimented in college with pot, speed, LSD, and mescaline and ended with, "I don't regret anything."

Mother had kept everything away from father over the years to protect Rachel and to avoid a conflict. When asked what he would have done had he known about these things, she stated "I don't know. I wasn't going to give him a chance! The girls have accused me of being manipulative and maybe I am but I have to be." She spoke of the many disagreements between her and her husband, describing a longstanding conflict because of her closeness with her parents.

At the end of the session, after consultation with the team, I told Rachel and her mother we felt we did not have enough information at this point to make any suggestions and would like to delay our comments until we had met with other members of the family. Rachel agreed to try and get Clare to come to the next session but Sandy was still recuperating from the birth of her baby.

In the following session, Clare, a thin, attractive woman, fashionably dressed, was more than happy to give her impressions of Rachel and other family members. She described Rachel as being "very difficult" and her family as being one in which it was difficult to become independent, as her mother was controlling and "throws guilt around a lot." Both she and Rachel had rebelled against her mother's control, but Sandy "is the model daughter, model sister, model grandchild and, now having had a baby, will be the model mother. She never displeases anyone. She is the buffer, the peacemaker."

Both Rachel and Clare spoke of their being afraid of their father when they were growing up. He was very conservative and strict about dates, two-piece bathing suits, boyfriends, hours, and so on. The mother, more lenient, took this opportunity to say that she was also afraid of his wrath and stated pathetically, "Thank God he never hit me." She compared him unfavorably with her own father and started to cry. "I tried very hard to get my family to help me, and my father would talk to my husband in a gentle manner and say how precious a wife is, how nothing really was as precious as a wife, and really she's the only one who is most important in life. But my husband would become antagonistic toward such conversations." She went into individual therapy at the recommendation of her doctor when she developed stomach trouble, and her doctor put pressure on her husband to go with her. Both blamed him for her physical problems.

Rachel and Clare defended their father and accused their mother of being overly close to her family and rubbing the father's nose in it. Rachel then spoke of her father and her as being the "underdogs in the family. We're ostracized by the rest of them." Rachel had given me the first clue as to how she fit into the power struggle between her parents: She identified with the father's underdog position. I now wanted to know the function of this identification: how it was used in the ongoing day-to-day battle between the parents and how the sisters responded to it. The following dialogue was included to demonstrate how these questions were explored.

Peggy: So you feel you're the bad guy and your father is the bad guy in the family. In what way do you feel you can bring comfort to your father?

Rachel: Because I can understand his viewpoint.

Clare: If there are two bad guys, then you both share the burden?

Rachel: There's company.

Peggy: How do you go about giving him company?

Rachel: We have a lot of common interests, we both like cars and nature and the Bronx Zoo, and we have a good time. We go across the country together.

Peggy: What do you think his life would be like if you weren't around?

Rachel: I don't know—I guess he'd survive.

Peggy: Do you think he'd be lonely?

Rachel: Maybe, sometimes—I'm nice company for him.

Peggy: Then who would there be around to really understand him?

Rachel: (*Long pause.*) I don't know.

Peggy: You don't think your mother could understand him?

Rachel: She will never ever. I shouldn't say that, but as far as I can see, it'll be a very tough thing for my mother to ever understand how my father feels about her family. She will never ever see how he feels about her.

Mother: But who do I think of when I want somebody to make nice to me? I go right back to the womb. On Tuesday I spent the day with my mom and dad and it was a good day. It was a hard day. I took them shopping. They're very old.

Peggy: Do you feel they're the only ones who nurture you?

Mother: (*Nodding.*) Who really take care of me. I don't want anyone here to feel bad, but Sandy also takes care of me.

Rachel: But you demand too much. You're very hard to give to when you demand.

Peggy: Let's see then. When you feel ganged up on by Rachel and your husband, you then go for nurturing to your parents. And who does your husband go to?

Mother: There's always been a young man in his life who treats him like God. Now it's Roy.

Peggy: You're saying that he always finds someone who is like a son to him?

Mother: Yes, Roy is like a son.

Peggy: Was he disappointed he didn't have a son?

Mother: (*Whispers.*) Very.

Peggy: You whispered that "very." You don't want the girls to hear that?

Mother: (*Emphatically.*) Very displeased that he didn't have a son.

Peggy: Do you think they don't know that?

Rachel: I'm daddy's son.

Peggy: In what way have you been his son?

Rachel: Just—my interest in things which aren't typically feminine. I'm not scared of bugs, little things like that. Cars. Daddy asked me to cook hamburgers on the barbecue pit because I can handle it. (*She imitates a boy.*)

Peggy: What's that like for you to be his son?

Rachel: I kinda like it. (*She laughs and acts like a boy again.*) I don't mind, but I don't think he thinks of me as a boy.

Peggy: Do you think of yourself as a boy?

Rachel: No. I was saying that I felt so independent on this move. It always bugs me to depend on people.

Peggy: What do you think it's going to be like for him, your moving out?

Rachel: I think it's going to be all right for him. Already they're talking about switch-
          ing homes with me.
Peggy: Do you think he's going to miss you?
Rachel: Maybe. He said he was going to miss some things but not others.
Peggy: Well do you think your mother's going to be able to take care of his
          loneliness?
Rachel: Not unless she starts to look at him from a more objective point of view.
Peggy: Do you think you can teach her?
Rachel: I try, I really try. Then she accuses me of ganging up on her.
Clare: (*Defending mother.*) Daddy's not nice all the time, either.

Step 2: Connecting the Symptom with the Family System

After this exchange, the therapist left the session to have a consultation with the group.
We formed a hypothesis based on answering the following questions:

What function does the symptom serve in the system? We speculated that Rachel
was starving herself in order to remain a son to her father and fill up the emptiness
in his life that she perceived was left by her mother. By not eating, she kept herself
looking like a boy, prevented herself from maturing into womanhood, and implicitly
promised to remain the guardian of her parents' marriage. The symptom served to
keep her at home where she could continue to serve as her father's ally in his battle
with her mother and to give her mother a reason for remaining close to her family.
By identifying with her father as the underdog in the family, she formed a coalition
with him in the service of fighting against her mother's control. The symptom also
served the function of freeing the other sisters to establish independent lives outside
the family, since Rachel had accepted the responsibility of mediating the parents'
marriage.

How does the family function to stabilize the symptom? When mother and father
became involved in a power struggle that they could not resolve, mother moved closer
to her parents and compared father unfavorably to her own father. Father retaliated by
siding with Rachel against his wife, and Rachel joined him to get back at her mother.
She became involved in masculine activities to please her father, knowing he felt alienated in a family of women. She cannot give up the symptom as long as she believes she
is needed to be a son to him. The power struggle between mother and Rachel has taken
many forms over the years, including Rachel's taking drugs, quitting jobs, leaving school,
dating non-Jewish boys, and disassociating herself from the family's religious beliefs, as
well as her present symptom of self-starvation.

What is the central theme around which the problem is organized? The central
theme in this family seems to be control—who is going to control the beliefs and values of the others. This is a conventional family that places high value on conformity,
respectability, achievement, duty, and family loyalty. Mother is less concerned about
some of Rachel's other activities than she is about her not accepting the tenets of the
Jewish faith. She complains that her husband rejects her father's value of a wife as being something "precious."

Since we have not yet seen father and Sandy, we are unable at this point to obtain a
complete picture of the way each individual operates to maintain control around these
central issues.

What will be the consequences of change? If Rachel stopped being a son to her father, she would have to abandon him to what she perceives to be an unloving wife, and
she would also be robbed of her major weapon against mother. If she left home, mother
and father would have to face their conflicts alone and would probably create a triangle

involving Sandy or Clare. Mother might move even closer to her own parents and father closer to his surrogate son, Roy. This would widen the breach between the parents. If father agreed to come for therapy in order to try and resolve these issues, he would lose a major battle with his wife regarding the value of therapy.

Rachel would have to confront the outside world and its relationships rather than centering her life on the family. This would mean her taking responsibility for becoming an adult woman sexually, professionally, and socially.

What is the therapeutic dilemma? The family must decide between Rachel continuing to be symptomatic or facing the above consequences.

STAGE II
SETTING THE TERMS FOR THERAPY

Step 1: Defining the Therapeutic Dilemma

Our first intervention consisted of setting the terms for the therapeutic contest that was to follow by defining the problem as a family dilemma. The family had defined the problem as an individual one—Rachel's rebelliousness, her obsessions, rigid expectations, and self-starvation all were seen as being disconnected from the family. In defining the problem as a dilemma, we connected the symptom with the system.

Peggy entered the session with the following message:

Peggy: (*Sighs.*) We are stuck.

Mother: So are we.

Peggy: We are in a bind and I don't know what to do about it except just be very honest and open and tell you what we're stuck with. Rachel, we are very hesitant to help you in the way we were planning therapy to take, which would be to help you think and feel more like a woman, to gain weight, to have curves, to menstruate, to go out with boys, and to just be yourself. Because, you see, we are concerned about what will happen to your father, that he will become more isolated in a family of women, that he will turn more to his surrogate son, Roy, leaving your mother more alone, so that she will turn more to her own family. We are worried this will create an irreparable distance between the two of them.

Clare: It's a vicious cycle, isn't it?

Peggy: And, you see, we are concerned about all the members of your family, and when one person in the family changes, that changes the relationship of everybody.

Rachel: (*Long pause.*) I don't think I want to sacrifice myself for my parents. I don't think I care that much. I want to help myself right now.

Peggy: (*Still posing the dilemma.*) I can understand how you feel. I just want to make sure you are aware of the effect it will have. . . . Well, think about these things and decide what you want to do.

Clare: (*Suddenly becoming aware of the implication of the terms I have set.*) I want to say that I got very angry about what the group said. That you decided to change your tack. I think that is wrong. (*She bursts into tears.*) I'm worried about Rachel and that's not the thing to do for her.

Peggy: You feel that we should help her—?

Clare: Yes, that's terrible! How can you say because it will affect other members of the family—what should she do—starve herself?

Peggy: (*Puzzling over the dilemma.*) Well, you know, I think that has to be Rachel's decision and all we can do is—

Clare: But you function in that decision. You are here to help her.

Peggy: Well, you see, Rachel is so close to her family that—

Clare: I think that's terrible! (*She strides across the room and grabs a Kleenex.*) I obviously don't understand what's behind it. I think it's awful.

Peggy: We feel responsible—we feel obligated to let you know what we think the consequences of change will be and to prepare you for them.

There was a knock on the door and the group summoned me out for a brief consultation.

Step 2: Setting the Terms for Change

Rachel and Clare had reacted against the therapist's homeostatic position and were pressing for change. We decided to use this as an opportunity to bargain with them over the conditions of change and set the price as Rachel's agreement to turn the burden of her parents' unhappiness over to me. We were aware that the father might not agree to do this since he was boycotting therapy. However, it was our way of dramatizing the connection between Rachel's problem and her parents' unhappiness.

Peggy: (*Entering the session.*) The group wanted to let you know that they heard what you said and that they take it very seriously, and perhaps there is a way I can help you. (*Turning to Rachel.*) If you would be willing for me to see your parents together and for me to take on the responsibility of what will happen to them if you change, then perhaps you could begin to eat. Could you allow me to take on that responsibility rather than your shouldering it?

Rachel agreed to do this and mother was more than willing to have her husband brought into therapy.

Peggy: My group feels that then it would be safe for you to become a woman. And I will handle the consequences of that with your father and mother.

I informed them I would call father and ask him to attend the next session. To summarize the terms of therapy:

1. We defined Rachel's symptom as her remaining at home and failing to become a woman in order to stabilize the relationship between her parents.

2. We defined the relationship between her parents as not being able to tolerate her absence.

3. We defined the therapeutic dilemma as having to choose between helping Rachel to become a woman and preserving the stability of her parents' relationship.

4. We defined the solution and therefore the terms for change as Rachel's agreeing to pass the responsibility for preserving her parents' relationship to us. This set up the following situation: If the parents allowed us to help them with their relationship, thus releasing Rachel, she would be relieved of her burden and able to leave home. If they did not, we would ask someone else in the family to take on the burden, or else pass it back to Rachel. By making a hot potato of the parents' unhappiness and passing it around to various members of the family, we would dramatize the therapeutic dilemma.

STAGE III
PUTTING THE THERAPEUTIC
CONTRACT INTO OPERATION

Step 1: Involving Father in the Therapeutic Dilemma

After this session I telephoned Sam, the father, and told him I respected his wish not to be involved in family therapy but since his wife had probably given me a one-sided view of the family situation, I would like to get his impressions over the telephone. He was more than willing to share these and spent the next half hour talking about how his wife put too many expectations on Rachel at too early an age, pushed her to leave home and go away to college at 16, and how he had nothing to say about it because his wife controlled the children and paid no attention to his opinions. He ended the conversation by saying he would be willing to come in for a session if it would help Rachel. I told him I would let him know when I thought it would be helpful, not wanting to seem overly eager about his becoming involved.

A week later Rachel moved away from home into her own apartment and I asked the father to come in for a session. He agreed, but only if Rachel and his wife were present, as he didn't want to be in a session with four women. His terms were accepted, and I began by informing him that we had discovered that Rachel was reluctant to leave home for fear he might be lonely if left alone with his wife. He initially scoffed at this idea, but as I began to discuss the family dinners in which Rachel sided with him against mother and her family, he validated the hypothesis. He admitted that he and Rachel had a lot in common. "We identify in certain ways, we understand each other." Rachel agreed with this.

Peggy: What else do you understand about each other?

Father then described a family dinner held with his wife's family at which he sat next to Rachel for comfort and mother had commented, "Like Robin Hood and his men, they gang up and snicker."

Peggy: What will happen at these dinners when Rachel is not there anymore? I worry about what will happen to your father when you're not there. He will be losing an ally.
Rachel: He won't assimilate.
Father: I don't understand what's going on. I don't think she's worried about me in every situation. Do you think about me when there's a party?
Rachel: Of course I'm concerned about you. It makes me feel bad when you're both unhappy.
Peggy: How do you know when either of them is unhappy? What are the signals?
Rachel: When I speak to mother I hear about things that aren't happy in her life, and vice versa. I don't think either of you should keep me out of it, though. You shouldn't try to hide it.
Peggy: Do you think you can be helpful to them?
Rachel: I could be—I don't think they think I care.
Mother: I don't think she doesn't care about us. She cares desperately. She's been very helpful, she picks up my spirits, talks to me when I'm feeling down.
Peggy: I guess you're not only worried about what will happen to your father when you're not there, but to your mother also.

Rachel agreed with this, and mother and father began to quarrel about their respective needs and sensitivities.

Peggy:	(*Again using parental conflict as an opportunity to define why Rachel cannot leave home.*) What will happen when Rachel is not there?
Father:	She's not there now.
Peggy:	What is happening?
Father:	We're having a bad time the last few months.
Peggy:	Maybe you'd better go back home, Rachel.
Rachel:	I'm not going home.
Mother:	I don't want her home. We can straighten out our lives better without her there.
Peggy:	Can you? Can you do it?
Father:	But if she wanted to be home—I don't think we would—I don't—right, Helen?
Peggy:	(*To Rachel.*) It's a tremendous temptation, isn't it?
Rachel:	No. I don't really want to go back there. I don't.
Mother:	I'm glad.
Peggy:	I don't know. How are the two of you going to make it on your own?
Mother and Father:	(*Together.*) I don't know.
Rachel:	Do you think it's going to go on like this forever?

Father said again that it was no concern of hers, but Rachel kept insisting it was and that they try and work it out.

Rachel:	I'd like it if you could both be happy.
Father:	How could we do that?
Rachel:	I don't know, but you're certainly not trying.

At this point I explained to father that during a previous session the group had counseled me not to help Rachel unless she agreed to release the responsibility of their unhappiness to me. I asked if he would be willing for me to take on that responsibility and he refused my offer. Mother then put pressure on father.

Mother:	You see how Sam calls the shots? When you say you won't come here to help us, I'm at your mercy.
Father:	I didn't want to start in the beginning. I've been through this and it didn't help.
Peggy:	Yes, you told me that.
Mother:	What bothers you? Do you feel vulnerable? Do you feel it is an undue expenditure? What is more important—an undue expenditure or our happiness?
Father:	Why do I have to be put in the position of choosing on the basis of what is important?
Mother:	There we are!
Father:	So it's therapy or nothing?
Mother:	Of course. It's not important—we're not important.
Peggy:	You may be able to work it out without therapy, but what concerns me is are you going to be able to work it out without Rachel?
Mother:	We should be able to go hang ourselves and have it not affect Rachel.
Peggy:	But how are you going to keep Rachel out of it?

The parents argued and Rachel tried to mediate. The therapist took a break to have a consultation with the group.

Step 2: Dramatizing the Therapeutic Dilemma

The group agreed that if I continued to pressure father to come into therapy I would be siding with mother and he would resist more and more. We decided the group should support his autonomy and recommended that the burden of the parents' unhappiness should be passed to Sandy. Since Sandy was considered a superhuman being and this was a superhuman job, she seemed the appropriate person. I read the following message:

> The group, not having met Sam before, is impressed with his ability to take care of himself. Somehow, the family mythology had led us to believe otherwise. We trust mother has the strength to do the same. As for Rachel, she has carried the burden of her parents' unhappiness long enough and should now pass the burden to Sandy.

All three burst into laughter. Father asked if I had met Sandy, and I replied, "No, but I'm looking forward to it." Rachel said they were just talking about what a super person she was, and I replied, "Then we've chosen the right person for the job."

Father offered to keep coming to the sessions on the basis of helping Rachel but not to work on his relationship with his wife. Sandy accompanied the family to the following session.

STAGE IV
COPING WITH THE FORCES OF CHANGE

Step I: Defining Change Within the Therapeutic Contract

Rachel began the session by reporting a sudden and unexpected change. She had started menstruating for the first time in a year and a half and gained several pounds. Following through on my definition of the problem, I gave father credit for convincing Rachel he could manage his life without her.

Rachel: I have to tell you something exciting that's happened. I got my period. It's very exciting.

Peggy: You did?

Rachel: Yes, at my sister's surprise party. (*Much laughter.*)

Peggy: Is this the first time?

Rachel: In a year and a half. I stopped expecting it.

Peggy: You've decided to become a woman?

Rachel: (*Laughingly.*) I'm considering it.

Peggy: You'd better think this over carefully.

Rachel: I know it's a big step.

Peggy: (*To the parents.*) Well, how do the two of you feel about what's happening to her?

Father: Very much relieved that she's on her own path. Things are becoming more normal—not altogether, but approaching it.

Peggy: You're not afraid you're going to lose your companion?

Father: No, I'm praying for it. (*Laughter.*) I was pleased that Rachel is approaching normalcy. She also said she gained three pounds. She is very happy about it. Didn't seem to worry about the three pounds.

Peggy: I think you did a very good job.

Father: I did?

Peggy: Yes, I think you did a very good job. Last time you were here you convinced Rachel you could manage your life without her, that you would be okay, that even if your marriage wasn't the greatest or if you didn't stay together that—

Father: Well, we didn't tell these kids that yet. (*Referring to the other sisters.*)

Peggy: Well, but you told that to Rachel and I think you did an excellent job in assuring her you're going to be okay and that it's okay for her to become an independent woman.

Father: And in the last two weeks things are even better between Helen and me.

Sandy was informed of our having designated her to relieve Rachel of the burden of the parents' unhappiness. Everyone reacted with amusement. Sandy refused, saying she had a new baby and besides the parents seemed to be handling their own burden now.

STAGE V
COPING WITH THE FALLOUT FROM CHANGE

Step I: Defining Resistance Within the Therapeutic Framework

Neither Rachel nor her family were prepared for this amount of change and Rachel suffered a relapse. We immediately realized our mistake in not anticipating the consequences of change and predicting a relapse to lessen the chance of its occurrence. The family used the Jewish holidays as a way of recreating the family turmoil, with Rachel at the center. By refusing to go to synagogue on Passover, she created a minor crisis. Mother reacted in her characteristic fashion by provoking guilt, father tentatively supported Rachel, and Rachel became depressed to keep attention focused on her. She tearfully complained about her apartment, her job, the classes she was taking, and ended with: "There's nothing good about my life right now."

The whole family became involved in trying to analyze Rachel's depression and giving her helpful advice about how to pull herself out of it. Father brought up the inflammatory subject of Rachel not having gone to temple on Passover and asked if her depression was related to her feeling guilty. She denied this, and father stated: "That's good." Mother vehemently disagreed with him. During the following exchange they spoke simultaneously.

Mother: I don't think that's good, that's my problem. I see it as bad that Rachel, who loves us and whom we love, can do something to make us feel badly continuously and continuously—

Father: That's something for us to get used to—

Mother: When it would be good if she would do something to make us feel good.

Father: Helen—no—that's—(*Indecipherable.*)

Rachel: How can you expect me to do something I don't believe?

Father: Helen, that's something—(*Indecipherable.*)

Mother: But you do believe. You've told me you believe.

Father: Helen, she believes in a different way.

Rachel: But I don't. I believe in my fashion. I don't believe in keeping kosher, I don't believe in going to temple, I don't believe in dating Jewish boys, I don't believe that!

Mother: All right. And I believe, Rachel, that it is a sign of not quite loving us enough! I see it as a very selfish kind of act. You have no consideration. She's liable to do exactly what she wants to do because she doesn't want to please us. She's very rebellious.

Mother then went into a long harangue, giving a history of Rachel's rebelliousness. She ended up talking about how important the Jewish tradition was to her.

Mother: I've cried about the continuation of our Jewish tradition.

Rachel: I'm sorry, Mommy; you can cry and cry, but I'm not going to become more Jewish because you cry.

Mother: Therefore, then I don't think that you love us very much.

Rachel: Well, Mommy, if that's your criteria, then I really can't help you.

Mother: Okay, these are my feelings. That's my criteria. Yes.

Peggy: If she really loved you enough, she'd believe what you believe?

Mother: No, dear, no; because I know she believes. She's told me she believes. She believes in God. She says the most important prayer in our religion every night of her life, which I don't do.

Rachel: Why not? Don't you love me?

Mother: Rachel, stop shouting at me.

Peggy: You didn't answer her.

Mother: Why don't I say that prayer? Have you ever asked me to join you in that prayer?

Rachel: No, it's a private prayer. You're supposed to say it by yourself.

Mother: So why are you shouting at me?

Rachel: Why don't you say that prayer? You love me?

Mother accused Rachel of being sarcastic. I asked father if he felt the same way as mother about Rachel's not going to temple. He said he would like her to attend but didn't feel as intensely as his wife. I then asked Clare and Sandy if they had a problem becoming independent in this family, and both answered in the affirmative, describing the pressure and guilt that were applied to them throughout their lives. Asked how they dealt with this, Clare replied she didn't let her parents know about half of what she was doing, and Sandy said she always did what she wanted to do. Both parents were attacked for their rigidity, and the session ended with everyone quarrelling over who was most to blame.

The group was not present during this session and the family was told they would receive a message from them after they had seen the tape. In a consultation with the team, I defined the relapse as a systems problem rather than an individual one and sent the following message:

> It is the conviction of the group that Rachel has wisely decided she has not yet finished her job of diverting her parents from their unhappiness. Since Sandy and Clare have refused to accept this job, she should return home until it is completed.

It was then agreed that at the next session I would take a more lenient position regarding this message, encouraging Rachel's independence in opposition to an adamant position from the group, thus intensifying the triangle between therapist, family, and group.

Step 2: Shifting the Definition of the Problem

In the following session, Rachel adamantly refused to return home and the parents insisted they did not need her anymore to solve their marital problem. Rachel reacted to this exclusion by complaining about every aspect of her life—her job, her apartment, her boss, her feelings of isolation and loneliness. As she enumerated her complaints, the family, following their characteristic pattern, gave her "helpful" advice replete with platitudes about how to pull herself up by her own bootstraps.

We saw Rachel's litany of complaints as a reaction to giving up her important job of repairing her parent's marriage and decided to ask the family to allow her to mourn her leave taking rather than trying to cheer her up. This was impossible for them to do.

Peggy: The group has observed that Rachel's unhappiness seems to be a reproach to you and you're not allowing her to be unhappy. Rachel, they want to say that it's very important that you are unhappy and that your family allow you to be. How can you get them to allow you to be unhappy?

Rachel: I'll just have to keep away from them, I guess.

Father: Then we would worry about her.

Mother: I worry about my children, especially when they're alone.

Peggy: This is supposed to be a happy family, so it's difficult for you to allow anyone in the family to feel unhappy.

Mother: Are you speaking about a facade, Peggy?

Peggy: All families are supposed to be happy. This is a very close family, so it is very important for you to feel that everyone's happy. And when anyone is unhappy (*Mother sobs*), it's really hard, isn't it? How can you get mother to allow you to be unhappy?

Rachel: I don't know. I can't reassure her.

Mother: (*Sobbing.*) I worry about you every day.

Clare then jumped in to say she never told her mother her problems because she didn't want this kind of reaction. Mother and Clare became involved in a heated argument. Mother stated she couldn't help crying over her children's problems. I then focused the issue between the parents.

Peggy: Do you also cry over Sam's unhappiness?

Mother: Yes, a little bit. I do. He doesn't even know it.

Father: I don't believe it. I really don't believe it.

Mother: So I don't tell him.

Father: I don't believe it. (*The parents begin to argue.*)

Peggy: When do you cry over his unhappiness?

Mother: When I see that he is unhappy in his business, that he's unhappy with his partners, if I see he's unhappy in community situations, when he's hurting himself and feeling terrible about it. When I see he's unhappy in relation to Clare's husband and himself, when I see he's unhappy about his mother and sick brother-in-law, my heart hurts—and it's very hard for me to let him know it bothers me, and so I do it in my own little corner.

Peggy: (*Sympathetically.*) You cry over him without letting him know?

Mother: Cry tears? No. For my children I cry tears.

Step 3: Prescribing Enmeshment

The group discussed the futility of persuading mother to allow any of her children to be unhappy. Worrying over her children was an important life job. Rachel knew this and kept her mother involved with her by continually giving her something to worry about.

Rather than trying to diffuse this intense involvement, we decided to prescribe the family's enmeshment—but in a way that would involve father in the transaction. We added a task that shifted some of mother's involvement with her children toward her husband. Our purpose in doing this was to test the parents' readiness to bridge the gap in their relationship left by Rachel's departure.

Peggy: It is the group's conviction that I am asking the impossible by asking a mother with a heart as tender as Helen's to allow her children to suffer. (*As an aside, I say, "There are a lot of Jewish mothers out there." Mother waves in recognition.*) It is equally impossible for Rachel to break her mother's heart. We, therefore, recommend that Rachel call every day and tell her mother about her unhappiness. Mother should then share this with Sam, who should then comfort her. (*Mother cries, father reacts negatively.*)

Father: I don't want that kind of scene. I don't want her to call every day and make Helen unhappy and I don't want her to confide in me. I don't see anybody getting better from a thing like that.

Peggy: You won't do that for your wife and Rachel?

Father: (*Laughs.*) It's like a prescription.
Peggy: That's exactly what it is—a doctor's prescription.
Father: That's terrible, that's very bitter tasting.
Mother: Why is it so hard to comfort me?
Father: Helen, the whole idea doesn't—
Mother: Why, honey? The only thing that's changed is the comfort, because she does call every day and unburden herself and I do listen.
Father: (*Surprised.*) You do call every day?
Mother: And I don't share it with you because I get the . . . (*She indicates with her thumb a downward movement.*) The only difference would be you would put your arm around me. (*She caresses him.*)
Clare: It would be nice if you were on mummy's side a little bit.
Father: I'm not not on her side.
Peggy: (*Earnestly.*) Sam, this is very important. Can you do that for Rachel—and for your wife?
Father: Sure I can do it.

Rachel did call her mother every day as requested, but mother became bored with her complaints, stopped trying to cheer her up and give her advice, and finally told her she would have to solve her problems herself.

After this session, the parents took a month vacation, cutting the bond with Rachel more decisively. Threatened by this separation, Rachel moved back to their home where she felt isolated and lonely without her old job of mediator. She fell into a morose state and complained endlessly about her feelings of unhappiness and failure.

There is a myth in our profession that if parents get together and free the child from the position of mediator, the child will automatically spring forth mature, well adjusted, and symptom-free. This rarely happens since the child's social development has been retarded through his/her preoccupation with the parents' problems. The child usually goes through a period of feeling a loss of identity as he/she relinquishes this very important family position.

Our next task was to help Rachel find a different position for herself. But this could not be done in the same way the family had tried, through encouragement and helpful advice, since she only rebelled against this. We decided instead to use her rebellious streak in the service of change and to define her unhappiness and failure as her way of differentiating herself from her family, which placed such a high premium on happiness and success. We decided to enlist her sisters in helping her to accomplish this task. Rachel had never felt supported by them in her attempts to establish her autonomy, as the sisters often took the side of the parents in haranguing and pushing her. The support she received from them in this new alliance proved to be enormously beneficial.

STAGE VI
ENLISTING THE SIBLING SUBSYSTEM

Step 1: Forming a Coalition with the Sisters

The sisters were more than happy to continue to meet without the parents and quickly joined me in my position that Rachel needed to keep rebelling in order to establish her independence. In the following session, I continually reframed Rachel's complaints within this framework.

Rachel: I feel sapped at this point.

Peggy: Well, your parents certainly wouldn't approve of that.

Rachel: No. I have to keep going.

Peggy: That's right, and by being completely sapped you're saying no to them, which takes a lot of guts.

Sandy: (*Wistfully.*) That's really true.

Rachel: But I have no self-respect.

Peggy: Do your parents want you to have self-respect?

Rachel: I think so.

Peggy: And you're saying you don't have self-respect. You say your parents want you to be happy and you're saying, "I'm unhappy."

Rachel: My parents want me to gain weight.

Peggy: And you're staying thin.

Rachel: I've gained five pounds and I'm very upset about it.

Peggy: I can understand that because you feel you're losing ground with them, that you're doing something they'd like you to do, which makes you feel a nonperson.

Rachel: I should move to Kalamazoo, get the hell out of New York, and not even think of pleasing my parents.

Sandy: (*Now in full support.*) Listen to what Peggy is saying. You are living your life to displease them.

Rachel: I want to please myself.

Peggy: Well, you are because you're displeasing them. The most important thing in your life right now is to say no to your parents, and you've found many ways of doing that.

Rachel: I want to please me.

Peggy: Well, you are because you're displeasing them.

The session ended with the group suggesting that Rachel enlist the sisters' help in the planned rebellion, saying it was too much of a burden for her to think up these elaborate schemes herself. The sisters eagerly agreed, with Sandy stating that it would be good training for her.

Step 2: Differentiating from the Sisters

We failed to anticipate that Rachel would sense her sisters' help at pressuring her to change, since it was being given within the context of therapy. Before forming an alliance with them, she made it clear that she had to first rebel against their expectations of her progress in therapy. She did this by remaining depressed and making veiled suicide threats. I defined these threats as her way of differentiating herself from her sisters' expectations.

Clare: I feel angry. What Rachel is doing is hostility, talking about killing herself. Besides the fact I love her, I'm angry at her for doing it to me.

Rachel: Then maybe I'll just make believe things are okay.

Clare: Why can't I say what I feel?

Rachel: Maybe I have to work it out away from my family. There are too many expectations and pressures.

Clare: Who puts expectations on you?

Rachel: You all do. You all expect me to deal with my problems in a certain way.

Peggy: (*Supporting her attempt to differentiate from her sisters.*) I think that's true. You do expect her to deal with her problems in a particular way and Rachel is saying no to all of you. Not only no to her parents but to her sisters.

Rachel:	I don't think so—maybe if I were getting pleasure out of it, I could think so.
Peggy:	I know you're not getting pleasure out of it, that's not the purpose.
Rachel:	What is the purpose?
Peggy:	The purpose is to establish who you are, and that you are the one who says no to expectations.
Clare:	You really calm down when we get upset, don't you?
Sandy:	I noticed that last time. As soon as we get upset, you sit back. Maybe this is what you want. Maybe we have to prove we're so concerned, or maybe you want to shake us up.
Rachel:	I'm not doing it to be dramatic.
Clare:	Look at you. Five minutes ago you were crying and saying how miserable you were.
Rachel:	(*Coolly.*) It doesn't take that much to make me go one way or the other. I don't know what it takes.
Clare:	(*Heatedly.*) Bullshit! (*They argue.*)
Peggy:	(*Defining this again as Rachel's way of rebelling against her sisters.*) I can understand why you're feeling better now, because you've just said no to your sisters and their expectations of you. I think you need to just keep doing that, Rachel, and to find other ways of doing it.
Rachel:	I really don't get this whole thing.

I then enlisted the sisters in trying to think of more constructive ways for Rachel to rebel and asked about some of the ways they had successfully rebelled. Clare listed her rebellious acts as going out with married men, dating non-Jewish boys, letting her parents know when she was having sex, not joining B'nai B'rith, and so on. Rachel joined in listing her accomplishments, such as going without a bra, wearing pantyhose without panties, raising her voice in public. Sandy suddenly burst out with, "I enjoy talking about these things. It makes me feel good." The tense atmosphere changed to one of camaraderie and laughter as they banded together in discussing acts of "disloyalty."

Some questions might be raised as to the advisability of encouraging sisters to band together to form a coalition against parental control. The fact that the sisters were all adults rather than young children who are financially, physically, and emotionally dependent on their parents was a determining factor in this intervention. We would refrain from doing this with younger children with whom obedience to parental control is age appropriate.

Rachel's rebellious acts had always been accompanied by enormous guilt, and she therefore failed in each endeavor to become independent. By bringing her rebelliousness out into the open, planning it, condoning it, and scheduling it with the help of her sisters, we stripped off its more toxic aspects. Note that she then chose to rebel in relatively benign ways rather than those destructive to her health and well-being.

The parents returned from their vacation, and I telephoned to let them know we had not forgotten about them but had found the sessions with the sisters so helpful to Rachel we wanted to continue them for a while longer. I assured them they would be involved later on.

In the following sessions, I pushed the sibling alliance further and suggested Sandy teach Rachel how to become self-indulgent since Rachel emulated her father by being rigidly self-denying and frugal. Sandy coached her by instructing her to buy things she would never think of buying, such as expensive perfume, luxurious underwear, silk suits, jewelry, expensive cosmetics, and so on. I warned Rachel against indulging in food, however, and cautioned her against gaining too much weight. I set the limit at what Sandy weighed, nine pounds heavier, and thus, while seeming to restrain her, I actually encouraged her to gain. As they continued to discuss different modes of self-indulgence, some of the suggestions became outrageous, and I joined them in their frivolity and laughter.

The group interrupted to restrain me and to point out that the kind of rebellion I was suggesting was too enjoyable. I agreed with them that it was too soon to stop pushing the unhappiness prescription and I returned with the following message:

Peggy: (*Looking contrite.*) I have been reprimanded by my group.

Sandy: (*With dismay.*) Again, Peggy? You're doing badly.

Peggy: Yes, but I can see their point. They feel I got swept away in talking about things that would make Rachel happy, like being self-indulgent, buying expensive perfume, underwear, indulging in sex, because, Rachel, that would make you happy. And your parents would know you were happy.

Sandy: That makes sense to me. Does it to you, Rachel?

Rachel: It doesn't make sense to me. How does it make sense to you?

Sandy: Because if you're happy, Mummy will do what she did to me. She'll make you want to puke. She'll make more fuss over that than she does over you now. If you're unhappy on your job, you can quit, and that will make them unhappy. As the job goes on, you make a list of all the things that you can complain about, so even if you have some happy moments, don't talk about those. Go home and tell them about all the lousy things that happened to you today, and make their evening miserable, and that will make you miserable too.

Peggy: Good, good, very good.

At the end of the session the sisters gave the first indication of how they saw me in relation to the group. Although I had consistently told Rachel she must remain unhappy, they perceived me as being on Rachel's side. They picked up the second level of the paradoxical message.

Sandy: You have children, don't you Peggy?

Peggy: Yes. I have a son, 17, and a daughter, 21.

Sandy: Is your daughter why you keep on wanting Rachel to be happy? Do you identify a little? The group keeps reprimanding you for being too soft-hearted.

Peggy: I don't know. I'll think about that. It's hard for me to tell Rachel to be unhappy. (*To Rachel.*) Do you know that? (*I reach out a hand and touch her.*) It's hard for me to tell you to be unhappy—but I know they're right. When I think about it and I'm objective, I know that's what you must do.

Sandy: I guess that's what's good about having a group. They keep you objective.

Peggy: That's right.

STAGE VII
SAYING NO TO THERAPY

Step 1: Pushing the Prescription to the Breaking Point

This next session was the most crucial session in therapy, marking the turning point of a lasting change. Before Rachel could become a truly independent woman, she had to be able to say no to therapy and to the absurd task we had given her of keeping herself miserable. She had been conscientiously trying to follow it, but she was becoming more and more dissatisfied with living with her parents and remaining unhappy. During this session, I pushed the prescription to the point where Rachel said no to therapy.

Peggy: (*To Rachel.*) Well, Rachel, are you being unhappy, covering up what is pleasurable? How well are you doing that?

Rachel: I'm trying to cover up whatever's pleasurable.

Peggy: Good. How well are you doing in that?

Rachel: I'm trying to say no to all my mother's suggestions, and I hate it there. (*She cries.*)
Peggy: You're supposed to hate it there. Of course you hate it there.
Rachel: I feel so out of it there, I really can't stand it.
Peggy: You're going to be unhappy as long as you're at home.
Rachel: So why do I have to be there? I don't want to be there. I have this chance to sublease this apartment and I think I'm going to do it, if it works out.
Sandy: They're telling you to do something and if you're planning to rent an apartment in April you're just not listening again. And just like mother's going to have to be unhappy for a while until things get better, maybe you're going to have to be unhappy for a while.
Rachel: Why can't I get out of there? I want out.
Sandy: Well, you can't. So it's just too bad.

Rachel moans and groans and ends up looking imploringly at me with big, wet eyes, asking, "Why can't I sublease the place for just six months?"

Peggy: The harder it is for you now, the better.
Rachel: I don't understand it, and I can't go on like this.
Peggy: You won't understand it right now.

The sisters supported me and Rachel argued, finally screaming, "I can't stand it, and why do I have to force myself to be there?"

Peggy: (*Kindly but firmly, like a doctor administering medicine.*) For the time being, the worse it is, the better it will be. The worse it is now and the more unhappy you are, the better it is. So have your sisters been helping you with that?
Rachel: With being unhappy? No.
Sandy: We were supposed to—if she felt guilty doing something, she would call us.
Clare: She hasn't been calling me.
Peggy: How come you haven't been calling your sisters?
Rachel: Sometimes I don't feel like it because I'm frustrated and I don't like this. I feel like evaluating the situation and how to make things better, and instead I'm told to make things worse, and I can't stand that. I can't go against my instincts any longer.
Peggy: For the time being, Rachel, you have to make things worse.
Rachel: Well, I can't, Peggy. I want to go out and get a better job and I want to make myself happy. I can't make myself get a bad job and I can't make myself more unhappy.
Sandy: Is it necessary for her to stay with her present job to make her more unhappy?
Peggy: She should make herself unhappy in every way possible.
Sandy: Why?
Peggy: Because only in that way is she going to be able to find herself.
Clare: She is making my parents so dissatisfied with her they both stood there and smiled at me like dummies, they were so happy to see me. They never did this before. I looked so good in comparison with Rachel.
Peggy: Don't you appreciate what she's doing for you?
Clare: Yes. I felt I didn't deserve it.
Peggy: She's giving you a gift.
Clare: I guess so, so I shouldn't be mad. I feel guilty when I get mad at Rachel. This is my baby sister.
Peggy: No. Anything you can do to help Rachel be unhappy is fine.
Clare: Rachel is so self-involved right now.

Peggy: But she needs to be self-involved in her unhappiness. She should be totally preoccupied with it.

Rachel: (*Crying.*) I can't deal with people on that basis. This totally isolates me from the entire world. It's a ridiculous request to make. How am I supposed to relate to friends when I'm unhappy? Who the hell wants to be with me?

Peggy: (*Sympathetically.*) I know this is hard.

Rachel: This is crazy! Not hard—crazy! This means you're asking me to exist alone, to lock myself in my parents' basement and exist alone, because no one is going to want to be with me and I don't want to be with myself when I'm like this. It doesn't give me any reason for doing anything—any purpose for wanting to exist. It's making my existence so much more miserable.

Step 2: Escalating the Therapeutic Triangle

Peggy: Let me talk to my group a minute. Maybe they will allow you to do something that will relieve you a little bit. You seem to get into trouble, though, every time I relent . . .

The group decided not to relent but to take a position of consternation in relation to Rachel's rumbling of rebelliousness.

Peggy: The group says it sounds like you're not only saying no to your mother but you're getting ready to say no to me, and they are quite appalled. Are you saying no to me?

Rachel: (*Hesitates, and then blurts out.*) Yes, I am. (*Changes her mind.*) Not to you, to the group. (*She is not quite brave enough to risk alienating me, but she feels it's safe to take a position against the group since she knows I have sometimes disagreed with them.*) I'm fed up. I don't know what to do. My human instincts tell me to do something to make things happier, and you people are telling me to be unhappy, and I don't know how to relate to other people on that basis.

Peggy: (*Acting puzzled.*) That was the way you were relating to them for quite a while. Can't you just go back to that? Or stay there?

Rachel: No, I can't. I can't sit around and complain.

Peggy: But you have been doing that, so it's hard for me to understand what would be intolerable about it now, since you were doing that for quite a while. What's different about it now?

Rachel: Because I see it differently now. I see the world is not interested in me and my problems and it's not appropriate.

I dismissed myself to talk to the group, thinking it might be time for me to take a position in favor of change. It is decided I should first explore what Rachel would do if she were allowed to change.

Rachel: I don't know. All I know is I've really been trying the past few weeks to do what you told me to do and really work at it between sessions, and Peggy, I can't stand it! And I can't stand living with my parents. I'm regressing.

Peggy: (*Pursuing the question of change.*) What would happen if you said no to them and me? What would you do?

Rachel: I'd try to do what the rest of the world does—break away from home, become an adult, get a job, find my own place to live, find my own circle of friends.

Peggy: (*Challenging her to prove herself.*) But that's just what we're afraid of, Rachel. You know the consequences of that. You know what's happened every time you've attempted to do that. The results have been disastrous for you. You've felt you couldn't do it, felt like a failure, something has always gone wrong, you've felt lonely, isolated, that you were going crazy, the noises bothered you—it was a disaster, and we're trying to save you from that.

The group called me out and we decided it was time for me to side with Rachel against the group and push for change. When given her freedom to go forward, Rachel hesitated. The medicine I had been prescribing, despite its bad taste, was a comfort to her, giving her a sense of security. The sisters also registered some apprehension as to Rachel's ability to assume responsibility for her own happiness.

Step 3: Opposing the Group

I entered the room and asked Rachel to support my opposition to the group.

Peggy: Rachel, you want to help me say no to the group? I just had a big fight with them. I can't budge them. Let's you and me say no to the group.

Rachel: (*Tearfully.*) I was afraid when you went out there I was going to hear my sentence for the week.

Peggy: Are you ready to say no to them with me?

Rachel: What do they say?

Peggy: They're adamant. I cannot budge them. They say absolutely you should stay at home. You should be unhappy, should not make your life any better, should stay miserable, isolated, complain, not look for a job.

Rachel: Forget that. Forget that right there.

Peggy: (*Extending her hand.*) Thanks, thanks. I told them you had suffered enough, been unhappy enough, said no to Mother enough, and enough is enough. And you have the right, if you feel you can do something different, to try. And I want to say, "Go ahead."

Rachel: With what?

Peggy: With whatever you want to do. Whatever you want to do to make yourself happy, and we will know whether or not I'm right or the group is right.

Rachel now had a choice of siding with me by changing or letting the group win a victory by remaining the same.

Rachel: How about saying no to my parents?

Peggy: I think you've had enough of that.

Clare: Can't she say no when she wants to say no?

Peggy: Oh, that's fine; if you want to say no or if you want to say yes, feel free at this point to do whatever you want to do.

Rachel: (*Stunned at this sudden shift and not knowing how to respond.*) Are you sincere?

Peggy: I am.

Rachel: (*Apprehensively.*) What do they feel I'm going to gain from doing things their way? Because, Peggy, the only thing is that when I'm unsure and don't know what I'm doing I can say, "Well, my therapist told me to do this, so it must be what I'm supposed to do." So I just don't know.

Clare: You're taking all the supports away from Rachel by saying do whatever you want to do.

Peggy: You mean you feel the group is right?

Clare: I would say it's all right to say, "Do whatever you want to do" in certain directions, but I think you're pulling all the props out from under her by putting all the responsibility on Rachel. I feel she's not ready.

Peggy: What do you think, Sandy?

Sandy:	I'm a little bit afraid for her.
Peggy:	Do you think the group's right, too?
Sandy:	I think they are too extreme.
Peggy:	Maybe I just had a reaction against them.
Sandy:	I think gradually. I look back on her life as being too much at one time and see her doing the same thing again. She'll have too many demands on her and expectations will be too great.
Peggy:	Actually, then, the two of you are taking a position between me and the group.
Rachel:	I'm also taking a position between the two.

Step 4: Supporting Autonomy

I then took the position that Rachel had the right to decide on her own how fast she should change.

Peggy:	I think you're right. My position is extreme. I lost my head and got angry. I admire the fact that you were able to say no to the group and also to me just now, and to stop me from going too far. I think your judgment will guide you now as to how much pleasure and progress you allow yourself.

Her task had been changed from being unhappy and saying no to deciding on how rapidly to say yes. Thus, she was placed in charge of her own change.

STAGE VIII
SOLIDIFYING CHANGE

Step 1: Anticipating and Rehearsing a Regression

Having defied the therapists, Rachel took a giant step toward independence and in the following session described her new life. The group reminded me to schedule a regression in order to solidify change.

Clare and Sandy arrived for the session without Rachel, who was late for the first time having gone for a job interview. Sandy burst out with: "She's so happy. She's always happy. I've been under pressure lately, I've had a lot on my mind, and there's Rachel off being so happy, and I'm saying to myself, 'Goddammit, enough of this already with the smile.'"

Peggy:	That must be quite an adjustment for you.
Clare:	Even my mother and father commented on how happy Rachel is. I'm giving my parents problems now, so it takes the pressure off Rachel.
Peggy:	That's terrific. What kind of problems?

Rachel entered, elegantly dressed and looking radiant.

Rachel:	(*Glowingly.*) I'm having such a good time, Peggy. I can't believe it. I bought myself this silk suit. (*Proudly shows off an elegant and stylish suit.*) A hundred and fourteen bucks. I want to start being really good to myself.
Peggy:	(*Cautiously.*) I'm afraid to be too enthusiastic because of my group.
Rachel:	I'm afraid to be too enthusiastic too. I'm so happy I began to be afraid it wouldn't last. I don't want to be devastated. I haven't been this happy in years.
Peggy:	What's making you so happy?

Rachel spoke excitedly about her new life. She was working on a magazine, getting published, meeting famous people, and doing something for the first time in her life that she really enjoyed. She had a chance to sublet an apartment for six months and was thinking about taking it. She felt she was making less frantic decisions, but looked apprehensively toward the mirror as she said, "I know the group won't like my moving." I said maybe they would change their minds now. She spoke about a new interesting man she was dating who looked like Woody Allen. I asked if her parents would approve of him and she said she was afraid they would. She discussed her problem of saying no to men for fear of hurting their feelings, and I asked her sisters to help her with this since they had had more experience. As I joined them in a humorous and intimate conversation, the group interrupted with a knock on the door and called me out to say they would like to take a position counter to the merriment and begin instead to worry about a regression. Passover was coming up and would probably create tension and conflict as it had last year. Also, Rachel was planning to move again and we could anticipate a recurrence of the former problems.

Peggy: The group is critical of me again. They feel we're having too good a time. (*The sisters boo.*) They are worried about what is going to happen on Passover or if you attempt to move again.

Rachel said she had already told her mother that she was not going to go to Seder on Passover. I asked her to anticipate her parents' reactions so she could be prepared for the worst. How might they draw her back into the fight between them? How could she deal with her guilt? How would she keep from siding with one against the other? What would happen to father at the dinners when she wasn't there to side with him against mother's family? Rachel replied, "I'll just have to give up that quest to please him." We went over all the possibilities carefully and Rachel said she was confident she could handle them.

Before the session ended I came back with one last warning from the group against premature optimism.

Peggy: The group is not as optimistic as we are. They anticipate you will get depressed again, and this will probably occur around Passover or if you move. They recommend, therefore, that you deliberately allow yourself to get depressed on those two occasions.
Rachel: What if I'm not?
Peggy: Try to feel that way. Try to go back to the way you were feeling or—(*Loud groans and laughter from everyone.*) You don't have to go all the way back.
Rachel: You don't know what you're asking. I want to be able to deal with these times.
Peggy: Then practice them.
Rachel: Okay.

We decided it was time now to involve the parents again as we anticipated they would have a reaction to the new Rachel.

The whole family was convened for this session. Rachel looked stunning with a new hairstyle, new clothes, new makeup, and a radiant expression on her face. She began the interview with:

Rachel: I'm great. I've never been greater.
Peggy: Tell me about it.
Rachel: Number one—I'm in love.
Peggy: In love? Not with a man? (*Laughter.*)
Rachel: Yes, with a man—with a really nice man.
Peggy: Jewish?
Rachel: (*Chagrined.*) Yes. That's his only drawback, but he didn't want a Jewish woman either, so we decided we'd overlook it. We don't have those attributes we were trying to avoid.

Peggy: Well, at least it's equal.
Father: Maybe you'll both convert. (*Much laughter.*)
Rachel: He's the one who looks like Woody Allen. Things are working out nicely. He's very kind and sensitive. Lots of fun. He loves me, and I'm living in Manhattan doing publicity work and I have a lot of promising job prospects.

Both parents expressed their pleasure over the changes in Rachel and only once attempted to use her new romance as a focal point for an old argument between the two of them.

Step 2: Redefining the Marital Relationship

It was quite clear now that the parents would never have a tranquil relationship but would probably go on fighting for the rest of their days. The important thing was that Rachel was no longer involved in their battles. She managed to stay out of this one and I described the parents' relationship as a profound and lasting bond between two stalwart, equally matched opponents who had strong and differing points of view and felt free to express them on every subject. Since it was their way of making love, they certainly didn't need any interference from anyone outside. Father, surprisingly, agreed, saying, "After all is said and done, we are meant for each other." And mother conceded that there must be something they enjoyed about fighting since they were always doing it.

An appointment was made for one month later, and I stated this would give us time to see if Rachel could stay out of her parents' love making. If she felt her parents needed a third party, she should call one of her sisters and ask them to be the third member. The sisters vociferously declined.

STAGE IX
PRESCRIBING A FAREWELL RITUAL

In a presession discussion we decided that if Rachel had managed to maintain her gains, we would ceremonialize her leave taking by prescribing a farewell ritual.

The family reported things *were* going well and the parents declared it was a relief to have Rachel out of the home as it was more peaceful. The session was spent giving the family credit for the changes that had been made, anticipating future trouble spots, and making some suggestions as to how to avoid them. The session ended with my suggesting they plan a farewell party to celebrate Rachel's becoming a woman and leaving home, and that father should propose a toast to send her on her way. They responded positively and Sandy suggested they have a broomstick for Rachel to jump over, as in Jewish weddings, symbolizing the beginning of a new life.

FOLLOW-UP

A one-, two-, and three-year follow-up revealed Rachel still in good spirits, living alone in her own apartment and loving it, excited about her new career, and dating several different men. The parents were still making love in their characteristic way, but the three sisters were staying out of it.

Editors' Introduction

Ruth Baer is one of the worlds's leading experts on mindfulness-based treatment approaches in psychotherapy, and she and two of her students wrote up these two cases to illustrate Roger Walsh's chapter on Contemplative Psychotherapies in Current Psychotherapies. *The two cases illustrate the utility of mindfulness in the treatment of Rachel, a woman who presents with generalized anxiety disorder (GAD), and Miranda, a more deeply troubled woman who presents with classic symptoms of borderline personality disorder (BPD).*

Mindfulness, acceptance, and dialectics have been described as the essential components of the "third wave" of cognitive-behavioral therapy, and it seems like a new book on the application of mindfulness to psychotherapy is published weekly. Why were psychology, social work and counseling professionals so slow to realize that Buddhist monks have been treating psychological problems for millennia using these methods, and to appreciate that these techniques and viewpoints can be integrated and included as primary approaches to therapy or as adjunctive therapies by practitioners trained in many different schools of therapy?

Both clients receive extensive psychological testing as a part of their treatment. Is this merely because they are being seen by student therapists in an academic setting? How valuable is psychological testing in developing treatment plans and assessing client progress?

It is sometimes challenging to introduce mindfulness to a deeply religious Christian or Muslim client. Would you use different terms to describe these techniques to avoid their historical link to Buddhist traditions and practices? Is it duplicitous to describe mindfulness as simply another way to reduce anxiety? How much training is necessary before one can include an approach like dialectical behavior therapy (DBT) in one's clinical practice? Are weekend workshops and reading sufficient, or is direct supervised clinical experience required? Have you had personal experiences with meditation or mindfulness? If so, how has your life been changed by these practices?

11 | USING MINDFULNESS EFFECTIVELY IN CLINICAL PRACTICE: TWO CASE STUDIES

Tory A. Eisenlohr-Moul, Jessica R. Peters, and Ruth A. Baer

THEORETICAL AND RESEARCH BASIS

Expanding the Cognitive-Behavioral Tradition in Psychotherapy: The "Third Wave" of Mindfulness, Acceptance, and Dialectics

Years of treatment-outcome research provide a solid foundation of empirical evidence for cognitive and behavioral psychotherapies (for meta-analytic reviews, see Butler, Chapman, Forman, & Beck, 2006; Olatunji, Cisler, & Deacon, 2010; Tolin, 2010). Because such treatment approaches usually focus on modifying behavior, cognitions, and emotions, they have been described as "technologies of change" (Dimeff & Linehan, 2001). Despite evidence that such technologies are effective at helping many individuals achieve symptom relief, they are not effective for all individuals and may not be comprehensive enough in their approach to preventing symptom relapse (Linehan, Armstrong, Suarez, Allmon, & Heard, 1991; Waters & Craske, 2005). Recently, a so-called third wave of treatment strategies have been developed that incorporate training in present-centered awareness, a nonjudgmental stance, acceptance of thoughts and emotions, and psychological flexibility into previously established technologies of change. Many of these "technologies of acceptance" have begun to demonstrate efficacy for treating previously untreatable or high-relapse disorders such as borderline personality disorder (BPD) (Linehan, et al., 1991), generalized anxiety disorder (GAD) (Roemer, Orsillo, & Salters-Pedneault, 2008), and even substance use disorders (e.g., Brewer et al., 2011).

Acceptance-based behavior therapy (ABBT) (Orsillo & Roemer, 2011) and dialectical behavior therapy (DBT) (Linehan, 1993) both belong to this new set of approaches. These treatments are particularly strong examples of integrating technologies of change with technologies of acceptance. Participants in these therapies learn traditional cognitive and behavioral methods for combating symptoms such as self-monitoring, shaping desired ways of thinking and behaving, and skills for avoiding problematic behaviors. However, they also learn to cultivate present-centered, nonjudgmental awareness of their experiences, acceptance of their experiences, and the ability to be flexible and effective in the face of more chronic symptoms. The two approaches are described in more detail in the paragraphs that follow.

DBT is a highly structured, multifaceted treatment designed originally for individuals with chronic self-harm and suicidality. It is most commonly applied to those with borderline personality disorder, a severe and prevalent disorder characterized by extreme emotion dysregulation, feelings of emptiness, stormy relationships, and impulsive or self-harming behaviors, among other symptoms. Based on a dialectical worldview in which acceptance and change must be balanced, this treatment mixes traditional approaches to behavior change with training in mindfulness and acceptance of the present moment. In its standard outpatient form, DBT includes weekly individual therapy sessions as well as group skills training organized around four modules that address symptoms in a broad variety of ways: (1) core mindfulness skills, (2) distress-tolerance skills, (3) interpersonal effectiveness skills, and (4) emotion-regulation skills. This treatment emphasizes the need to engage in dialectical thinking and flexible responding by selecting from the wide range of change-oriented and acceptance-oriented skills presented.

ABBT is a new mindfulness-based therapy for the treatment of generalized anxiety disorder, a disorder characterized by excessive worry, restlessness, sleep disturbance, fatigue, muscle tension, irritability, and impaired concentration. ABBT is based on an integration of cognitive-behavioral therapy (CBT) for GAD with mindfulness-based therapies such as acceptance and commitment therapy (ACT) (Hayes, Strosahl, & Wilson, 1999) and dialectical behavior therapy (Linehan, 1993). Drawing heavily on existing treatment protocols, ABBT emphasizes acceptance of internal experiences by increasing willingness to experience negative emotion while simultaneously decreasing efforts to control or change thoughts and feelings. Individuals with GAD may exert a large amount of energy toward efforts at experiential control; however, research consistently demonstrates the paradoxical results of these strategies. Therefore, ABBT draws heavily on ACT's notion of living a valued life despite negative internal experiences, shifting the focus from emotional and cognitive control to behavioral control, where it is more likely to be beneficial. To achieve behavior change, ABBT borrows techniques from traditional CBT while emphasizing the need for self-compassion and flexibility during the process.

Introduction to the Chapter

This chapter will describe the treatment of two individuals using mindfulness-based treatment approaches. One presents primarily with symptoms of GAD, and the second presents primarily with symptoms of BPD. The purpose of describing the treatment of these two individuals is threefold: (1) to provide examples of the usefulness of mindfulness-based psychotherapies, (2) to highlight variability in client reactions to these "technologies of acceptance," and (3) to demonstrate the flexible and effective application of these treatment approaches to individuals with both positive and negative initial reactions to the central concepts in third-wave therapies.

INTRODUCTION TO RACHEL

Rachel was a 23-year-old Caucasian female. She had a master's degree and was employed full time in an administrative position. She was engaged to be married and had no children. Rachel's daily life was somewhat restricted by her anxiety. She described spending large amounts of time at work and home preoccupied with health worries. She noted that although she had some friends, her anxiety often prevented her from spending time with them. She worried about the possibility of feeling sick or panicky. Rachel was also afraid of being outside alone at night, so when an outing required her walking to a car alone, even for a short distance in a likely safe environment, she would typically stay home instead. While at home, she spent most of her time on the computer, watching TV, and in other sedentary and solitary activities.

Rachel's Presenting Complaints

Rachel presented with several concerns. She reported a wide range of anxiety symptoms, including intense worry, social anxiety, health anxiety, and numerous specific phobias. She had previously been diagnosed with irritable bowel syndrome, which she reported was aggravated by stress. She reported insomnia, which involved waking up multiple times a night and falling back asleep with difficulty. She described troubles in her relationship with her mother and people in general, particularly in regard to asserting her own needs. She described a tendency to always try to please others, even when an event was focused on her, such as when choosing what restaurant to go to for a birthday dinner.

Rachel's History

Rachel reported struggling with self-directed negative feelings and anxiety ever since she was a child. She described her family as less sensitive emotionally than she was, which resulted in her mother often brushing off her feelings and fears as overreactions.

The client presented with a long-term history of medical problems, including irritable bowel syndrome, hypothyroidism (treated), and chronic problems with muscle tension and pain. The client described numerous frustrating experiences with the medical system trying to find answers for her symptoms, many of which remained unexplained. Rachel had no prior experiences with therapy, although she had attempted psychiatric treatment for her anxiety, on the recommendation of her general physician, two years before entering therapy. She reported that she had been prescribed a selective serotonin reuptake inhibitor (SSRI) medication and experienced side effects. Rather than reducing the dose, the physician abruptly discontinued the medication, and the client terminated treatment. The client was not on medication when therapy began.

Assessment of Rachel

The client completed a Beck Anxiety Inventory (BAI) (Beck & Steer, 1990) and a Beck Depression Inventory (BDI-II) (Beck, Steer, & Brown, 1996) before the session and demonstrated extremely high levels of anxiety symptoms (BAI = 27) and moderate levels of depressive symptoms (BDI-II = 18). The client also completed the Minnesota Multiphasic Personality Inventory (MMPI-2) (Butcher, 2001) between her second and third sessions. She noted that completing the MMPI-2 brought to her attention her many fears, including fears of cats and of being out alone at night. She reported finding those two fears to be problematic for her, and they were added to the list of issues to address in therapy.

On the MMPI-2, the client had elevations on scales 1, 2, 3, 6, 7, and 0 and on the anxiety, health concerns, and low self-esteem content scales. She did not have a defined code type; however, these elevations suggested a tendency toward physical symptoms and concerns; depressive symptoms, including low energy, sleep disturbance, self-depreciation, and guilt; and anxiety symptoms, including worries and fears. Her scores also suggested a tendency to react to stress by developing physical symptoms, to be excessively sensitive and overly responsive to the opinions of others, and to be introspective, plagued by self-doubts, and perfectionistic. Her responses also indicated likely strengths, including tendencies to be persistent, reliable, and conscientious. The client agreed with these interpretations and reported finding it validating.

For the first several weeks of therapy, the client also completed anxiety records. She noted episodes of heightened anxiety and recorded relevant physical symptoms, thoughts and imagery, and behaviors. When reviewing the sheets in session, the client and therapist identified three major problems—health anxiety, social anxiety, and phobias—and they identified rumination and judgmental thoughts as part of the maintaining mechanism for all three. The client reported that she was most distressed by recurring ruminative worries about potential health problems and wanted to make this aspect of her anxiety a high priority for treatment.

Case Conceptualization for Rachel

The client was an emotional and sensitive person with a history of invalidating feedback from her family about her temperament. She had learned to be excessively judgmental about her emotions and thoughts, especially when negative, and to try hard to avoid them or make them go away. This cycle created intense anxious and self-critical rumination, preventing the client from engaging in her life in ways that might lessen her anxiety via exposure. In addition, the high level of arousal created by the constant worry likely exacerbated her physical symptoms, including gastrointestinal problems and muscle tension, which in turn provided more stimuli to worry about. The worry appeared to underlie her insomnia and depressed mood.

The client's tendency to engage in rumination and self-judgment suggested that a mindfulness-based treatment might be useful. Learning to engage with her experiences in a present-centered, nonjudgmental way was expected to target the underlying mechanisms behind her broad range of anxiety symptoms and help increase her acceptance of the emotions, thoughts, and physical sensations she experienced. Engaging more directly with her experiences, including both external stimuli and internal responses, would also function as a form of exposure to feared stimuli, eventually reducing her anxiety.

Structure and Course of Treatment for Rachel

Treatment was conducted at a university-based outpatient mental-health clinic operated by a doctoral program in clinical psychology. The therapist was a graduate student in clinical psychology who was supervised by a licensed clinical psychologist. Formal supervision meetings took place once a week and included discussion of session content, a review of videos of sessions, and treatment planning. Therapy sessions lasted 50 minutes and included homework review, discussion of new concerns from the past week, discussion of assigned reading, practice of exercises during the session, discussion of exercises, and collaborative planning of homework for the next week. Homework assignments typically included reading and regular practice of some form of the exercise practiced in session. Although Rachel expressed some anxiety about specific components of treatment, she was committed to therapy and highly motivated to change.

Treatment of Insomnia

For several reasons, therapy began with a behavioral approach to the treatment of insomnia in conjunction with pharmacological treatment provided by a psychiatric resident affiliated with the clinic. The client's sleep deprivation likely contributed to her anxiety and depressed mood, so improving sleep was a way to begin improving symptoms while further assessing the nature of her anxiety. Working on sleep skills first also allowed the client and therapist to build greater rapport before addressing the anxiety. Basic sleep hygiene tips were reviewed in session, and Rachel was given a sleep diary to track her sleep habits. Rachel was also prescribed 25mg of Trazadone to take before bed. The following session, we reviewed her sleep diary, which showed a dramatic improvement and good sleep efficiency, with an average of only two brief periods (10–15 minutes) of waking during the night. Rachel reported that taking the Trazadone was helping and that she was feeling only minimal grogginess in the morning. Because her sleep had improved so quickly, no additional insomnia treatment was conducted. Rachel continued monitoring sleep via the diary for another week, during which she experienced only one night with any sleep disturbances. Sleep monitoring was discontinued with the plan that further improvement would likely come from working on her anxiety but that she would start again if her sleep became more disturbed in the future. Sleep quality continued to improve over the course of treatment, and insomnia did not recur.

Treatment of Anxiety Using Acceptance–Based Behavior Therapy

Treatment was based on the book *The Mindful Way Through Anxiety*, which presents ABBT in a self-help format (Orsillo & Roemer, 2011). Rachel purchased the book and read relevant chapters before sessions. The initial several sessions of mindfulness-based treatment for anxiety focused on introducing the concept of mindfulness, which is defined as observation of present-moment experiences with a nonjudgmental and self-compassionate stance. Rachel continued tracking her anxiety. In session, she generated a list of self-compassionate responses to say to herself during anxious moments. Examples included "It makes sense that I feel the way I do," "I can feel anxious and also be a strong person," and "Everyone feels anxious sometimes." The therapist and client discussed what the experience of practicing mindfulness involves, including examples of different forms of meditation and how activities in daily life could be practiced in a mindful way. In session, the therapist led the client in mindfulness exercises, which were followed by extensive discussion of the thoughts and feelings that had occurred during the experience. The first exercise was a mindful breathing exercise. During the exercise, Rachel's face tensed and frowned, and she reported that the mindfulness exercise was more difficult than she had anticipated. She described feeling anxious while observing her breath and having the thoughts that she could not keep focused. Expectations for mindfulness practice were also discussed, including that her mind would inevitably wander and that the goal is just to do the exercise, not to expect to be able to do it easily or have any particular outcome. The latter point was particularly emphasized given this client's tendency toward perfectionism. Rachel and the therapist discussed what it would be like to bring mindful attention to daily activities. Rachel expected activities that brought attention to physical sensations, such as brushing her teeth, might be more anxiety inducing, but she was eager to try mindful awareness of sitting on her porch and observing nature. The client agreed to a homework plan for engaging in five minutes of mindful breathing or mindfulness of an activity each day and to record her observations.

In the next session, mindful progressive muscle relaxation (PMR) was introduced. Like standard PMR, mindful PMR involves a systematic inventory of the body's muscles, during which the client flexes and then relaxes individual muscles or muscle groups. In mindful PMR, the goal is increasing awareness and acceptance of the experience. The client is encouraged to notice what the process of tensing and releasing each muscle feels like and to accept the observations. Although the process will likely induce relaxation, the primary goal when practiced mindfully is increasing mindful awareness, so clients are reminded to notice and accept all sensations, including discomfort or tension. The client expressed anxiety about attempting this because of concerns about noticing pain that might trigger health-related worries. The client identified her arms as an area of the body that she felt least likely to be anxious about, so the initial practice was limited to her arms. The client reported less anxiety during the practice than she had anticipated and that she was willing to add it to her home practice.

The client practiced her mindfulness homework regularly and approached the exercises both in session and at home with interest despite some initial anxiety. Each time she discovered that she was able to do an exercise, it seemed to increase her willingness to try other potentially daunting activities. When practicing progressive muscle relaxation, she noticed she was often tense and began working on relaxing whenever she could in daily life. Rachel began practicing with her leg muscles as well as her arms. She also started choosing to engage in exposure activities with some of her feared stimuli, such as sitting next to cat on a couch. Although she described still feeling some anxiety, it subsided to a large extent as she used her mindfulness skills to notice any feelings, thoughts, or sensations without trying to change them and returned to focusing on her breath and the details of her surroundings. She also reported being able to be more mindful when a wasp was in her office, which allowed her to leave the office slowly and deliberately instead of panicking. Rachel also began exercising, engaging in a gradual but increasingly rigorous running program. She reported "feeling silly" at first, although using mindfulness skills helped her be self-compassionate and have the thought that most people likely feel silly when beginning new things. She continued running after therapy ended.

In later sessions, the client expressed concerns about body-image issues. She described specific, vivid memories from the past that continued to arise for her and distress her, such as when family members had said critical comments about her appearance and weight. Rachel reported that those memories tended to come up when she was paying attention to her appearance, and she was concerned that they might cause distress for her at her wedding. She agreed to try an exercise in which she remembered one of those incidents, but she did so mindfully, initially in session and then independently for homework. The client reported that after practicing the inductions, she found them still unpleasant in the moment but increasingly tolerable and temporary in their effects. Rachel expressed increased confidence in her ability to have a memory occur without becoming overly distressed by it.

As Rachel practiced mindfulness skills, she reported feeling "more like herself" on her own but noticed some patterns in her friendships she found frustrating. Rachel described a tendency for her interactions to focus strongly on the other person, such as conversations with a friend who talked about her own problems at length while never asking about Rachel's life. Rachel described her own behavior in these situations as passive and accommodating, and she said she typically felt concerned about the other person's reaction to her. The therapist and client discussed what it would be like to be more mindful in social interactions, including awareness of her own emotions, thoughts, and sensations, instead of only focusing on the responses and behaviors of others. The therapist and client also discussed specific skills she could try to be more assertive in her relationships, and the client practiced expressing what she observed about her own thoughts, feelings, and desires in session. Rachel said she felt ready to try being more direct about her needs with her friends. When exploring the possible outcomes of that in session, she could not see any significant downsides except potential short-term anxiety, which she was now willing to endure. Rachel practiced these skills and found that, for the most part, her friends responded well and expressed interest in what she shared. The client also decided that she would be willing to limit friendships if people did not respond well.

This section of therapy continued over several sessions. Rachel found it easier to apply the skills with friends but more challenging with her family. Given the propensity of Rachel's family to invalidate her emotions, the therapist suggested the client focus on aspects of the interactions under her own control rather than trying to elicit particular responses from her family. Rachel had expressed concerns about interactions with family at her upcoming wedding, and she agreed to visit her grandmother as an exposure exercise and a chance to practice using her mindfulness skills in that type of interaction. When her grandmother said things that frustrated her, such as ignoring Rachel's accomplishments when talking about those of her cousin, Rachel reported that being aware of her own thoughts and feelings during the interaction allowed her to validate her feelings and say self-compassionate things internally. She was able to reduce her distress in the experience independently of her grandmother's response, which further lowered her anxiety because she then felt she could choose whether or not to address the situation and that her emotional well-being did not hang in the balance.

The client participated in the mindfulness-based therapy eagerly, completing homework assignments and reading and participating in discussions and exercises in session. The client brought a high level of intelligence and insight to her work and was able to progress at a rapid pace, often choosing to engage in exposures to feared stimuli on her own volition as treatment progressed. The focus of therapy eventually expanded to include relationships and values before termination. All of the client's symptoms remitted by the end of treatment.

Complicating or Treatment-Promoting Factors for Rachel

The client initially expressed anxiety about initiating treatment and trying any new exercises. She was highly motivated to change, although this desire was paired with high expectations for herself. When beginning mindfulness practice, most individuals, including Rachel, tend to feel uncertain and uncomfortable with the new way of approaching experiences, and she reported anxiety and distress as expected. Despite this discomfort, Rachel demonstrated a high level of perseverance. The creation of explicit self-compassionate mantras for use during practices helped her continue practicing new skills independently.

The client's history of physical problems and health-related anxiety also required that the progressive muscle relaxation exercise be modified to be less anxiety inducing initially. By limiting focus to parts of the body that she typically did not worry about, the client was able to practice with and increase feelings of mastery of the technique of attending to bodily sensations before bringing awareness to more challenging areas of the body.

Despite her anxiety, which had limited her ability to explore her world, Rachel also was a highly curious, intelligent person. The conflict between these two sides of her personality had created great distress for her before therapy, but she thrived when encouraged to be curious about experiences within the safety of therapy.

Follow-Up for Rachel

After four and half months of therapy, the client no longer met criteria for any anxiety or other psychological disorders. The client was administered a BDI and BAI and scored a 0 and 2 on them, respectively, indicating minimal levels of depression and anxiety. The client also completed the MMPI-2 again and demonstrated no clinical elevations. The client chose to discontinue the Trazadone, with no noticeable effects.

At the final session, the client reported that she was continuing to do well, despite having faced several obstacles and stressful situations in the past couple of weeks. For example, she had met with her mother and sister to work on her wedding plans, and she was able to tolerate disagreements and voice her own opinions. She said that before treatment, her priority when planning her wedding had been minimizing potential conflict at all costs and that she dreaded the process; however, now she felt excited about planning the wedding she actually wanted. She expressed relief at knowing that she was able to handle those types of situations with her current skills. The therapist and client discussed how she might cope with difficulties in the future, including strategies such as trying to deal with problems early on, reducing her expectations for herself, and asking for help from others. The client identified several goals for herself for the future, including professional development, volunteer work, continuing to practice mindfulness skills, and setting aside time for herself and her needs. The client made tremendous progress in a relatively short time in therapy, and she achieved all of her goals for therapy. She reported functioning better than she has in many years, and at termination she appeared happy, confident, and engaged with her life.

INTRODUCTION TO MIRANDA

Miranda was a 29-year-old multiracial female. She lived with her husband of 7 years; they had no children. She had a master's degree, was employed full time, and appeared to be functioning adequately professionally. Her day-to-day life was characterized by constant work; Miranda noted that although she sometimes made time for pleasurable activities, there was insufficient energy and money for her to do anything other than watch TV and do "busy work" on the couch in the evenings. Her husband was currently unemployed, so they were struggling financially. She reported that they were fighting constantly and had recently quit couples counseling after deciding that it was not helpful for them.

Miranda's Presenting Complaints

Miranda came to the clinic seeking dialectical behavior therapy for symptoms of borderline personality disorder. Specifically, she reported intense mood swings; fluctuations in her appraisals of others as good or bad; suicidal urges; frequent temper outbursts; related relationship problems with family members, friends, and her husband; impulsive spending on things she couldn't afford; and engagement in several types of self-injury, including punching and scratching herself. She also described long-standing feelings of depression, stress-related fatigue, pain, and insomnia; highly critical thoughts about herself and others; social anxiety; and difficulty with assertiveness. She stated that her feelings of social rejection as well as her tendency to procrastinate when upset were impairing her work, where she felt pressure to "be brilliant and helpful" at all times. Notably, she felt that she was constantly falling short of such expectations. She also noted that her impulsive and self-injurious behaviors while at home were contributing to her ongoing marital difficulties, and she was concerned that she and her husband would not be able to remain together if she didn't address her emotional and behavioral problems.

In addition, she reported having been molested when she was a young adolescent, and she felt this event was plaguing her by causing low self-esteem, feelings of worthlessness, and intense shame over episodes of sexual abuse that she considered to be "her own fault," all of which made her unable to trust others. The client communicated a desire to stop self-injuring, to learn new ways of coping with her intense negative emotions and urges, and to learn more effective methods of communicating her needs and opinions to both her husband and her colleagues.

Miranda's Family and Personal History of Psychopathology and Treatment

The client described a family history of mental illness on both the maternal and paternal sides. She noted that both of her parents, who divorced when she was just five years old, had displayed various symptoms of mental illness. Her mother had moved away when she was young, leaving Miranda and her siblings to be raised by their father. The client noted that both of her parents had been diagnosed with both psychiatric and substance use disorders at some point in their lives. The client further explained that, though she felt strongly that her five siblings also met criteria for borderline personality disorder, she was unaware of them receiving any diagnosis or treatment. At the time of therapy, the client reported having "almost no contact" with her parents, though she noted that she spoke with her siblings about once per year.

The client also described a long personal history of psychopathology. She noted that she could not remember a time when she was not depressed, and so she assumed that she had suffered from depression her entire life. She also described a history of post-traumatic stress disorder (PTSD) symptoms following repeated sexual abuse by a male relative as a teenager. She reported a history of chaotic interpersonal relationships in which she alternated between idealizing and devaluing her partners, friends, and family, as well as self-injurious and suicidal thoughts and behaviors beginning at age 12. She stated that a school counselor who had noticed signs of cutting on her arms diagnosed her with borderline personality disorder at the age of 14; at that time, she had looked up the diagnosis and felt it fit her very well.

Despite receiving what was probably an accurate "prediagnosis" at age 14, the client's therapeutic history suggested that her previous treatment had been unsuccessful. The client had received treatment for depression (and not specifically for symptoms of BPD) from five other therapists and four different prescribers of medication (e.g., psychiatrists or other medical doctors) since she was 14. She reported that each of her previous therapeutic experiences had lasted for between six months and one year, but that no therapy had been very helpful for her. She noted that some of her current medications (citalopram and Trazadone) had "taken the edge off" her depression and insomnia. However, she stated that previous therapy, which had been cognitive or Rogerian in nature, had only made her more frustrated. Miranda's most recent mental-health treatment had come one year earlier when she had checked herself into the hospital for four days after her fourth unsuccessful suicide attempt. Though the client displayed optimism about the current therapeutic endeavor, she also expressed a strong undercurrent of pessimism about the outcome of therapy given her previous experiences, saying, "Everyone says cognitive therapy is scientifically supported. So if it didn't work for me, I must be beyond help." When asked more specifically about her experiences with cognitive therapy, the client noted, "it was all about how I was thinking wrong, and since I really deeply believe those 'wrong' things, that just made me feel completely out-of-control."

Assessment of Miranda

Initial Consultation

Miranda requested specifically to be admitted for treatment in the clinic's dialectical behavior therapy program. In accordance with the clinic's standard procedures, she attended an initial appointment to determine her eligibility and review her presenting complaints, her social and psychological history, and her goals for therapy. In addition to these basic consultation procedures, the DBT-focused consultation also included the BPD section of the Structured Clinical Interview for DSM-IV (SCID) (First & Gibbon, 1997), a psychoeducational review of the nature of BPD, and a discussion of the purposes and structure of DBT. Miranda met all nine criteria for BPD, including frantic efforts to avoid real or imagined abandonment, a pattern of unstable and intense interpersonal relationships characterized by idealization and devaluation, identity disturbance, impulsive eating and drinking alcohol, suicidal ideation and attempts, chronic feelings of emptiness, intense anger and difficulty controlling anger, and transient, stress-related paranoia. Miranda was also questioned about other symptoms and met criteria for dysthymic disorder, posttraumatic stress disorder, and secondary insomnia.

Formal Assessment

The client completed the BAI, the BDI-II, the MMPI-2, and the NEO Personality Inventory–Revised (NEO-PI–R) (Costa & McCrae, 1985), a personality inventory, during the first four weeks of therapy. Miranda's score on the BDI-II was 46, and her score on the BAI was 33, placing her well above the cutoff for the "severe" category for both depression and anxiety. On the MMPI-2, Miranda's validity scores indicated that she approached the test in a valid manner; however, she had elevated scores on six of the clinical scales (scales 1, 4, 6, 7, 8, and 9). She did not have a defined code type; her highest elevation was scale 1, suggesting the presence of a variety of stress-related physical symptoms; this elevation was consistent with her self-report of chronic generalized physical discomfort, and the way in which her depression often manifested as physical fatigue. Elevations on this scale have also been associated with difficulty expressing oneself verbally when emotional; this is also a symptom that Miranda had mentioned on several occasions. Her second highest elevation was scale 4, which likely reflected Miranda's self-reported difficulty incorporating the values and standards of society into her own life. Her next highest elevation was scale 8, which may reflect not only a somewhat nontraditional lifestyle and nontraditional interests but also self-doubt, social withdrawal because of feelings of being misunderstood, acute psychological turmoil, and avoidance of difficult situations. Miranda elevated several other scales: scale 6, which likely reflects sensitivity and reactivity in interpersonal situations; scale 7, which likely reflects anxiety, self-doubt, and high standards; and scale 9, which may reflect emotional instability and a tendency to become bored and restless. Her elevation of scale 9 may have also reflected, to some degree, the ways in which her depression and relationship difficulties frustrate her self-reported desire to be active and engaged in social activities.

Miranda's NEO-PI-R scores revealed a pattern of personality traits consistent with her previous diagnosis of BPD (see Lynam & Widiger, 2001). Her Neuroticism score fell within the very high range, suggesting that she was much more prone to experiencing negative affect than the average person; however, her impulsiveness and vulnerability facets were both in the average range, suggesting that she may be resilient under stress and able to control her urges reasonably well. Her extraversion score fell within the average range; however, her gregariousness facet fell within the very high range, suggesting that she has a great desire to be around others, and her positive emotions facet fell in the very low range, suggesting that she experiences very few positive feelings.

Openness was in the very high range, suggesting Miranda enjoys fantasy and art, is receptive to her internal experience, and is willing to consider new ideas and values. Miranda's agreeableness score was in the very low range, but there was a great deal of variability between the facets; although her trust, straightforwardness, altruism, and tender-mindedness facets were all low or very low, her compliance was average, and her modesty was very high. Her very low facet scores on trust, straightforwardness, altruism, and tender-mindedness suggest that Miranda may have reservations about the goodness or kindness of others, may be willing to stretch the truth in social situations when it is advantageous, may be reluctant to help others in need, and may make decisions based on hard logic rather than the emotions of others.

Her very high score on modesty suggested that she is humble and self-effacing. Her conscientiousness score fell in the low range, suggesting that she may be unorganized, unreliable, or careless; tends to be casual about morality and rules; may tend to procrastinate; and may speak or act without considering the consequences. However, her compliance and achievement-striving facets were both in the average range, suggesting that she sets goals for herself and is able to follow basic guidelines to achieve those goals. Based on behavioral observations of Miranda during treatment, it appears that Miranda's conscientiousness score may be artificially low, and it may have been based more on her own negative self-evaluation as opposed to actual behavioral tendencies.

Case Conceptualization for Miranda

Because Miranda met criteria for BPD, it was expected that a DBT treatment framework would be most helpful for reducing her symptoms. Consistent with Linehan's biosocial theory of BPD, Miranda's symptoms were conceptualized as arising from emotion regulation difficulties caused by the interaction of her emotionally vulnerable temperament with invalidating and abusive experiences she had growing up (Linehan, 1993). DBT conceptualizes sexual abuse as an extreme example of invalidation. Notably, Miranda stated that her father had praised her only when she brought home perfect report cards from school, and he would punish her harshly for anything less than a 4.0 grade-point average. Miranda's history of being invalidated by others when upset was seen as a major contributor to her pattern of self-judgment and self-invalidation. In addition, her unstable, invalidating home life growing up and history of molestation were likely linked to her difficulty trusting others as well as her lack of skill in asserting her own needs in relationships. Furthermore, her father's pattern of largely ignoring her except to reinforce "perfect" academic behavior and punish imperfect but good behavior likely contributed to the client's depression, tendency to seek approval from others with the expectation of falling short, perfectionism and unrealistic standards for herself, and self-judgment.

Miranda reported a variety of rigid cognitive patterns that may have been more proximally tied to her difficulties. She reported believing that the world was dangerous and that she was defective. Such beliefs are characteristic of victims of abuse and individuals with BPD and were conceptualized as promoting self-injurious patterns and interpersonal chaos. In addition to distorted thought content, Miranda's problematic *relationship* to her thoughts was also believed to play a central role in her difficulties; that is, her inability to notice her experience without immediately becoming fused to her thoughts and the underlying beliefs (e.g., about defectiveness or trust) that they activated left her unable to choose different responses to her life. Miranda's inability to trust others was complemented by a tendency to cling to primary intimate partners. For example, her feelings toward and thoughts about her husband seemed to fluctuate between the extremes of trusted caregiver and hated abuser. Her difficulties with that relationship in particular appeared to perpetuate and amplify her distress and urges to self-harm. When Miranda's husband expressed doubt about the relationship, she experienced frantic feelings of self-worthlessness and despair, often threatening to leave preemptively or harm herself. Although the client appeared to have adequate self-control to avoid harmful behaviors much of the time, the client judged herself harshly for her failure to perfectly control her emotions, thoughts, urges, and behaviors. Such judgment perpetuated her feelings of defectiveness.

The structure of DBT case conceptualization and treatment is based on the hierarchy of targets, which delineates the order in which various categories of behaviors are "targeted" in treatment. First, life-threatening and self-harming behaviors are treated because they may lead to serious injury or death. Second, DBT focuses on the treatment of behaviors that may interfere with the client's ability to engage with therapy (e.g., skipping sessions, lack of homework completion) because such behaviors may prevent the client's progress in any number of important treatment areas. The third step of the hierarchy is to address skills deficits related to quality of life and managing emotional states such as depression. PTSD symptoms are not treated until emotion regulation and distress-tolerance skills are sufficient for managing the distress elicited by discussing past traumas. Because case conceptualization is an ongoing process during DBT treatment, further case conceptualization is integrated into the treatment section that follows.

Structure and Course of Treatment: Miranda

Treatment was conducted at the same clinic described previously. The therapist was a graduate student in clinical psychology who was supervised by a licensed clinical psychologist. Formal supervision meetings took place once a week and included discussion of session content with a focus on adherence to DBT principles and identification of optimal strategies for teaching the client to apply skills.

Treatment included group and individual DBT sessions once per week. Weekly skills group lasted 2.5 hours and was comprised of homework review, presentation of new skills, and in-session practice. Skills are organized in four modules: core mindfulness, interpersonal effectiveness, emotion regulation, and distress tolerance. Completion of all modules generally takes six months; therefore, the standard one-year commitment to DBT skills group allows the client to go through all modules at least twice. Weekly individual therapy sessions were 50 minutes and included diary card review, homework review, and discussions about how DBT skills could be applied. Initial sessions of individual therapy focused on orientation to treatment, assessment of motivation, and goal setting. The client expressed a strong motivation for completing DBT.

Treatment of Self-Harm and Impulsivity Using Dialectical Behavior Therapy

After reviewing the hierarchy of targets, it was decided that treatment would begin with a focus on reducing Miranda's self-harming behavior, which currently entailed two acts of cutting, scratching, or punching herself per week. To gain a clearer understanding of the causes and contexts of the client's self-injury, the therapist introduced a diary card—a central self-monitoring tool in DBT that allows the therapist and the client to accurately track the daily co-occurrence of mood, urges, problematic behavior, and skill use. The client's original diary card included the experience of basic emotions, urges to self-harm, and instances of self-harm. As the client progressed in learning DBT skills, spaces were added where the client could indicate whether or not she practiced each skill daily. Per DBT protocol, the client was instructed to complete this diary card every day and bring it to session each week.

During the time in which self-injury was the focus of treatment, individual sessions proceeded in a highly structured format. First, the diary card material was reviewed, and specific instances of self-harm were noted. Next, a behavioral chain analysis was conducted in which the therapist helped the client detail the progression of thoughts, feelings, sensations, and behaviors that occurred before, during, and after an episode of self-injury. Finally, the therapist coached the client in the use of DBT skills—especially mindfulness and distress-tolerance skills—that were expected to be helpful for disrupting the chain of events leading to self-injury.

For the first four weeks, the client continued to report one or two episodes of self-scratching and self-punching per week and strong urges to engage in cutting, scratching, and punching behaviors numerous times per day. After conducting a few behavioral chain analyses, some typical patterns of conditions and events surrounding the client's self-injurious behaviors became clear. Specific risk factors were identified: The client was more likely to respond to negative events with extreme distress if she was tired, hungry, or had forgotten to take her medication. Specific instigating events were also identified: The client was more likely to have urges to self-harm in addition to being distressed if she perceived rejection from others or if she felt ashamed. It became clear that the client experienced the vast majority of her social interactions as episodes of social rejection and was therefore feeling distressed and having strong urges to self-harm for a large portion of the day. However, the client was not typically acting on these feelings, and the therapist praised her for this pattern of adaptive responding. When the client did end up self-harming in these situations, she noticed that it was generally when she was at home and without the distractions provided by the presence of others.

Therefore, the therapist introduced the distress-tolerance module skills, and a great deal of time was spent brainstorming specific distress-tolerance behaviors that could be used to foster distraction from, self-soothing in, and acceptance of the present moment when she was experiencing an urge to self-harm. The client was encouraged to focus on monitoring the use of these skills on her diary card. The client focused primarily on distraction and self-soothing skills; particular distress-tolerance skills that were useful for the client included taking a cold shower, lighting a candle in her room, playing video games with bright colors, and calling a friend; the client was also encouraged to pay close attention to the sensations associated with these behaviors. Though the client had been hesitant to use any of the distress-tolerance skills that incorporated mindfulness specifically, she did acknowledge that she was interested in fostering "acceptance of the pain" in the present moment because she realized that this was central to avoiding self-harm. The client applied the distress-tolerance skills quickly and effectively; she was able to identify situations in which she was losing control and insert these behaviors in the place of self-harm. By the fifth week of treatment, the client reported no self-harm. Self-harm urges and episodes were continually monitored for the rest of the therapeutic year. The client continued to report a declining number of urges to self-harm, and she reported no episodes of self-harm after the fourth week.

Treatment of Depression Using Behavioral Activation Techniques and Mindfulness

When appropriate, DBT allows for the integration of additional empirically supported treatments for specific problems or disorders. As the client was experiencing symptoms of both major depressive disorder and posttraumatic stress disorder, the client and therapist discussed the relative priorities of treating these two problems. The client expressed a strong interest in improving her mood and felt that she was not yet "stable enough" to deal with the negative feelings that exposure-based PTSD treatment was likely to bring up. Therefore, it was decided that we would start behavioral activation therapy for the treatment of her depressive symptoms. This treatment began with the client tracking her activities for a week and rating her mood during each activity. The client reported a variety of interesting patterns surrounding her mood; in particular, she noted that she felt more depressed when she was sitting around at home in the evenings. The client also noted that nearly 90 percent of her waking hours were spent working and that she had stopped doing nearly all leisure activities. For the next four weeks, sessions emphasized scheduling new activities. The client completed a wide variety of behavioral experiments designed to diversify her experiences and test her ideas about her ability to experience pleasure and interest. Miranda noted great improvements in her mood when she engaged in these alternative behaviors, and this improved mood extended to a general feeling of mastery. The client became more active in applying DBT skills during this time; in particular, she began to work very diligently on the application of interpersonal effectiveness skills to her relationships with colleagues and her husband.

During the period of treatment in which depressive symptoms were the target of treatment, the therapist also often encouraged the client to use mindfulness skills learned in DBT group for observing and describing depressive thoughts and other symptoms in a nonjudgmental manner. The therapist explained that using these skills may help the client's depression by reducing the likelihood that negative thoughts would escalate into episodes of depressive rumination. However, whenever the therapist brought this up, the client responded with annoyance and anger, often stating, "I *hate* mindfulness." When asked to elaborate, the client explained that the mindfulness module had been her least favorite skill module in group because she felt that the mindfulness skills seemed "new-agey," "illogical," and "faddish." More problematic, however, were the client's rigid beliefs that the practice of mindfulness was an unethical attempt to divorce oneself from the genuine guilt and concern that one should feel as a human being and that nonjudgmental self-observation equated to "running away from the genuine depravity of [her] humanity." On numerous occasions, the therapist attempted to engage the client in an intellectual discussion about the possibility of ethical motivations for and empirically verifiable positive ethical consequences of mindfulness practice; however, the client was firm in her rejection of mindfulness practice as a treatment tool. On the other hand, the client admitted that she had experienced increased "awareness" of her emotions, thoughts, sensations, and experiences through DBT skills training, and she felt she had benefited from this increased awareness. Therefore, at this point in the treatment, the topic of mindfulness was dropped.

Though the client's mood had improved a great deal over the course of behavioral activation treatment for depression, the therapist noticed that the client had avoided completion of many behavioral experiments that were designed to take place outside her home. When the therapist inquired as to the reason for this, the client responded that, though she was feeling less depressed since she started experimenting with new activities as home, she was feeling more and more anxious and mistrustful of others, particularly when outside the home. She also noted that she was now having recurring nightmares of being raped, short flashbacks to her experiences of sexual abuse, and more frequent fears of being sexually abused by strangers she met. The therapist attempted to shape the client's behavior by reinforcing even small attempts to engage in new activities outside the home; however, the client expressed extreme fear and resistance. Because the client's mood had improved and because the client had demonstrated mastery of skills for coping with unpleasant emotion, it was decided that treatment for PTSD would be the next therapeutic task.

Treatment of PTSD Using Exposure–Based Cognitive Processing Techniques

The client was now much more emotionally stable; however, the therapist prefaced the exposure-based cognitive processing therapy for PTSD (Resick & Schnicke, 1992) by reviewing distress-tolerance skills to ensure that initial exposure to memories of being sexually abused would not cause a relapse in self-harm behavior. This particular treatment for PTSD is composed of three main components: psychoeducation about PTSD, exposure and reprocessing of traumatic episodes, and cognitive restructuring of cognitive rules or beliefs that the client has acquired as a function of the abuse. Treatment began with psychoeducational material about PTSD. The client identified strongly with the desire to avoid all reminders of her sexual abuse and with the idea that her avoidance was causing symptoms of intrusive reexperiencing of the event.

The next task in this treatment is to help the client identify cognitive rules and beliefs that have arisen as a function of their abuse. Miranda identified several cognitive rules and beliefs: "Trust no one," "All people, especially men, are dangerous and should be avoided," and "I am to blame for the abuse because I didn't make a big enough deal about it." Next, the therapist and client worked together to generate evidence for and against these beliefs. The client was highly defensive about generating alternative ideas because she was thoroughly convinced that these beliefs were absolutely true and appropriate. Given the client's previous negative experience with cognitive therapy, such a response was not unexpected. In addition, it seemed to highlight the importance of eventually addressing not only the content of the client's thoughts but also her relationship to them (i.e., fused to and overidentified with thoughts).

Next, we progressed to the exposure therapy portion of the treatment. Here, the client was asked to recount on paper two or three of the most salient traumatic episodes. Then, over the course of six weeks, she was asked to read each story several times per week as well as several times during each session. At first, the client reported feelings of numbness or feelings of intense shame after reading the stories out loud. The therapist validated and normalized such feelings and encouraged the client to continue with exposures at home. The client reported that she was generally able to complete about two to four exposures per week during this phase of treatment. Although symptoms spiked after the first week, the client reported a rapid decline in all symptoms of reexperiencing and avoidance after the second week. For example, she stated that she no longer had intrusive thoughts about her episodes of abuse, no longer felt overwhelmed by these experiences, and began to attend a few social functions and go shopping for groceries on her own. The client was pleased with these results; however, she noted that on the rare occasions that she did think about the abuse, she continued to feel intense shame and engaged in a great deal of rumination about the abuse being her fault.

The final stage of PTSD treatment was to attempt once again to examine and challenge the cognitive rules and beliefs that the client reports as related to the traumatic experiences. As noted previously, the two main beliefs that appeared to be problematic for the client were (1) that she was defective because she caused the abuse and because the abuse occurred and (2) that no one was trustworthy and the world was therefore a dangerous place. As before, the therapist aided the client in enumerating evidence for and against these beliefs. The client was now able to acknowledge that she had not been 100 percent at fault for the abuse. However, it became clear that such a shift in understanding did not alleviate distress for the client, who then reported feeling "deeply saddened and upset" to think about her male relative as a "bad person." The therapist then encouraged the client to examine the costs and benefits of such dichotomous thinking; the client seemed to understand but did not seem to feel better. The client continued to assert that there was no evidence that the world was not a dangerous place and that people could be trusted in general; however, these beliefs no longer elicited the intense fear of venturing out of her house that they once had. The client asserted that these beliefs were simply true and that no amount of rationalization would change the fact that all of humanity was essentially defective.

Treating Cognitive Rigidity by Fostering Mindful Cognitive Decentering and Experiential Acceptance

The client had made functional gains both socially and occupationally by applying DBT skills, experimenting with new behaviors that alleviated her depression, and overcoming her symptoms of PTSD. However, she was still experiencing a great deal of distress related to her chronic and intense self-criticism. In addition, she remained strongly suspicious of the motives of others. Such beliefs and the automatic thoughts to which they frequently led to episodes of rumination. The client noted often that she still disliked herself and feared others and that constant rumination on these themes and on her own suicidal urges caused her a great deal of distress.

Because the client was relatively unresponsive to cognitive restructuring or challenging her beliefs, it was felt that her remaining symptoms would be best treated through mindfulness training. However, as noted previously, the client actively disliked and objected to the mindfulness skills as presented in DBT, so it was decided that alternative methods would be used to encourage the client to foster mindfulness. First, the therapist practiced acceptance of the fact that the word *mindfulness* was not currently useful to the client and that using it would reduce therapeutic effectiveness. Therefore, the word *mindfulness* was no longer used in session. Instead, the therapist presented the highly related skill of cognitive defusion from acceptance and commitment therapy (Hayes & Smith, 2005). *Cognitive defusion* is described as the ability to notice thoughts and feelings as mental events rather than reifying them as absolute truth or overidentifying with them. Great care was taken to explain this skill as fostering a "healthy psychological space and flexibility." As homework, the therapist asked Miranda to practice a variety of cognitive-defusion techniques from the ACT manual (Hayes & Smith, 2005). For example, the client practiced restating her experiences using defused sentence stems such as "I'm having the thought that . . ." or "I'm having the sensation of . . ." She also practiced saying "Thank you, mind" when having strong thoughts or emotions rather than automatically believing her thoughts and feelings, and she imagined her unpleasant mental events as a little monster that walked around beside her at all times but did not control her behavior. Miranda successfully completed these exercises and reported that she liked this new type of awareness. Homework assignments focused on practicing cognitive-defusion skills as a way of improving her ability to respond rather than react to life circumstances. The client was diligent in completing the homework, and reported that defusion made her psychological reactions to events much more bearable because she was able to see them as "just thoughts" or "just feelings" rather than absolute truth. The related concept of experiential acceptance—that is, being willing to experience one's thoughts, emotions, and sensations rather than suppressing or avoiding them—was also presented, and the client reported that a commitment to experiential acceptance rather than avoidance was helpful for fostering the motivation to use cognitive defusion.

During the time cognitive defusion was the focus of treatment, the therapist also used several other strategies to encourage the development of mindfulness without explicitly referencing it. First, the therapist demonstrated a mindful stance by reframing things that the client noticed in a nonjudgmental way. For example, the client often noted that, even though she knew they were harmless because she had no longer had any interest in acting on them, she was ashamed of and concerned about her frequent thoughts of suicide. Whenever the client noted this, the therapist said, "So it sounds like when you have thoughts about killing yourself, you notice that you have some mental reactions to that which are unpleasant for you: feelings of shame and thoughts about how you're not normal." Second, the therapist praised the client when she expressed nonjudgmental or one-mindful awareness of her experience. Third, the therapist asked the client to practice defusion techniques in session. For example, when the client expressed strong negative emotion about her relationship with her husband, the therapist sometimes encouraged the client to restate her feelings in a defused way. For example, rather than "I am trapped with this frustrating person," she was encouraged to say, "I am having the thought that I am trapped with my husband and am experiencing frustration quite frequently when I'm with him." The client was initially hesitant to do this;

however, such in-session practical work and feedback was important because the client had little previous experience with relating to her negative intense feelings and thoughts as simply mental events.

Complicating or Treatment-Promoting Factors for Miranda

As a client, Miranda had many strengths. Although her NEO-PI-R scores suggest low conscientiousness, Miranda repeatedly demonstrated high conscientious and an ability to work hard to learn new skills. In addition, her strong intellectual abilities allowed her to thoroughly understand skills. She was generally quite agreeable in session, but her willingness to be disagreeable about things that simply did not make sense to her was actually a strength; had she been unwilling or unable to express her ethical concerns regarding mindfulness, for example, her failure to truly integrate these skills into her life may have "slipped beneath the radar." Her willingness to try a variety of treatments in order to address her numerous concerns was also a strength, and it was likely the primary reason that treatment was so successful.

Follow-Up for Miranda

Following this part of the treatment, Miranda reported that she was feeling very well and felt ready to terminate her treatment. In a final session, the client and the therapist reviewed what the client had learned and discussed plans for addressing future issues. The client no longer met criteria for any disorder. However, the client still reported experiencing some strong negative emotions and painful or difficult thoughts every day (e.g., about committing suicide or about being rejected by others). Though the frequency of these experiences had reduced somewhat and the content of these experiences had shifted slightly, only the nature of her *relationship to these experiences* had changed dramatically over the course of treatment. She was now able to see these experiences as passing thoughts and feelings rather than absolute truths demanding strong reactions in the moment, and this change appeared to be responsible for her newfound sense of stability and well-being.

USING MINDFULNESS EFFECTIVELY: REFLECTIONS ON TWO CASE STUDIES

The two case studies presented here demonstrate the effective use of mindfulness-based interventions, the wide variety of client reactions to such treatment modalities, and the need to be flexible in tailoring the semantics of mindfulness-based interventions to particular client needs. Though Rachel and Miranda both benefited from mindfulness practice, their pathways to practice differed because of their different levels of interest in and resistance to mindfulness. Both therapists demonstrated flexible application of mindfulness-based treatments that also allowed for the use of more traditional CBT techniques. In both cases, clinical outcomes were excellent. These cases suggest the importance of therapist flexibility while using mindfulness-based treatments, as well as the need for assessment of client attitudes toward mindfulness and mindfulness practice at the outset of therapy.

The results of both cases are consistent with relevant treatment-outcome research that demonstrate positive outcomes associated with training in both experiential acceptance and behavioral regulation. In the case of both DBT and ABBT, treatment focuses on striking a balance between accepting unpleasant experiences and shaping behavior to create a higher quality of life. In the case of Rachel, her response to ABBT and the mindfulness skills involved was positive, leading to a self-compassionate orientation toward her anxiety that allowed her to experience symptoms without dwelling on them or letting them derail her from desired goals. Rachel's new ability to tolerate anxiety allowed her to develop awareness of other components of her experience, including her somatic sensations, emotions, and desires, most of which she had previously ignored in efforts to avoid triggering anxiety. Mindful awareness of her experiences allowed her to be more flexible in pursuing a life that she valued.

Miranda's response to DBT was similarly positive. Though Miranda was extremely resistant to practice mindfulness, she diligently practiced distress-tolerance skills that fostered experiential acceptance and learned a variety of cognitive-defusion skills that changed her relationship to her experience in helpful ways. Although Miranda continued to experience a variety of painful emotions and even frequent suicidal thoughts, her ability to notice these experiences in nonjudgmental ways using awareness and defusion skills allowed her to engage in more constructive behaviors that improved her mood and decreased feelings of hopelessness and shame.

In general, Rachel was very enthusiastic about mindfulness, whereas Miranda strongly objected to it. Nevertheless, they were both able to benefit from cultivating an ability to attend to present-moment experiences in accepting ways. Clinicians who meet resistance when attempting to teach mindfulness skills may benefit their clients by making a commitment to flexibility and effectiveness (in contrast to rigidity) while applying these concepts. Many authors have noted that mindfulness is a heterogeneous construct with multiple aspects (e.g., Baer, Smith, Hopkins, Krietemeyer, & Toney, 2006). Having specific knowledge about the key behavioral components of mindfulness may make it easier to quickly adapt concepts and skills into concrete language that is most likely to be effective given an individual client's particular strengths and level of openness to mindfulness.

REFERENCES

Baer, R. A., Smith, G. T., Hopkins, J., Krietemeyer, J., & Toney, L. (2006). Using self-report assessment methods to explore facets of mindfulness. *Assessment, 13,* 27–45.

Beck, A. T., & Steer, R. A. (1990). *Beck Anxiety Inventory: Manual.* San Antonio, TX: Psychological Corporation.

Beck, A. T., Steer, R. A., & Brown, G. K. (1996). *Manual for the Beck Depression Inventory–II.* San Antonio, TX: Psychological Corporation.

Brewer, J. A., Mallik, S., Babuscio, T. A., Nich, C., Johnson, H. E., Deleone, C. M., . . . & Rounsaville, B. J. (2011). Mindfulness training for smoking cessation: Results from a randomized controlled trial. *Drug and Alcohol Dependence, 119*(1), 72.

Butler, A. C., Chapman, J. E., Forman, E. M., & Beck, A. T. (2006). The empirical status of cognitive-behavioral therapy: A review of meta-analyses. *Clinical Psychology Review, 26,* 17–31.

Butcher, J. N. (2001). *MMPI–2: Minnesota Multiphasic Personality Inventory–2: Manual for administration, scoring, and interpretation.* Minneapolis: University of Minnesota Press.

Costa, P. T., Jr., & McCrae, R. R. (1985). *The NEO Personality Inventory manual.* Odessa, FL: Psychological Assessment Resources.

Dimeff, L., & Linehan, M. M. (2001). Dialectical behavior therapy in a nutshell. *The California Psychologist, 34,* 10–13.

First, M. B., & Gibbon, M. (1997). *User's guide for the structured clinical interview for DSM-IV axis I disorders SCID-I: Clinician version.* Arlington, VA: American Psychiatric Publications.

Hayes, S. C., & Smith, S. (2005). *Get out of your mind and into your life: The new acceptance and commitment therapy.* Oakland, CA: New Harbinger.

Hayes, S. C., Strosahl, K. D., & Wilson, K. G. (1999). *Acceptance and commitment therapy: An experiential approach to behavior change.* New York: Guilford Press.

Linehan, M. M. (1993). *Cognitive Behavior Treatment of Borderline Personality Disorder.* New York: Guilford Press.

Linehan, M. M., Armstrong, H. E., Suarez, A., Allmon, D., & Heard, H. L. (1991). Cognitive-behavioral treatment of chronically parasuicidal borderline patients. *Archives of General Psychiatry, 48*(12): 1060–1064.

Lynam, D. R., & Widiger, T. A. (2001). Using the five-factor model to represent the DSM-IV personality disorders:

An expert consensus approach. *Journal of Abnormal Psychology, 110*(3), 401.

Olatunji, B. O., Cisler, J. M., & Deacon, B. J. (2010). Efficacy of cognitive behavioral therapy for anxiety disorders: A review of meta-analytic findings. *Psychiatric Clinics of North America, 33*(3), 557.

Orsillo, S. M., & Roemer, L. (2011). *The mindful way through anxiety: How to break free from chronic worry and reclaim your life*. New York: Guilford Press.

Resick, P. A., & Schnicke, M. K. (1992). Cognitive processing therapy for sexual assault victims. *Journal of Consulting and Clinical Psychology, 60*(5), 748.

Roemer, L., Orsillo, S. M., & Salters-Pedneault, K. (2008). Efficacy of an acceptance-based behavior therapy for generalized anxiety disorder: Evaluation in a randomized controlled trial. *Journal of Consulting and Clinical Psychology, 76*, 1083–1089.

Tolin, D. F. (2010). Is cognitive-behavioral therapy more effective than other therapies? A meta-analytic review. *Clinical Psychology Review, 30*(6), 710–720.

Waters, A. M., & Craske, M. G. (2005). Generalized anxiety disorder. In M. M. Antony, D. R. Ledley, & R. G. Heimberg (Eds.). *Improving outcomes and preventing relapse in cognitive behavioral therapy* (pp. 77–127). New York: Guilford.

Editors' Introduction

This case study illustrates the ways in which assessment can facilitate psychotherapy; more importantly, it demonstrates how the assessment of specific character strengths and virtues can be used to supplement more traditional measures of personality, deviance and psychopathology such as the Minnesota Multiphasic Personality Inventory (MMPI). The senior author of this chapter coauthored the companion chapter on Positive Psychotherapy (with Martin Seligman) in Current Psychotherapies, *and he believes this is the best available case study to supplement his chapter.*

Students interested in learning more about their own profile of character strengths are encouraged to assess their own signature strengths by taking the VIA Inventory of Strengths survey online. There is no charge for taking or scoring the VIA-IS, and the inventory has been translated into 17 languages and taken by more than two million people. The VIA-IS can be found at viame.org.

Do you agree with the listing of your own strengths? How will these strengths facilitate your work as a therapist? What will you do to cultivate those character strengths that are are less well developed in your own life? Do you agree with the authors' contention that viewing films is a powerful way of exposing your clients to positive role models and that doing so will help them cultivate these strengths? Can you think of examples of important and powerful films that illustrate each of the 24 character strengths?

Numerous reviews of Positive Psychology films can be found on the PsycCRITIQUES Blog (psyccritiquesblog.apa.org). Additional Positive Psychology assessment tools are available at www.tayyabrashid.com.

Will you include the assessment of strengths into your own work as a therapist or counselor? What other psychological tests will you give up in order to make time for this additional level of assessment? Is the payoff from assessing and discussing strengths sufficient to justify additional costs to the client? Does Positive Psychotherapy reflect a genuine paradigm shift that will change the way we understand and treat our clients?

12 | STRENGTH–BASED ASSESSMENT IN CLINICAL PRACTICE

Tayyab Rashid and Robert F. Ostermann

Assessment, whether formal or informal, objective or projective, is an inherent part of clinical practice. Traditionally, clinical assessment has explored the southern side of mental health by identifying symptoms, deficits, and disorders. Our central point in this article is that clinical assessment can also expand northward to incorporate strengths. To make our case, we underscore the utility of deficit-oriented assessment, highlight its shortcomings, describe strength-oriented assessment, and present concrete ways of incorporating strengths into clinical practice.

Undoubtedly, negatives fascinate us. Negatives are pervasive and potent. Deviation from norms attracts our attention more than adherence to them. Negative impressions and stereotypes are quicker to form and more resistant to disconfirm. Negative emotions, sour interactions, and bad feedback affect us more than their positive counterparts (Baumeister, Bratslavsky, Finkenauer, & Vohs, 2001). Clients seeking psychotherapy have often experienced the potency and pervasiveness of negatives. They often ruminate about negative emotions for months or even years. They easily recall negative events, setbacks, and failures. By assessing and treating negatives, psychotherapy has made huge strides. Rigorous studies have demonstrated that assessment and treatment of psychopathology helps significantly more than placebos do and often the effects last far longer than the effects of medications (Seligman, 1995; DeRubeis, Gelfand, Tang, & Simons, 1999).

Exclusive focus on negatives, however, has often the effects last far longer serious shortcomings. First, there is an untested assumption that symptoms are authentic and central ingredients that ought to be assessed carefully, whereas positives are by-products of symptom relief or clinical peripheries that do not need assessment. So entrenched is this assumption about the assessment of symptoms that the *Diagnostic and Statistical Manual* (DSM-IV) labels *affiliation, anticipation, altruism,* and *humor* as "defense mechanisms" (American Psychiatric Association, 2000, p. 752). Altruistic behavior is often considered a coping mechanism to counteract guilt. By contrast, we believe strengths are as real as human weaknesses, as old as time, and valued in every culture (Peterson & Seligman, 2004). In clinical assessment, strengths contribute to well-being in the same way that weaknesses contribute to psychopathology.

JOURNAL OF CLINICAL PSYCHOLOGY: IN SESSION, Vol. 65(5), 488–498 (2009) © 2009 Wiley Periodicals, Inc. Published online in Wiley InterScience (www.interscience.wiley.com). DOI: 10.1002/jclp.20595. Reprinted by permission.

Second, a deficit-oriented model of assessment reinforces a fundamental negative bias (Wright & Lopez, 2002). In other words, if symptoms stand out saliently and if these are regarded as negative (as they usually are) and if context is vague or sparse, then the perception of the individual will likely be negative. This was demonstrated in a study specifically designed to explore the clinical impact of the negative bias (Pierce, 1987). Participants in this study, simulating the role of a clinician, were asked what they would like to know about a client. The client, Jane, was identified as either just having been released from a psychiatric facility (salient negative) or just having completed her undergraduate studies (salient positive). In both instances, she was described as seeking help because she was "feeling somewhat anxious and uncertain about her future, including her job and her and other issues in her life." The research participants selected 24 facts they would like to know about Jane from a list of 68 items, half of which were positive (e.g., "Is Jane intelligent?") and half negative (e.g., "Is Jane cruel?"). Significantly more negative items were selected in the case of the former psychiatric patient than the college graduate. This experiment demonstrates that if a clinician elicits only negatives, then a fundamental negative bias is likely to color his or her perception.

Third, deficit-oriented assessment reduces a holistic view of clients and may compartmentalize them into synthetic labels and DSM categories. Sophisticated objective and projective measures are used to validate the existence of these categories. So pervasive have these labels become that often clients, after a Google search, come to psychotherapy prepared to fit themselves in these categories. Arriving at an accurate diagnosis, which should be a careful and discerning process, frequently becomes an exercise in labeling. Labeling itself is not undesirable. Labels categorize and organize the world, but reducing or objectifying clients to labels of psychopathology may strip them of their rich complexity (Szasz, 1961). In turn, they may think of themselves as deeply disturbed, anxious, or depressed—characteristics frequently associated with diagnostic labels.

Fourth, the role of clinician in deficit-oriented assessment inevitably becomes that of someone with expertise to diagnose and treat symptoms and weaknesses. This may create a power differential in which the client is more likely to passively comply with clinician's perception and works toward correcting deficits or managing symptoms. Refusal to share a clinician's perception could be perceived as resistance or denial. The clinician is generally perceived as more empathic and attuned by clients if he or she can accurately list deficits and locate them in a coherent personality structure.

Deficit-oriented models of assessment, in our view, paint an incomplete picture of the client, reducing clarity, information, and completeness. Clinical assessment should be a hybrid endeavor: exploring strengths as well as weaknesses. The focus of assessment should be collecting not only stories of unmet needs but also tales of fulfillment. Assessment should explore not only conflicts but also compromises, transgressions as well as acts of compassion, selfishness affecting others and also genuine actions of sharing, grudges as well as expressions of gratitude, and episodes of vengeance as well as instances of forgiveness. It is about exploring in an authentic way hubris as well as humility, haste as well as self-restraint, hate as well as love, and the pain of trauma as well as growth from it.

STRENGTH-BASED ASSESSMENT

Although strength-based assessment finds its contemporary thrust in positive psychology and solution-focused therapy, humanistic psychology has long advocated that psychological assessment should accommodate core elements, such as growth orientation, personal agency, subjective experience, and the development of personhood (Friedman & MacDonald, 2006). Similarly, Marie Jahoda (1958) made a persuasive argument that well-being should be assessed along six dimensions: acceptance of oneself, growth and becoming, integration of personality, autonomy, accurate perception of reality, and environmental mastery. These six components have been operationalized and empirically examined (Ryff & Singer, 1996). Unfortunately, assessment and treatment of deficits has become the primary function of clinical practice. During the last century, the study of character strengths was phased out because of increasingly pragmatic specializations and tightening of disciplinary boundaries (Sloan, 1980). These factors combined to push strengths out of the clinical picture and training of clinicians, especially in psychiatric facilities run on the deficit model, which focused on honing diagnostic skills to uncover deficits.

Assessing strengths can provide the clinician with a powerful tool to understand a client's skill repertoires, which can be effectively utilized to counter troubles. Considering what strengths a client brings to effectively deal with troubles stimulates a very different discussion and therapeutic relationship from a deficit-oriented inquiry asking, "What weaknesses or symptoms have led to your troubles?"

What is strength-based assessment? It essentially involves exploring *what's strong* to supplement traditional digging for *what's wrong* (Duckworth, Steen, & Seligman, 2005). Strength-based assessment is a multimodal endeavor that explores clients' strengths as well as weaknesses. The strength-based model of assessment is about not only strengths, as the name may imply, but also understanding the client in an integrated way so that strengths can be marshaled to undo troubles.

Concurring with this notion, Epstein and Sharma have defined the strength-based assessment as follows:

- The measurement of those emotional and behavioural skills, competencies and characteristics that create a sense of personal accomplishment; contribute to satisfying relationships with family members, peers, and adults; enhance one's ability to deal with adversity and stress; and promote one's personal, social, and academic development (1998, p. 3).

The four-front model of positive assessment gives serious attention to the following areas: (1) deficiencies and undermining characteristics of the person (what deficiencies does the client contribute to his or her problems); (2) strengths and assets of the person (what strengths does the client bring to deal effectively with his or her life); (3) deficits and destructive factors in the environment (what environmental factors thwart clients' development); and (4) resources and opportunities in the environment (what environmental resources facilitate positive human functioning) (Wright & Lopez, 2002).

Strength-based assessment also invites interesting alternative hypotheses about psychopathology. For example, depression may not be just a cluster of symptoms described in the DSM-IV, but it can also reflect a lack of positive emotions and meaning in a client's life. Strengths, from this standpoint, serve us best not when life is easy, but when life is tough. With a depressed client, the clinician can explore and work on strengths such as perspective, zest, and gratitude. Shoring up social strengths of the client such as teamwork, social intelligence, and kindness could be a viable way of counteracting depression. Similarly, anxiety may represent worrying, feeling restless, fidgety and impulsive behavior, as well as a lack of focus; however, it can also reflect a lack of purposeful goals, actions, and habits that utilize clients' strengths and absorb him or her immensely.

Some clinicians are concerned that assessment of strengths may either reinforce narcissistic attitudes for some clients or distract them from serious problems that need immediate attention. We reiterate that the goal of a strength-based assessment is neither to create Pollyannaish or Panglossian caricatures of clients nor to inflate grandiose egos of clients. Of course, in assessing strengths, the goal is never to minimize or mask negative experiences such as abuse, neglect, and suffering.

We would also distinguish the differences involved in assessing strengths, talents, and abilities. For example, intelligence, melodic voice, and athletic ability are talents that are different from strengths in the sense that strengths fall in the moral domain but talents and abilities do not. Strengths are valued in their own right and are not tied to other variables.

CONDUCTING STRENGTH-BASED ASSESSMENT

In our clinical work, we have successfully used several strategies, some of which have been empirically tested (Seligman, Rashid, & Parks, 2006), to integrate strengths in clinical assessments. Here are 10 concrete strategies:

1. A number of assessment scales, inventories, and interviews have been developed to assess positive emotions, strengths, meaning, and a host of strengths-related constructs. Clinicians can choose validated instruments to assess specific positive constructs. *Positive Psychological Assessment: A Handbook of Models and Measures* (Lopez & Snyder, 2003) and *Handbook of Methods in Positive Psychology* (Ong & Van Dulmen, 2006) provide reproducible measures that can be used in clinical practice. Among our favorite are the Positive and Negative Affect Schedule, Hope Scale, Life Orientation Test–Revised, Satisfaction with Life Scale, Love Attitudes Scales, and Heartland Forgiveness Scale.

2. Most measures of psychopathology are expensive and require completion in clinical settings. Strength measures developed by practitioners and researchers of positive psychology are readily available online without any charge—for example, the Authentic Happiness Inventory, Fordyce Emotions Questionnaire, General Happiness Questionnaire, Gratitude Questionnaire, and the Grit Survey at www.authentichappiness.sas.upenn.edu. This Web site provides instantaneous feedback about strengths or positive attributes. The personal website of the first author (www.tayyabrashid.com) offers useful clinical measures such as Positive Psychotherapy Inventory, Signature Strengths Questionnaire (SSQ-72), and a measure to assess engagement and flow. Clients can complete these measures at home and can bring printouts of results to therapy. These measures could also be used to track changes over the course of psychotherapy.

3. Interviews guided by research can also be used to assess strengths. If a clinician prefers not to use formal assessment, then he or she can use questions during intake or evaluation that elicit strengths, positive emotions, and meaning. Some of the questions we use are: "What gives your life a sense of meaning?" "Let's pause here and talk about what you are good at"; "Tell me what you are good at"; "What are your initial thoughts and feelings when you see someone doing an act of kindness or courage?"

4. To help clients to discern and identify their own strengths, clinicians can also use icons of certain strengths (e.g., Gandhi, Mother Theresa, Nelson Mandela, Martin Luther King, Jr., Albert Einstein, Aung San Suu Kyi, Ken Saro-Wiwa) real-life narratives, and popular films (*Pay It Forward, Forrest Gump, My Left Foot, Precious, To Kill a Mockingbird,* etc.). By using strengths displayed by specific icons and film characters, the clinician can discuss with clients whether they partly or fully identify with these icons and characters and, if so, which conditions clients see to display these strengths maximally and what might be some of the consequences of displaying these strengths. (For a comprehensive list of films, please see Snyder & Lopez, 2007; Niemiec & Wedding, 2013.)

5. Clinicians can also seek collateral information from family members, colleagues, and friends about the strengths of their client as well as strengths of concerned

individuals as they relate to the client. This is particularly helpful in assessing and identifying social and communal buffers. For example, in addition to inquiring about problems with family members, clinicians may also assess attachment, love, and nurturance from the primary support group. Instead of looking for problems related to social environment, a clinician can ask clients to describe humor and playful interactions, connectedness, and empathetic relationships at work.

6.   Clinicians can also use standardized as well as informal measures to assess strengths of the client displayed during challenges and trauma. A number of psychometrically sound resilience measures are available (see Tedeshi & Kilmer, 2005, for a review). Informally, clinicians can ask questions such as, "Tell me about a challenge you handled adaptively?" or "What have you done to overcome a serious difficulty?" or "Tell me about a setback from which you learned a lot about yourself?" Discussing critical items from various resilience and posttraumatic growth scales can also facilitate these lines of inquiry.

7.   We recommend that clinicians assess strengths early in the therapeutic process. After establishing rapport and empathically listening to the concerns that brought the client to therapy, the clinician can mindfully explore strengths. We realize that during the course of treatment as usual, most clinicians become aware of their clients' strengths. But it is also possible that this vital information never becomes available during a crisis, and most clients don't know how to use their strengths to cope with the challenging situation. Along with the assessment as usual profile, clinicians are encouraged to assess the criteria for *flourishing*, which involves assessing the following parameters (Snyder & Lopez, 2007):

A. Individual must not have had episodes of major depression in the past year.

B. Individual must possess well-being defined by meeting all three of the following measures.

  1.   High psychological well-being, defined by four of six scale scores on appropriate measures falling in the upper tertile:

      a. Positive affect

      b. Negative affect (low)

      c. Life satisfaction

  2.   High psychological well-being defined by four of six scale scores on appropriate measures falling in the upper tertile:

      a. Self-acceptance

      b. Personal growth

      c. Purpose in life

      d. Environmental mastery

      e. Autonomy

      f. Positive relations with others

  3.   High social well-being defined by three of five scales scores on appropriate measures falling on the upper tertile:

      a. Social acceptance

      b. Social actualization

      c. Social contribution

      d. Social coherence

      e. Social integration

8. Assessment of strengths provides the clinician with a powerful mechanism with which to encourage clients to pursue absorption and deep engagement. Clients can be encouraged to use and further develop strengths such as creativity, curiosity, appreciation of beauty, love of learning, and social intelligence, or they can tweak activities to experience more engagement. Engagement can be especially beneficial for clients who have concentration difficulties, boredom, and listlessness. In addition, strengths-based engaging activities are also likely to reduce brooding and rumination.

9. Clinicians, who, for practical and clinical reasons, prefer not to use formal measures of strengths, can use a narrative strategy, which we have found to be very helpful in eliciting strengths. This strategy is called Positive Introduction. In this assessment strategy, after listening to the account of troubles, the clinician encourages the client to introduce himself or herself through a real-life story (about 300 words, with a beginning, a middle, and a positive end) that shows the client at his or her best or during a peak moment of life. The clinician discusses the story with the client in detail in terms of what strengths are displayed and whether they are accurate descriptions of the client's current functioning. Clients having difficulty writing a story or identifying specific strengths may be encouraged to ask family members and friends to tell a story depicting her or his strengths. This strategy reveals the client's strengths to the clinician as well as to significant others.

10. Finally, clinicians can assess whether the client is currently able to translate abstract strengths into concrete actions, behaviors, and habits. This assessment is important because real-life challenges rarely come in neat packages with labeled instructions such as "When depressed, use zest and vitality." Challenges and hassles often occur amidst a dizzying jumble of emotions, actions, and their effects. The role of the clinician is to assess and gently guide the client to use his or her strengths to solve a problem. Strengths elicited from the Positive Introduction or from measures of character strengths or talents (e.g., SSQ-72, VIA-IS, Strength Finder, etc.) are used to reframe problem solving skills. This narrative becomes dynamic and can assist clients to visualize a rich, full, rewarding and meaningful life. For instance, a clinician may say to a client, "Let's discuss the strengths that you displayed in your positive introduction. What role might they play in this challenging situation?" This exercise provides rich data on the client's past and current strengths and weaknesses.

In using one or more of these 10 strength-based strategies, we are mindful that not all have been the subject to the same empirical and psychometric validation as their deficit-oriented counterparts. Compared to the existing sophisticated taxonomy of psychopathology and the hundreds of measures to assess it, the classification and measures of strengths are few and far between. The first serious classification of strengths, *Character Strengths and Virtues* (Peterson & Seligman, 2004), has only recently been published, whereas five editions of DSM have appeared so far.

Many clients feel a depleted sense of worth before coming to a clinician. When weaknesses and strengths are assessed and discussed in an integrative manner, clients are likely to find psychotherapy to be affirming, empowering, and even motivating (Saleebey, 1996). Such integration may reassure clients that their unique, holistic selves are recognized beyond their diagnostic profiles. Thus, the strength-based assessment process, entirely independent from its outcome, can bring substantial benefits. Furthermore, attending to the whole individual can foster a different than usual therapeutic relationship that balances the power differential between the client and the clinician and positively affects the therapeutic alliance (Harris, Epstein, Ryser, & Pearson, 1999). In turn, the client sees that the clinician is trying to understand him or her as a whole person, not just a bundle of problems.

CASE ILLUSTRATION

Client Description and Presenting Problem

Riba, a 38-year-old married woman, presented with significant symptoms of depression that were affecting her functioning at home and work. She lived with her husband and a 10-year-old son. Riba works for an information technology firm. At the time she entered treatment, Riba reported being sad; feeling empty and slow; having diminished appetite, low libido, and sleep disturbances; worrying a lot; and feeling anxious. These symptoms had been ongoing for the last 5 months and became severe enough that Riba was unable to continue her job and had to take a sick leave. Riba described her marriage as stable but somewhat "empty and lacking intimacy." She often felt alone as her husband traveled a lot for his work. She sometimes worries about her son's academics, although her son is doing well. Riba has not socialized with her close friends lately. Riba's health is generally good and she is currently not taking any medications. This was the first time Riba sought psychotherapy.

Course of Assessment and Treatment

From a deficit-oriented model, Riba was administered the Minnesota Multiphasic Personality Inventory-2 (MMPI–2) and Beck Depression Inventory (BDI). Her scores on MMPI–2's depression scale and BDI were significantly elevated. She did not endorse any thoughts of suicide. Based on the clinical interview and the test results, the clinician (first author) determined that Riba's mood was consistent with the DSM-IV diagnosis of major depressive disorder.

Our first two sessions were devoted to establishing rapport, exploring Riba's history of depression, understanding the family dynamics, and assessing her perception of problem and her reasons to seek therapy. In the third session, the clinician and Riba discussed her clinical profile from a deficit-oriented perspective, underscoring patterns of symptoms and the course of depression and its consequences. Speaking in a soft tone and making little eye contact, Riba endorsed her profile and expressed feelings of hopelessness about her ability to get better. Toward the end of this session, Riba was gently asked to introduce herself through a real-life story that would show her at her best. Reluctant initially, Riba agreed to give it a try. In the next session, she brought her story. She was encouraged to read it. Riba read:

> I was in tenth grade when my family moved across the country. I loved my previous high school and had a lot of friends. I missed it greatly and did not feel like going to my new school, but I had to. Class work was less painful but the lunch was the worst because I didn't have anyone to eat with and I felt like a lonely dork. During the second week, sitting alone, I was staring at my salad and almost believing that onion cuts formed the word "loser" when I heard some students laughing hysterically at the next table. At first, I thought they have read what was written on my salad. I hunkered down and dared not to look at them but soon I figured out that their laugh was not directed at me or my salad. I turned and looked at this was a bunch of kids who seemed quite cool. Soon, I noticed that they were all laughing at this boy who sitting alone at an adjacent table and there seemed something not alright with him. I didn't know then, that Harris had a tic disorder which made him to jerk his head involuntarily. It was quite obvious that he was not doing this on his own. Clearly, he seemed embarrassed and confused. I thought it was very mean of these kids to make fun of him. I felt very sad. For a moment I thought I should stop them but then I thought, they are the "cool" kids and if I did that I will never be able to make any friend at this school. But this selfish impulse passed quickly and I

started feeling angry. Without thinking much, I just got up and walked to them and in a single breath I shouted, "I don't know you, and I don't know him, but whatever you are doing is sick. I thought I was a loser here for not having any friend but I think you are much bigger losers." I came back to my table and felt good.

Riba finished the story with misty eyes but with her face lit up. Upon prompting, Riba identified courage and fairness as salient strengths displayed in her story. She was then asked to complete the online Values in Action–Inventory of Strengths (VIA-IS) and bring the printout of her feedback to the next session.

In the following week, Riba brought the printed VIA-IS feedback. Interestingly, neither courage nor fairness were included among her top strengths. From a list of 24 core strengths, capacity to love and being loved, creativity, social intelligence, appreciation of beauty, and spirituality were her top strengths. Courage and fairness was in the middle of the list, and zest and self-regulation were found toward the end. During next three sessions, the clinician and Riba discussed wholeness and the relationship between her symptoms of depression and her profile of strengths.

In the light of her positive introduction, we also discussed how Riba's self-identified strengths of courage and fairness might still serve her during tough times. The notion of using her top strengths and working on her weaker strengths, such as zest and self-regulation, was discussed in detail.

Combining her strengths was discussed with the help of a metaphor: an *orchestra of strengths* that is constantly changing and adapting its tempo and tune in accordance with changing circumstances. The change and adaptation was particularly highlighted because strengths have their shadow sides. In Riba's case, one of her top strengths of social intelligence helped her at work as she used her acute awareness of emotions and intentions of others and made every attempt to make everyone feel comfortable. However, at the same time, in making everyone feel comfortable, Riba took too much responsibility on her shoulders and did not say no. Similarly, at home she understood her husband's work demands but took on more work herself than she could comfortably handle. Consequently, she felt that she understood everyone but not many understood her. This feeling not only saddened her but also left her feeling helpless.

After thorough discussions on integration of strengths, Riba decided she would work on them, at the same time she was working to decrease or eliminate her depression. Riba began with appreciating beauty by actively searching glimpses of natural and artistic beauty everyday and journaling about these experiences. She also decided to use her creativity to experience flow. For example, Riba loved cooking. Every Sunday, she started enjoying a long, slow dance of chopping, grating, stirring, simmering, tasting, seasoning, and sharing the wonderful meals she cooked with her family. She also decided to work on self-regulation; she joined a gym and worked out three times a week.

In this process, Riba's symptoms were not ignored. She had good and bad days. Whenever she brought forth these struggles with depression, her concerns were validated but her attention was gently guided to negotiate with them by mindfully working on her strengths.

Outcome and Prognosis

Assessment and leverage of strengths helped Riba shift her focus from deficits and helplessness to what was right about her. She learned ways to use her deepest psychological resources to manage her sad mood. Using strengths through concrete actions helped her reeducate her attention and memory to notice genuinely good aspects of her life. After about 20 sessions, both measures of psychopathology and strengths were administered again. Riba's scores on depression decreased significantly, and she no longer met criteria for the diagnosis of major depressive disorder. Her strengths profile remained largely similar, with the exception of self-regulation, which moved from bottom of the pack to the middle. In addition, she also returned to her work.

CLINICAL ISSUES AND SUMMARY

In many ways, Riba represents a typical depressed client whose progress in therapy could have been reduced significantly if she was perceived only through a deficit-oriented assessment. However, close to the onset of therapy, the clinician included assessment and diagnosis of strengths into therapy, and this helped to forge treatment collaboration. Strengths elicited from both the positive introduction and the VIA-IS helped Riba internalize the notion that, despite her depression, she possessed strengths that could be used to overcome her struggles. Assessment of Riba's deficits *and* strengths helped her to understand herself more fully and structure a life that included enhanced pleasure, engagement and meaning.

Assessment of Riba's strengths enhanced the work of therapy in this case as, in our experience, it does in the vast majority of cases. However, we are mindful that the complexity and time of clinical assessment increases when strengths are incorporated along with deficits. We recommend that clinicians adopt a flexible approach of strengths assessment, incorporating both qualitative strategies and objective measures and integrating strengths with weaknesses.

REFERENCES

American Psychiatric Association. (2000). *Diagnostic and statistical manual of mental disorders* (4th ed., text rev.). Washington, DC: Author.

Baumeister, R. F., Bratslavsky, E., Finkenauer, C., & Vohs, K. D. (2001). Bad is stronger than good. *Review of General Psychology, 5,* 323–370.

DeRubeis, R. J., Gelfand, L. A., Tang, T. Z., & Simons, A. D. (1999). Medications versus cognitive behavioral therapy for severely depressed outpatients: Mega-analysis of four randomized comparisons. *American Journal of Psychiatry, 156,* 1007–1013.

Duckworth, A. L., Steen, T. A., & Seligman, M. E. P. (2005). Positive psychology in clinical practice. *Annual Review of Clinical Psychology, 1,* 629–651.

Epstein, M. H., & Sharma, J. M. (1998). *Behavioral and emotional rating scale: A strength-based approach to assessment.* Austin, TX: Pro-Ed.

Friedman, H. L., & MacDonald, D. A. (2006). Humanistic testing and assessment. *Journal of Humanistic Psychology, 46,* 510–529.

Harris, M. K., Epstein, M. H., Ryser, G., & Pearson, N. (1999). The behavioral and emotional rating scale: Convergent validity. *Journal of Pychoeducaitonal Assessment, 17,* 4–14.

Jahoda, M. (1958). *Current concepts of positive mental health.* New York: Basic Books.

Lopez, S. J., Synder, C. R., & Rasmussen, N. H. (2003). Striking a vital balance: Developing a complementary focus on human weakness and strength through positive psychological assessment. In S. J. Lopez & C. R. Snyder (Eds.), *Positive psychological assessment: A handbook of models and measures* (pp. 3–20). Washington, DC: American Psychological Association.

Niemiec, R., & Wedding, D. (2013). *Positive psychology at the movies: Using films to build virtues and character strengths.* Gottingen, Germany: Hogrefe.

Ong, A. D., & van Dulmen, M. (Eds.). (2006). *The Oxford handbook of methods in Positive Psychology.* New York: Oxford University Press.

Peterson, C., & Seligman, M. E. P. (2004). *Character strengths and virtues: A handbook and classification.* New York: Oxford University Press.

Pierce, D. L. (1987). *Negativity bias and situation: Perception of helping agency on information seeking and evaluation of clients.* Unpublished master's thesis, University of Kansas, Lawrence.

Ryff, C. D., & Singer, B. (1996). Psychological well-being: Meaning, measurement, and implications for psychotherapy research. *Psychotherapy and Psychosomatics, 65,* 14–23.

Saleebey, D. (1996). The strength perspective in social work practice: Extensions and cautions. *Social Work, 41,* 296–305.

Seligman, M. E. P. (1995). The effectiveness of psychotherapy: The consumer reports study. *American Psychologist, 50,* 965–974.

Seligman, M. E. P., Rashid, T. & Parks, A. C. (2006). Positive Psychotherapy. *American Psychologist, 61,* 774–788.

Snyder, R. C., & Lopez, R. J. (2007). *Positive Psychology: The scientific and practical explorations of human strengths.* Thousand Oaks, CA: Sage.

Sloan, D. (1980). Teaching of ethics in the American undergraduate curriculum, 1876–1976. In D. Callahan & S. Bok (Eds.), *Ethics teaching in higher education* (p. 30). New York: Plenum Press.

Szasz, T. (1961). *The myth of mental illness: Foundations of a theory of personal conduct.* New York: Harper & Row.

Tedeshi, R. G., & Kilmer, R. P. (2005). Assessing strengths, resilience, and growth to guide clinical interventions. *Professional Psychology: Research and Practice, 36,* 230–237.

Wright, B. A., & Lopez, S. J. (2002). Widening the diagnostic Focus: A case for including human strengths and environmental resources. In C. R. Snyder & S. J. Lopez (Eds.), *Handbook of Positive Psychology* (pp. 26–44). New York: Oxford.

Editors' Introduction

Although some therapists still adhere dogmatically to the theoretical model in which they were trained, an increasing number of therapists simply identify themselves as eclectic. In short, they do what works, and when what they are doing doesn't work, they try something else.

Larry Beutler and John Norcross coauthored the chapter on Integrative Psychotherapies for Current Psychotherapies. *Dr. Beutler is a master therapist and one of the world's leading psychotherapy researchers. In the following case, he demonstrates the application of systematic treatment selection (STS), an eclectic methodology for therapy in which patients are thoughtfully and scientifically matched with a variety of specific therapeutic approaches. Beutler applies STS to a deeply troubled client with a serious addiction to heroin and cocaine and concomitant marital and financial problems.*

This case study illustrates the way in which behaviorally oriented therapists still use and benefit from psychological tests, such as the MMPI-2, and the ways in which these assessments can be used to guide treatment. It shows how homework assignments can benefit clients and demonstrates the utility of medication as an adjunctive treatment. Most important, it demonstrates the apparently seamless integration of diagnosis with assessment of stages of change, coping style, resistance level, and the patient's personal preferences.

Will you be comfortable with an approach to treatment like the one outlined by Larry Beutler, or will you be more likely to identify with a particular school of therapy? Is it reasonable to assume that any given theoretical approach can be applied to every patient who walks in the door? If psychologists are licensed to prescribe medications— like the antidepressants used to treat this patient—will you make psychopharmacology a part of your practice?

13 | INTEGRATIVE THERAPY WITH MR. F. H.

Larry E. Beutler

Our approach to psychotherapy is broadly characterized as integrative and specifically labeled *systematic treatment selection,* or STS. Concisely put, we attempt to customize psychological treatments and therapeutic relationships to the specific and varied needs of individual patients, as defined by a multitude of diagnostic and particularly nondiagnostic considerations. We do so by drawing on effective methods across theoretical schools (integrative), by matching those methods to particular cases on the basis of empirically supported principles (treatment selection), and by adhering to an explicit and orderly (systematic) model.

Systematic treatment selection is a flexible system whose principles have identified a number of dimensions on which patients and treatments and relationships may be matched and customized. The actual number of dimensions that have received research support for their ability to optimize treatment outcomes surpasses that which can easily be applied by a clinician operating in the absence of a computer-assistant program. Such programs exist (e.g., www.systematictreatmentselection.com), but for convenience of the current illustration, we have selected some of the more common dimensions used in treatment planning and have applied them to the current case.

Systematic treatment selection (Beutler & Clarkin, 1990; Beutler, Clarkin, & Bongar, 2000) embraces two basic assumptions: (a) no treatment methods work well on all patients and (b) most treatment methods work well on some patients. The effects of most (if not all) treatments range from very positive to at least mildly negative depending on the patient observed. STS seeks to identify which patients will respond positively to various mixes of interventions from different treatment models.

Contemporary efforts to construct research-informed guidelines do not address the commonalities among treatments, preferring instead to think of each treatment as a discrete and identifiable entity that can be applied to all patients who are assigned a given diagnosis. However, the presence of a shared diagnosis occludes the presence of important differences among patients. Thus, the appropriateness of any given treatment depends on both the pattern of methods used and the fit of these methods to both the diagnostic and nondiagnostic characteristics of the patient.

In contrast to the broad-grain approach of fitting a treatment solely to a patient's diagnosis, STS seeks to identify multiple patient dimensions that best fit with corresponding treatment strategies and a therapist's particular relationship style. Rather than identifying treatments purely in terms of global theories (e.g., cognitive therapy, psychoanalytic therapy, interpersonal therapy) or specific techniques that comprise it (e.g., interpretation, thought records, evidence analysis), STS is constructed around research-informed principles of behavior change. These guiding theorems of change and relationship cut across theoretical orientations and can be applied by individual therapists from different perspectives (Beutler et al., 2000).

The principles and applications of STS were developed through a four-step process (Beutler et al., 2000). The first step was a series of literature reviews to identify predictors and moderators of therapeutic change. The second step was to collapse and combine these variables into a smaller set of clusters, each of which identified a particular fit or match between patient qualities and treatment strategies that reliably relate to change. Our third step was to develop means for measuring the patient qualities and treatment strategies that emerged from the prior steps. The fourth step was to test hypotheses extracted from the reviews of literature, all of which bore on the question of what factors accounted for optimal therapeutic change.

In the following case, we apply some of the resulting STS dimensions to planning and conducting psychotherapy with Mr. F. H. He was a patient experiencing comorbid depression and substance abuse who was seen in a randomized controlled trial of the efficacy of STS predictions (Beutler et al., 2003).

CASE DESCRIPTION

Mr. F. H. is a 39-year-old Caucasian man with 14 years of education, married for about 3 years, and with no children. F. H. has just started a home-based business with his wife, after having changed several jobs in the last few years. He decided to consult a psychologist because he was undergoing severe financial problems due to his drug abuse (he had incurred a considerable debt by borrowing money to pay for his drugs) and his wife was threatening to leave him if he did not find a definitive solution to his addiction. He also reported symptoms of anxiety, feeling sometimes "overwhelmed by a lack of motivation," and talked about having "no desire to do anything," describing some severe episodes of depression. Now he is "tired of lying to himself and to others."

INITIAL INTERVIEW

F. H. appeared 15 minutes late for the first interview. His language was logical and coherent, even if sometimes distracted. He claimed slight memory impairment because of the drug use, and therefore, he was vague and found it difficult to remember some dates and events. The following information was extracted from the initial interview and administration of standardized intake procedures, which included the MMPI-2, STS Clinician Rating Form, and Beck Depression Inventory.

The client was taking both heroin, approximately one-quarter gram three or more times a week, and cocaine, approximately one-half gram almost every day. He reported using them together or alternatively and stated that he was able to stay clean from one drug or the other just for a few days. He was trying to self-titrate the doses, but he felt that he "cannot go any lower." He had been treated twice for drug abuse, one treatment consisting of detoxification only, but he was not able to remember the specific dates of such treatments. F. H. tried numerous "30-day" outpatient programs but never methadone because "it's just synthetic heroin, but with a third of the power. If I want that, I can just take less dope." He attended several AA and NA meetings, expressing a preference for the first. None had produced more than transitory relief from his addiction.

F. H. reported difficulties in various cognitive functions, such as concentration and decision making. He was experiencing frequent loss of appetite and insomnia, leading him recently to spend an entire week without sleeping. Everything went from bad to worse after visiting his stepbrother. Nonetheless, he "didn't feel like going to a shrink" before the visit, and he tried to "get into a better mood" by consuming more drugs and alcohol.

Mr. F. H. was raised by his natural parents until the age of 14, when they divorced and he stayed with his mother. She remarried soon after the divorce; meanwhile, his father disappeared, and the client has never known if he is dead or alive. F. H. reported that his father was an alcoholic, and his mother possessed a "paranoid phobic" personality. He always suspected she was a prostitute, but he was not sure about this attribution. She committed suicide 16 years prior to this interview and only a couple of months after the patient had a terrible car accident. F. H. stated that she physically abused him and his brothers. He does not remember his father abusing him, but he was hurt for all the times the father ignored what the mother was doing to his brothers and him.

Mr. F. H. started drinking when he was a teenager, and he has continued to abuse alcohol since then. Sixteen years before entering treatment on the current occasion, and in reaction to both the physical problems that followed his car accident and the nearly concomitant suicide of his mother, the patient started using heroin to "get out from the physical and emotional pain." In a short period, he developed an addiction to heroin, and he started consuming regular amounts of cocaine as well. After 6 years of drug abuse, he was arrested for the first and only time, charged with drug possession. Following this event, he entered or was committed by the court to several 30-day outpatient treatment programs. He successfully stopped using drugs and remained "clean" for a period of 4 years, during which time he started seeing a psychiatrist. He was dissatisfied and left treatment without further benefit.

Seven months ago, F. H. went to visit J., the older stepbrother he had not seen for a long period. While there, his stepbrother helped F. H. remember some physical and emotional abuses they had both experienced in childhood at the hands of their parents, especially their mother. When he came back home, F. H. felt depressed and began having suicidal thoughts. He subsequently slashed his wrists in an attempt to kill himself. At the time of this evaluation, however, he reported no suicidal ideation. He did report continuing depression and anxiety and indicated that this had been relatively constant for a period of more than 6 months. He reported a recurrent fear that he might "go crazy."

F. H. has many friends among drug abusers but only "two good pals" who were not drug-related. These two friends and his wife were the only persons he could trust. One of these friends was a physician who had sometimes helped him by prescribing drugs during the patient's efforts to withdraw.

CASE FORMULATION

Most psychotherapies can be represented by mapping the therapist's actions against several dimensions (Beutler & Clarkin, 1990; Beutler et al, 2000; Castonguay & Beutler, 2006), including the following: (a) variations in intensity of treatment, (b) variations in the focus on insight versus behavior and skill change, (c) variations in the level of directiveness used, and (d) variations in the way that patient affect is managed. STS proposes that each of these variations in therapy implementation tends to be most suitable for a patient who has a particular and corresponding quality of personal or situational attribute. In other words, different folks need different strokes. Patient characteristics and environments serve as powerful indicators (and contraindicators) of different treatments. Below we present a sampling of five patient characteristics commonly used by integrative psychotherapists. These patient characteristics or variables guide us in identifying a beneficial "fit" between patient and treatment. As noted earlier, integrative therapists are not confined to these five considerations in making treatment decisions. The dimensions applied here serve to illustrate the process of clinical assessment and treatment matching in integrative psychotherapies.

1. Diagnosis and Functional Impairment

A patient's *diagnosis and level of impairment* serve as the basis for the assignment of an appropriate level of care. A thorough assessment of functional impairment includes a consideration of the patient's problem complexity (comorbidity and personality disorder), chronicity, and the available social support system. Level of impairment is considered a determiner of treatment intensity, which can be varied by increased length, the use of multiple formats, and increased frequency. Concomitantly, complexity—a condition indexed by comorbidity and related to level of impairment—is an indicator for the use of multiperson or family-based interventions.

F. H. displayed moderate impairment as indicated by his chronic history of multidrug abuse and alcohol abuse, both combined now with a diagnosis of depression and a previous suicide attempt. Additionally, his MMPI-2 Social Introversion (*Si*) and Paranoia (*Pa*) scales were elevated, indicating his feelings of alienation from others. Thus, current levels of social support were considered weak, and his problem was characterized as complex because it was impacting negatively on numerous areas of functioning, and at the time he sought treatment, he was in danger of losing both his job and his marriage. MMPI-2 scores and various indicators of work and family disturbance also suggested above average difficulties. Accordingly, the intake clinician gave F. H. a global assessment of functioning (GAF; American Psychiatric Association, 2000) rating of 56, indicating moderate disturbance in functioning.

Based on the conclusion of moderate impairment, treatment was scheduled at an intensity of twice a week, at least for the beginning 4 to 6 weeks of the therapy. Because of his low level of social support, high level of problem complexity, and sense of alienation from others, two of the early sessions were scheduled for work with his wife and him together. Some later sessions were also planned to include work with his wife (as it turned out, a total of 7 of the 15 sessions of treatment were with his wife). After an initial 4 to 6 weeks of treatment, if the patient had been adequately stabilized and symptoms had been addressed (e.g., the drug abuse noticeably declined, he was less depressed and anxious), then he may be able to decrease the frequency of the sessions to one a week supplemented by phone calls and emergency sessions if needed.

The primary goal of therapy and the initial focus of treatment were on reducing the risk posed by self-destructive behaviors (substance abuse and suicidal behavior). The principal means of accomplishing these aims was through increasing [the] level of felt support from his wife. The need to provide a protective environment was given serious consideration and remained an option throughout treatment, even though it was eventually decided that frequent outpatient visits would be adequate to the patient's needs.

Mr. F. H.'s level of functioning also suggested that the therapist assign and monitor his attendance at NA and/or AA meetings on a regular, perhaps daily, basis. His wife agreed to play an active role in helping him monitor these activities. Antidepressant medication was considered as an eventual adjunct to psychotherapy (specifically, an antidepressant that may also help reduce the patient's symptoms of general anxiety). In the long run, the recommendation encouraged the patient to employ psychological change procedures as a first-line treatment before applying biochemical agents, in an effort to help maintain the patient's focus on developing a chemical-free lifestyle.

In the service of achieving chemical-free living, the patient also was encouraged to decrease his use of substances based on a realistic schedule of substance use reduction/titration. A medical specialist in substance abuse was consulted with respect to the titration schedule, and a physical exam was conducted that cleared the patient for gradual withdrawal from drugs. Additionally, the patient and his wife were provided with educational material describing the possible withdrawal effects and specific behaviors (e.g., exercise, diet, vitamin supplements, sleep hygiene, stress management) that have proved helpful in reducing the negative aspects of the withdrawal process.

Because of the chronicity and complexity of the patient's problems, the STS model recommended long-term outpatient care. The frequency of treatment was adjusted as the patient succeeded in reducing drug use, but the therapist was encouraged to expect periods in which the patient's symptoms would become stimulated or activated, necessitating temporary increases in treatment frequency. During these times, work with the patient and his wife as a couple was also increased to both support his changes and to enhance the level of pleasure available in his relationship.

2. Stage of Change

The stages represent a person's readiness to change, defined as a period of time as well as a set of tasks needed for movement to the next stage. People progress across six stages: precontemplation, contemplation, preparation, action, maintenance, and sometimes termination.

Mr. F. H.'s substance abuse history is that of a chronic contemplator who occasionally enters the action stage for a few successful months or years but then returns to contemplation. People can remain stuck in the contemplation stage for long periods (i.e., years and even decades). But F. H. is now preparing to enter the action stage, largely at the insistence of his wife and due to his financial problems.

The patient's stage of change is an indicator for both treatment methods and relationship stances. As someone in the preparation or early action stage, F. H. is most likely to prosper from methods traditionally associated with the existential, cognitive, and interpersonal therapies. As he enters the later action stage and progresses to maintenance, then behavioral and exposure methods are probably most useful. Each therapy system has a place, a differential place, in the "big picture" of behavior change.

The therapist's relational stance is also matched to the patient's stage of change. The research and clinical consensus on the therapist's stance at different stages can be characterized as follows (Prochaska & Norcross, 2002). With precontemplators, the therapist stance is often like that of a nurturing parent joining with the resistant youngster who is both drawn to and repelled by the prospects of becoming more independent. With contemplators, the therapist role is akin to a Socratic teacher who encourages clients to achieve their own insights and ideas into their condition. With clients who are preparing for action, the stance is more like that of an experienced coach who has been through many crucial matches and can provide a fine game plan or can review the person's own action plan. With clients who are progressing into maintenance, the integrative psychotherapist becomes more of a consultant who is available to provide expert advice and support when action is not progressing as smoothly as expected.

3. Coping Style

An assessment of the patient's coping style informs the focus of treatment, encouraging the therapist to select methods that vary along a continuum from insight-focus to behavior-change-focus. In this, there are aspects of patient coping style that correlate with one's stage of readiness to change. Thus, coping style serves as a partial cross-check on the treatment decisions that arise from assessing a patient's stage of (or readiness to) change. For example, externalizing and impulsive behaviors (i.e., coping styles) indicate the value of problem and behaviorally focused methods, much as does the action stage of change readiness, whereas internalizing and restraining behaviors indicate the value of insight and emotional awareness, in a similar manner as indicated by a contemplative stage of change.

F. H. presented with a mixed pattern of internalizing and externalizing symptoms. He had a history of acting out (externalizing) through drug use and substance abuse. A history of suicidal acts accompanied by the self-reported claim of "interpersonal conflict" suggested the presence of impulsiveness, which accompanied a correlated pattern of self-blame emotional restriction. The MMPI-2 also confirmed the presence of mixed personality features, including both internalizing and externalizing behaviors. Specifically, F. H. produced not only elevations on several internalizing scales, like the Depression (D), the Social Introversion (Si), and the Anxiety (Pt) scales, but also elevations on two externalizing scales, the Impulse (Pd) scale and Paranoia (Pa) scale.

The symptoms that placed this patient at risk for continued drug use and for suicidal behavior were given priority and served as the initial focus of psychotherapy. Because he presented with both externalizing and internalizing coping patterns, short-term work focused directly on developing impulse control, while long-term goals included achieving insight into his motivations and awareness of his unmet emotional needs. This decision was consistent with that associated with the assessment of his contemplative and early action stage of change.

Initially, work with the patient and his wife aimed at identifying drug and suicide risk behaviors and at establishing a sense of emotional caring and support that could help him weather these occasions. Later, as the patient began individual treatment, the focus shifted more to the achievement of understanding and insight. The following exchange, which took place during his fourth session (two sessions after the two sessions in which he was seen with his wife), shows how the therapist tried to facilitate insight and personal and emotional awareness by teaching the patient (notice the focus on understanding and feeling identification):

T: When you take a lower dose, and you believe that nothing is happening and that you need to have another "hit," how do you feel?
FH: I don't know—helpless, I guess is the word.
T: Because that's actually what you are likely to feel when you are at the detox program. You are not going to get the feeling that you have to have your stuff to help you feel more powerful!
FH: That's true.
T: What do you think? What do you tell yourself, when you are in that spot? Something like, "the stuff is not working, I've gotta get more!"
FH: I don't know. Maybe.
T: Let's assume that this is the feeling and thought you have—of being helpless and needing something to pull you out of it. How does that sound?
FH: It's uncomfortable—I feel lost. I hate it.
T: It feels like you don't have any options at that point?
FH: It does! Yeah! Actually, I feel that way about a lot of things right now! I feel like my options are very limited, I feel helpless, and I don't like what I see. What I've been left with.
T: So, even though you feel helpless and don't like that, maybe there are some options, but you just don't like them!
FH: Probably. Yeah, you're right!

T: This is important because the more you can get an understanding of how those feelings make you do things, before going to the detox program, the easier it will be for you.

4. Resistance Level

An assessment of the patient's level of resistance informs the selection of the therapist's level of directiveness. High resistance is taken as an indicator for the use of procedures that deemphasize therapist control, and vice versa. Resistance is defined as the degree of patient opposition to perceived efforts on the part of the therapist to control the patient's behavior. Managing resistance by the selection of methods that are either nondirective or directive and skillfully adapting to changes in resistance levels will minimize the occurrence of negative interactions in therapy and enhance the development and maintenance of the therapeutic alliance.

At the beginning of treatment, and in his wife's presence, the patient expressed a strong desire to quit his drug abuse, and his motivation seemed to be quite high—good signs with respect to treatment compliance. Based on quantitative assessments early in treatment, F. H. scored just above average on a measure of resistance (Dowd Trait Reactance Scale; Dowd, Milne, & Wise, 1991), but he scored below the average on the MMPI-2 Readiness for Treatment scale (*TRT*). Taken together, these scores suggested that F. H. manifested low average resistance, therefore indicating the use of therapist-directed procedures.

For example, early in treatment, the therapist offered a directive homework task:

FH: Change apartments, go to work, talk to my doctor, detox. I should make a list! I keep making lists, but every time my priorities change.
T: Maybe you should make a short list and a long list. The long list is what you have to do in the next couple of weeks or so; the short list is what you have to do today.
T: Keep it simple. Just one thing at a time; commit to one thing each day. You have to say to yourself: "Today I'm definitely gonna do this for me!" Can you do that?
FH: Yeah.
T: So, what can it be today?
FH: Well, calling the detox program!
T: Okay. So next time you can tell me how it went and what's your next choice.

The patient's homework assignment was reviewed and monitored in each session. The patient's cooperation and compliance confirmed for the therapist that the client possessed a relatively low level of resistance. Thus, the patient continued to benefit from the structure and guidance provided by the symptom-focused strategies employed. Nonetheless, the therapist remained vigilant to any signs of increase in resistance level (e.g., patient is often late for therapy, patient becomes argumentative, homework is not completed) throughout the course of therapy and adjusted directiveness levels accordingly.

5. Patient Preferences

When ethically and clinically appropriate, we accommodate a client's preferences in psychotherapy. These preferences may be heavily influenced by clients' sociodemographics—gender, ethnicity, sexual orientation, for example—as well as their attachment styles and previous experiences in psychotherapy. These preferences may refer to the person of the therapist (age, gender, religion, ethnicity/race), therapeutic relationship (how warm or tepid, how active or passive, etc.), therapy methods (preference for or against homework, dream analysis, two-chair dialogues), or treatment formats (refusing group therapy or medication).

In this case, F. H. was interested in some work in couples therapy to improve the quality of the relationship with his wife and to lower her level of frustration with his many failed efforts to overcome his addictions. Thus, two early sessions included his wife. As she became more hopeful, we shifted more to an individual focus. This shift could only occur, however, when the patient was comfortable with the clinician, the therapeutic relationship, and the treatment plan offered. What was important to him was his level of emotional arousal in the therapy session. In psychotherapy, patients usually seek treatment to reduce the intensity of painful emotional states; however, if emotional arousal levels are too low, patients may lose their incentive to continue the therapy, and they may fail to persist in making positive changes in their lives. Conversely, when anxiety is high, the patient may be too distressed to approach treatment in a planned and receptive manner.

An examination of the patient's treatment history revealed that F. H. usually entered treatment in an acute state of anxiety that dissipated rapidly, after which he had little motivation for change. Based on this assessment, it was decided to employ a modest amount of confrontation to maintain the patient's anxiety and, hence, his motivation for change. F. H. preferred this strategy: one in which the therapist would take an active role in keeping him engaged in the therapeutic work, would not allow him to terminate prematurely, and would present him with new challenges every session or two.

A decrease in F. H.'s anxiety through the development of a supportive structure, the improvement in his relationship with his wife, and a safe psychotherapy environment were used to enhance the development of the therapeutic alliance—a necessity for continued involvement and successful treatment. The integrative therapist provided phone and pager numbers to the patient and encouraged him to contact the therapist anytime he felt the need to do so.

The following exchange, which occurred in session nine, illustrates the therapist's efforts to manage and control the patient's discomfort.

FH: I'm doing better. My work, my behavior, my being with other people, the sensation of being sober and clean instead of drug motivated.

T: When you say that you are doing better, I don't think that you completely believe that, but . . .

FH: I believe that I'm going in the right direction and I have more desire to get clean and sober. But, like you said, it's not entirely true.

T: What is really better right now?

FH: I have that desire and, at the moment, I'm off the coke, and right now it just disgusts me! You know, I disgust me! When I think about using it . . . I just wanna be out of that!

FH: Yes, physical and psychological.

T: Both. And your body is telling your brain: take more, use more, you need it! Our mind and our body tell us a lot of things. But we don't have necessarily to obey.

It is notable, from an integrative perspective, that one must balance and integrate the level of confrontation that produces arousal and the focus of treatment—in this case, the focus on insight and awareness of feelings.

T: These experiences have been really, really dramatic.

FH: You know, the drugs don't scare me one tenth as much as the idea of some of these [things] reoccurring.

T: The drugs have been an escape from those memories.

FH: I guess so. I don't remember the time when I was home.

T: Unconsciously, they have always been there.

FH: Sure. I would say that I didn't think about that until the day I talked to my stepbrother.

T: I think it's gonna take time to process all those memories.

COURSE OF TREATMENT

After the first four sessions, two of which had included his wife, F. H. and the therapist were able to start working on the establishment of self-awareness and insight, complemented by homework assignments that targeted specific behaviors such as drug abuse, impulse control, and the development of healthy interaction skills. At this point, the therapy was tailored to track the patient's drug use, drug cravings, and his unique pattern of depressogenic events, thoughts, and behaviors. Considering the client's low resistance, his preferences for guidance, and early action stage, the therapist used primarily directive interventions that combined insight and action goals. These included homework, the psychoeducation, scheduling of healthy (nondrug use) activities, and goal deadlines.

After 15 sessions, fewer than the scheduled 20 sessions of therapy, F. H. was able to begin a methadone detox program and attend NA meetings on a regular basis. By the end of this time, F. H. was abstinent from all drugs and was able to establish new social networks and increase his social contact within nondrug-using contexts. He successfully moved from his previous residence, and he started a new job in a new environment, the combination of which required that he terminate psychotherapy. In the final termination sessions, F. H. reported improvements in his marital relationship, and he had managed to eliminate his financial problems through careful counseling and skills gained in budget management and couples therapy. All these changes gave the therapist the opportunity to partially shift his attention to F. H.'s lifelong threatening memories and his history of losses and abandonment, very likely the primary causes of his depression and suicide attempt.

At follow-up 6 months after treatment, F. H. reported that he was "on the right track." He was abstinent from heroin and cocaine. He was not depressed. He acknowledged the therapist as an important and trustful figure. And impressively, he was ready to slowly discuss and face what he experienced in childhood.

SUMMARY

Systematic treatment selection, broadly integrative in nature, fits the treatment to the patient on the basis of research-based principles of change. This approach stands in contrast to many pure-form or brand-name systems of psychotherapy that tend to fit the patient to their particular treatment on the basis of preferred theory or personal bias.

STS fits the treatment to the individual patient and his or her singular situation on a host of interacting, empirically informed principles. The patient's functional impairment, for example, is used to set the treatment intensity. In the spirit of basing psychotherapy on principles rather than recipes, the way in which therapy is intensified will necessarily vary from patient to patient. In our case example, the therapist chose to vary the frequency of sessions, but one could add treatments, extend treatment, or do some combination of these things. The resistance level, another example, is used to select the therapist directiveness. The directiveness defines the therapist's role as either teacher and authority or collaborator and student. On one hand, the therapist may assume the role of authority as in behavioral or psychodynamic therapies, and on the other, he or she may assume a reflective and questioning role, much like that used by cognitive and client-centered therapists. In the case presented, the therapist adopted a largely teaching and guiding role with the patient, recognizing the patient's relatively low resistance. In many cases, of course, the therapist will adopt both strategies in a seamless and responsive manner.

Different folks require different strokes. The five client characteristics, as illustrated in the case of F. H., serve as reliable markers to systematically tailor treatment to the individual patient, problem, and context. Although these client characteristics are likely to evolve as research progresses, they are based on extensive reviews and meta-analyses of the treatment literature. These client characteristics, including but not limited to diagnosis, can be applied independently of a specific theoretical orientation. All of this is to say that psychotherapy has progressed to the point where clinically relevant and readily assessable patient characteristics can inform specific treatment plans and thereby enhance the effectiveness and efficiency of our clinical work (Norcross & Beutler, 2014).

REFERENCES

American Psychiatric Association. (2000). *Diagnostic and statistical manual of mental disorders* (4th ed., text revision). Washington, DC: Author.

Beutler, L. E., & Clarkin, J. (1990). *Systematic treatment selection: Toward targeted therapeutic interventions*. New York: Brunner/Mazel.

Beutler, L. E., Clarkin, J. F., & Bongar, B. (2000). *Guidelines for the systematic treatment of the depressed patient*. New York: Oxford University Press.

Beutler, L. E., & Harwood, T. M. (2000). *Prescriptive psychotherapy: A practical guide to systematic treatment selection*. New York: Oxford University Press.

Beutler, L. E., & Harwood, T. M. (2002). What is and can be attributed to the therapeutic relationship? *Journal of Contemporary Psychotherapy, 32,* 25–33.

Beutler, L. E., Moleiro, C., Malik, M., Harwood, T. M., Romanelli, R., Gallagher-Thompson, D., & Thompson, L. (2003). A comparison of the Dodo, EST, and ATI indicators among co-morbid stimulant dependent, depressed patients. *Clinical Psychology & Psychotherapy, 10,* 69–85.

Castonguay, L. G., & Beutler, L. E. (Eds.). (2006). *Principles of therapeutic change that work*. New York: Oxford University Press.

Dowd, E. T., Milne, C. R., & Wise, S. L. (1991). The Therapeutic Reactance Scale: A measure of psychological reactance. *Journal of Counseling and Development, 69,* 541–545.

Norcross, J. C., & Beutler, L. E. (2014). Integrative psychotherapies. In D. Wedding & R. J. Corsini (Eds.), *Current psychotherapies* (10th ed.). Belmont, CA: Brooks/Cole.

Prochaska, J. O., & Norcross, J. C. (2002). Stages of change. In J. C. Norcross (Ed.), *Psychotherapy relationships that work* (pp. 303–313). New York: Oxford University Press.

Editors' Introduction

Lillian Comas-Díaz is the leading proponent of multicultural psychotherapy in the United States, and this case study illustrates the benefits of culturally adapting mainstream psychotherapy for a Latina client. The case illustrates a variety of culturally specific techniques and methods with a woman (Alma) who presents with a concern that transcends culture: "I'm dead inside." However, despite the existential nature of the presenting complaint, we quickly see that this woman's concerns are deeply influenced by and embedded in a complex cultural matrix.

How does your program ensure that you receive the training necessary to deal effectively with clients with a variety of cultural backgrounds? Do you feel equipped to work with clients with a different ethnic background or sexual orientation? Should graduate programs require all mental health professionals to be bilingual? Is psychotherapy likely to be more effective when clients and therapist share the same cultural background? Why or why not?

14 | ALMA

Lillian Comas–Díaz

Alma—a 35-year-old single lawyer—entered therapy a year after her grandmother's death. A bilingual Mexican American, Alma frequently traveled to Mexico for business and pleasure. "I'm dead inside," was her presenting problem. Blanca, her grandmother, had been a positive maternal figure. Consequently, Alma felt guilty for "not being there" when Blanca died. "I'm an emotional orphan," Alma said. "My mother has been suffering from Alzheimer's for the past 10 years." Alma's parents divorced when she was six and her father kept no contact with them. She seemed to express her complicated bereavement through self-destructiveness. Alma experienced relational difficulties, drank too much alcohol (a bottle of wine with dinner), and smoked a pack of cigarettes daily. Suicidal and homicidal assessments were negative. Alma revealed that her grandmother Blanca, who drank alcohol and smoked "too many cigarettes," died of lung cancer. She connected the source of her self-destructive behavior to her identification with Blanca. During the initial stages of therapy, Alma became receptive to anxiety-reducing techniques.

I used relaxation techniques and systematic desensitization to help Alma regain a sense of agency and balance. Afterward, we addressed her negative cognitions regarding not being there for Blanca. Alma's self-destructive behavior decreased significantly. She seemed to develop trust in me (a middle-aged Latina psychologist) and in the psychotherapeutic process. At this point, Alma revealed that she had been self-medicating her sleeping problems with NyQuil. . . . Her sleep improved with the deep relaxation, and she stopped the over-the-counter medication. "*No hay aguacero que no escampe,*" Alma said when describing her mood. This *dicho* (The rain will eventually stop) signaled the beginning of Alma's recovery. Afterward, I suggested completing a cultural genogram. Among other things, the genogram revealed that Alma was named after Blanca's mother. The family genogram unfolded that Doña Alma immigrated when she was 20, married a Mexican American, gave birth to five children, and became a successful businesswoman. "I've not done enough," Alma concluded upon describing her great grandmother's accomplishments. I invited Alma to give a *testimonio*. She identified the burden to succeed created by bearing the name of her great grandmother. However, the narrative experience seemed to liberate her. Alma's *testimonio* helped her to "individuate" from the family expectation of being like her namesake. Interestingly, Alma was successful at work; she was partner at a prestigious law firm. Nevertheless, "I carry too many battle scars," she said, referring to her struggle against racism and sexism on her way up the

Excerpt from Comas-Díaz (2006). Latino healing: The integration of ethnic psychology into psychotherapy. *Psychotherapy: Theory, Research, Practice, Training, 4,* 436–453.

corporate ladder. We addressed her battle scars with CBT desensitization approaches. However, Alma did not find her career fulfilling. I used schema work combined with mindfulness to address this issue. We identified fear of abandonment and feelings of inadequacy as her main negative schema. Out of this experience, Alma started a daily mindfulness practice. She identified a lost love—volunteerism—and decided to reclaim it. "I have to give back to my community." Alma began to do legal *pro bono* work for immigrant Latinos. Beatriz, one of her *pro bono* clients, gave Alma an *arpillera*—a Latin American weaving. The tapestry was a rendition of Beatriz's disappeared relatives' arrival into heaven.

During this time, Alma reported a recurrent dream. She saw her *Abuela Blanca* transform herself into a crone. We analyzed the dream from different perspectives. Alma preferred a cultural interpretation: *Blanca* appeared as the Aztec goddess *Coatlicue*, who represents the cycle of creation and destruction of life, death, and rebirth. Alma interpreted her Abuela's manifestation as a message: "*Vive tu vida*" (Live your life). The dream analysis helped Alma with her fear of abandonment. She expressed feeling connected to Blanca in a deeper way. Through cultural resonance, I felt that something was missing and remembered Alma's godmother. Cultural resonance involves the ability to understand clients via clinical skill, cultural competence, and intuition. While completing her cultural genogram, Alma revealed that Guadalupe, her *madrina* (godmother), was a folk healer. I explored if she wanted to contact Guadalupe for a consultation. "How did you know also I had a dream with *Madrina*?" Alma replied. Indeed, Guadalupe had a message from *Blanca* to Alma. *Blanca* wanted her granddaughter to visit the Sanctuary of Chimayó, a peregrination site in New Mexico. Pilgrims complete a ritual of eating some of the church's dirt (earth) floor. Spiritual rituals and ceremonies reaffirm ethnic identity grounded in a collective self. According to Bolen (1996), a ritual is an empowering outer expression of an inner experience that infuses an act with deeper meaning. Along these lines, the ritual of Chimayó symbolizes the seeker's reconnection with mother Earth. Alma returned renewed from Chimayó. "I did not eat dirt, but felt connected to Abuela," she reported. Around that time, Alma consulted a Toltec oracle where she received an instruction to reconnect with mother earth. We continued to work on her complicated bereavement.

Alma discussed another recurrent dream after completing her bereavement. She reported that she was taking a bath at the top of an Aztec temple. Again, we analyzed the dream from diverse perspectives, but Alma preferred a cultural interpretation. Instead of being a sacrificial place, the top of the Aztec temple was the site of her initiation. "I felt baptized," she said. "Although I share the same name with my great grandmother, I have to honor my self," Alma said. "I need to take better care of my soul." Incidentally, the word *alma* means soul in Spanish. Besides doing mindfulness, Alma developed a spiritual practice blending Catholicism with Toltec philosophy. "It's a rebirth," she concluded. Alma expressed interest in working on romantic relationships. She discussed her breakup with Carlos, her ex lover. "When I first met him, he told me he was divorced. I was suspicious," Alma said, with tears in her eyes. "We even discussed marriage," Alma continued. "Later on, I found that Carlos was still married and living with his wife!" I replied: "*A la major cocinera se le escapa un tomate*." The *dicho*, loosely translated as "Even the best cook can lose a tomato," conveys that we all make mistakes, even the experts. This *dicho* facilitated a culturally sensitive therapeutic intervention—it is okay to miss something without feeling guilty, you don't have to be perfect (like Doña Alma appeared to be in her granddaughter's eyes) in order to be good. In response, Alma laughed and took a tissue from the box. "You're right," she said while blowing her nose. "Help me break the negative cycle with men."

I suggested the completion of a relationship inventory. Based on interpersonal approaches, this tool examines past relationships to ascertain patterns, dynamics, and other relevant issues. Alma's inventory yielded that she had replicated two types of romantic relationships: symbiotic and distant. Seeing her inventory's "checks and balances," as Alma put it, gave her the emotional stamina to initiate change in choosing potential partners. We continued our work to help Alma live her own life in the context of her family and community. "I want to fly," Alma declared at this point. Upon exploration, Alma revealed that she felt stagnated in her spiritual life. To address this issue I suggested guided imagery. Alma received this suggestion with enthusiasm and read several books on the topic. During one experiential session, she saw herself as Icarus with artificial wings. She became terrified of being burnt by the sun. "What do you need?" I asked her. "Reconnect with the Earth," she said. In her visualization Alma saw Quetzalcoalt, the Aztec feathered snake. The god asked Alma to plant her feet deeply into the earth. At that moment, Alma visualized herself growing real wings. She began to soar. "I'm alive inside." Two years into psychotherapy Alma met Miguel, soon after we completed treatment. A year and a half later, I received an email announcement: "Join me in welcoming my daughter Blanca Alma. Thanks for being my *comadre*."

RENACER: HEALTHY MIND IN HEALTHY BODY AND IN HEALTHY SOUL

I envisioned Alma's presenting complaint (I am dead inside) within a holistic perspective: *Mente sana en cuerpo sano y en alma sana* (Healthy mind in healthy body and in healthy soul). CBT approaches facilitated the development of our therapeutic relationship. Within this context I was able to "give" to Alma by helping her to reduce her anxiety. Additionally, I looked through La Raza's lens to conceptualize her treatment. In other words, instead of promoting personal agency and mastery, I encouraged integration and development. For instance, the teaching of relaxation and desensitization techniques was consistent with striving for *sabiduria*. Moreover, Alma's *familismo* allowed her to perceive me as a member of her extended family and thus, cemented the therapeutic alliance. Latino healing helped to integrate Alma's spiritual beliefs into therapy. Cultural communication with her dead grandmother allowed Alma to complete her complicated bereavement. I integrated magical realism into family therapy with one person. Alma's ability to mourn losses was previously compromised by unrealistic gender role expectations. Her namesake, Doña Alma, was an unreachable star in the family's firmament. Her message, "*Vive tu vida*," (Live your life), promoted Alma's consciousness. She challenged internalized expectations and reformulated her identity. My use of Latino healing facilitated Alma's ability to call back her spirit. The cultural interpretation of dreams was catalytic in her spiritual development. It helped Alma to connect with her ancestors through magical realism. Acting upon her grandmother's message, Alma visited Chimayó, a ritual that facilitated purification and reconnection with her ethnic roots. The mind-body approaches encouraged healing and liberation. More specifically, experiential approaches promoted Alma to transverse her spiritual path. Her dreams—spiritual initiation and "growing" real wings in order to fly—were emblematic of her liberation and spiritual growth. Moreover, the concept of *renacer*, (rebirth) became a banner in Alma's spiritual journey. Alma reformulated her identity from a sufferer to a seeker. I often function as a *comadre* to my clients. As her comother, *comadre*, I assisted her in her rebirth.

Alma's case illustrated the integration of ethnic psychology into mainstream psychotherapy. To increase their cultural competence with Latinos, therapists need to become familiar with collectivistic constructs such as *familismo personalismo* and others. In addition, they can complement mainstream psychotherapy with ethnic psychological approaches, such as *dichos*, *testimonio*, and Latino spirituality. Furthermore, when deemed appropriate, collaboration with folk healers could prove useful. In conclusion, therapists can enhance their cultural competence with collectivistic Latinos by working within contextualism, interconnectedness, and magical realism, while acknowledging the importance of spirituality.

ARPILLERA: **COMPOSING A LIFE**

Latino healing promotes transcendence and rebirth. I use the concept of *arpillera* as a symbol of this rebirth. Literally meaning cloth or weaving, *arpilleras* are folk tapestries that illustrate the stories of oppressed Latinos. To illustrate, Chilean women weaved their trauma stories of political repression and torture into these beautiful folk expressions. *Arpilleras* embody Latino resistance, cultural resilience, and transformation. They sublimate suffering into conscious art. To create an *arpillera* is empowering. Nowadays, *arpilleras* tell stories of all aspects in life.

For me, *arpilleras* symbolize the creative expression in composing one's life. Just as Mary Catherine Bateson found that women compose their life based on their gender-specific circumstances, many Latinos compose theirs by creating *arpilleras.* Latinos craft emotional tapestries in response to the challenges of living in the "cultural hyphen." Identity issues, cultural conflict, discrimination, and oppression are some of the threads in their weaving. Latinos weave *arpilleras* as they travel back and forth through the cultural *puente* connecting North and South. In their journey, they impart resilience, *mestizaje,* and creativity into the building of the American *arpillera.*

INDEX

A

Absolutisms, 53
Abuse, sexual, 2, 4, 183
Acceptance and commitment therapy (ACT), 174
Acceptance-based behavior therapy (ABBT), 173, 174, 177–179
Adler, Alfred, 12, 14
Adlerian psychology, 11–31
    antithetical modes of apperception, 21
    dreams, 29–30
    interpretations in, 14
    Life Style assessment, 15–19
    Life Style Summary, 16–18
    multiple psychotherapy, 15
    neurosis in, 14, 26–27
    overview, 12–13
    The Question, 14
    social interest, 12–13, 15, 29, 30–31
    spitting in the soup, 25
    tasks of life, 12, 14, 15
Agoraphobia, 13–15, 20, 24–25
Alcohol abuse, 17
Anorexia nervosa, 148, 149, 150–151, 153
Antidepressants. *See* Medications
Antithetical modes of apperception, 21
Anxiety, 6, 13, 77, 175–176, 177–179, 182
Arpilleras, 216, 218
Assessment, 15–19, 88, 147, 203. *See also* Strength-based assessment
    deficit-oriented, 193–194
Attunement, 129n
Authentic Happiness Inventory, 196
Authority, client-centered view of, 36–37

B

Baer, Ruth, 172
Barlow, David, 78
Bateson, Mary Catherine, 218
Beck, Aaron, 55, 87
Beck Anxiety Inventory (BAI), 175, 182
Beck Depression Inventory (BDI), 199, 205
Beck Depression Inventory (BDI-II), 147, 175, 182
Behavioral activation techniques, 185–186
Behavior therapy, 78–86
    dialectical, 172
Bereavement, 215
Beutler, Larry, 203

Body-image issues, 178
Borderline personality disorder (BPD), 115, 172, 173, 180–189
Boundaries, 9–10, 121, 129, 132–133, 136
Brodley, B.T., 38
Bulimia, 2, 3, 115

C

Cancer, 104–105
Case formulation, 34
Causation, unitary theory of, 34
Change, 19–23, 28–29, 141–143, 149, 150, 155, 158–162, 169–171, 208
Character Strengths and Virtues, 198
Client-centered therapy, 32–57
    case formulation, 34
    diagnosis in, 37–38
    living a lost life, 52–54
    means and ends, consistency between, 39–40
    nondirective attitude, 38–39, 44
    power and authority in, 36–37
    practice of hope, 54–55
    restoring self to congruence, 35–36
    therapy session, 40–52
    universal theory of psychological maladjustment, 35
Client-Centered Therapy (Rogers), 37–38
Cocaine, 205
Cognitive behavior theories, 34
Cognitive-behavior therapy (CBT), 174, 216, 217
Cognitive defusion, 188
Cognitive rigidity, 187–189
Cognitive therapy, 87–101
    alternative therapy, 90, 93–94
    closure, 90, 99–100
    collaborative empiricism, 101
    eliciting information, 89–92
    overview, 88–89
    patient's perspective, 89–91, 92–93
    suicide and, 87–89, 91, 95, 97, 100–101
    testing conclusions, 90, 94–100
Collaborative empiricism, 101
Comas-Diaz, Lillian, 214
Conditions of worth, 35
Conflicts, 143–147
Confluence, 136
Congruence, restoring self to, 35–36

Contact boundaries, 121, 129, 132–133, 136
Contemplative psychotherapies, 172–191
    acceptance-based behavior therapy, 173, 174, 177–179
    assessment, 175–176, 181–183
    behavioral activation techniques and mindfulness, 185–186
    dialectical behavior therapy, 172, 173–174, 184–185
    exposure-based cognitive processing techniques, 186–187
    mindful cognitive decentering and experiential acceptance, 187–189
    theoretical and research basis, 173–174
Coping style, 208–209
Countertransference, 2, 6
Covert sensitization, 78–86
Cultural differences, 3, 9, 214–218
Cultural genogram, 215

D
Deficit-oriented assessment models, 193–194
Denham-Vaughan, Sally, 114
Denial, 102, 111
Depression, 87, 89, 94, 98, 100, 115, 138–147, 159, 181, 182, 185–186, 195, 199
Desensitization techniques, 215, 216, 217
Diagnosis, 47, 207–208
    effects of, 119
Diagnostic and Statistical Manual (DSM-IV), 193
Dialectical behavior therapy (DBT), 172, 173–174, 184–185
Dissociation, 124–125, 128, 134
Distress-tolerance module skills, 185
Dream analysis, 2, 6–8, 29–30, 69–70, 102, 110, 216, 217
Dreikurs, Rudolf, 13
Drug abuse, 203, 205–212
Dying patients, 102, 104–113

E
Eclectic psychotherapy, 203
Ellis, Albert, 58
Empathic understanding, 42, 50–51
Empirically supported treatments (ESTs), 78
Enmeshment, 161–162
Existential psychotherapy, 102–113
    denial in, 102, 111
    dream analysis in, 102, 110
    with a dying patient, 102, 104–113
    in groups, 102, 103–109, 113
Experiential acceptance, 187–189
Exposure activities, 178

Exposure-based cognitive processing techniques, 186–187

F
Family therapy, 148–171
    coping with change, 149, 158–162
    farewell ritual, 150, 171
    follow-up, 171
    hypothesis forming, 149, 150–154
    saying no to therapy, 150, 165–169
    sibling subsystem, 150, 162–165
    solidifying change, 150, 169–171
    therapeutic contract, 149, 156–158
    therapeutic terms, 149, 154–155
Fear, 25–26, 60
Feminist psychology, 34
Field theory, 114, 119–121, 132–133
Fordyce Emotions Questionnaire, 196
Freire, Paolo, 40

G
General Happiness Questionnaire, 196
Generalized anxiety disorder (GAD), 172, 173, 174–180
Genogram, 215
Gestalt therapy, 114–137
    contact boundaries, 121, 129, 132–133, 136
    field theory and, 114, 119–121, 132–133
    labeling, 130, 132
    relational, 133
    repetitive and recursive loops, 127–131, 135–136
    retroflection, 120, 121–123, 135
    spontaneity, 125
    transitional objects, 121–122
Gratitude Questionnaire, 196
Greek Chorus, 148
Grit Survey, 196
Group psychotherapy, 102, 103–109, 113
Guided imagery, 217

H
Haley, Jay, 102
Handbook of Methods in Positive Psychology (Ong & Van Dulmen), 196
Heroin addiction, 205–212
Homework
    in Adlerian psychotherapy, 22–23, 29
    in behavior therapy, 82–84
    in contemplative psychotherapy, 176–179, 184–188
    in systematic treatment selection, 210, 212
Homosexuality, 4, 11, 24–25
Humanistic psychology, 194

I

Impulsivity, 184–185
Inclusion, 129
Incongruence, 35
Individual placement and support (IPS), 54*n*
Individual Psychology, 12
Insomnia, 175, 176–177
Integrative psychotherapy, 203–213
International Gestalt Journal, 114
Interpersonal disputes, 139, 143–147
Interpersonal psychotherapy (IPT), 138–147
Intervoice, 51
Irritable bowel syndrome, 175

J

Jacobs, Lynne, 114
Jahoda, Marie, 194
Josselson, Ruthellen, 102

L

Labeling, 130, 132
Latino healing, 214–218
Lear, Jonathan, 52–53
Life Style Assessment, 15–19
Linehan, Marsha, 183
Living with Christian (Wakefield), 55

M

Magical realism, 217
Meaning, loss of framework of, 52–54
Means and ends, consistency between, 39–40
Medical model, 34
Medications, 175, 176, 179, 181, 203
Mindful cognitive decentering, 187–189
Mindfulness, 172, 173, 177–178, 185–186, 216
Mindful progressive muscle relaxation, 177–178
The Mindful Way Through Anxiety, 177
Minnesota Multiphasic Personality Inventory-2
    (MMPI-2), 175, 182, 192, 199, 203, 205, 207
Mosak, Harold, 11
Multicultural psychotherapy, 214–218
Multiple psychotherapy, 15

N

Narcissistic grandiosity, 6
NEO Personality Inventory Revised (NEO-PI-R), 182
Neurosis, 14, 26–27
Nondirective attitude, 38–39, 44

O

Obesity, 17
O'Hara, Maureen, 40
Organismic valuing, 35
Outcome, defined, 34

P

Panic, 13–14
Papp, Peggy, 148
Paraphilia, 78–86
Pedophilia, 78–86
Perfectionism, 27, 28, 61, 68, 74, 183
Perls, Fritz, 136
Phobias, 175, 176
Plenty Coups, 52
Positive Psychological Assessment (Lopez & Snyder),
    196
Positive psychotherapy, 193–202
Positive Psychotherapy Inventory, 196
Posttraumatic stress disorder (PTSD), 181, 184, 185,
    186–187
Power, client-centered view of, 36–37
Pre-expressive, 55
Progressive muscle relaxation (PMR), 177
PsycCRITIQUES Blog, 192
Psychoanalysis, 3–10
Psychodynamic theory, 34
Psychological maladjustment, universal theory of, 35
Psychosocial rehabilitation (PSR), 54*n*

Q

The Question, 14

R

Radical Hope (Lear), 52
Rape, 102, 103–104, 107, 109
Raskin, Nathaniel J., 38
Rating System for Nondirective Client-Centered
    Interviews-Revised, 51
Rational emotive behavior therapy (REBT),
    55–77, 87
    attacking beliefs in, 61–64, 66–69
    dream analysis, 69–70
    questioning dialogue, 75
    repetitive teaching, 66–67
    symptom identification, 59–61, 71
    therapist-directed discussion, 64–66
    unconditional acceptance, 66, 73–74
Recapitulation of past in present, 2, 3–10
Regression, 169–171
Rejection, 24, 27
Relational Gestalt therapy, 133
Relationship inventory, 216–217
Relaxation techniques, 176–179, 184–189, 215–217
Repetitive and recursive loops, 127–131, 135–136
Repetitive teaching, 66–67
Resistance, 149, 159–160, 210
Retroflection, 120, 121–123, 135
Rogers, Carl R., 35, 36–38, 39, 40, 55, 66

S
Schizophrenia, 32, 33, 40–52
Self-criticism, 175, 178
Self-harm, 115, 123, 181, 183, 184–185
Self-object needs, 133
Semidelusional ideation, 4, 5
Sexual abuse, 2, 4, 183
Sexual identity, 11
Signature Strengths Questionnaire
        (SSQ-72), 196
Social anxiety, 175, 176
Social interest, 12–13, 15, 29, 30–31
Sommerbeck, Lisbeth, 47
Spitting in the soup, 25
Spontaneity, 125
Stolorow, R., 53
Strength-based assessment, 194–196
    case illustration, 199–201
    conducting, 196–198
    defined, 195
Stress management. *See* Relaxation techniques
Structured Clinical Interview for DSM-IV (SCID),
        181
Style of life, 12, 15–19
Substance abuse, 173, 203, 205–212
Suicide, 87–89, 94, 98, 100–101, 115, 123, 163, 205,
        209
Systematic treatment selection (STS), 203, 204–213

T
Tasks of life, 12, 14, 15
Technologies of acceptance, 173
Technologies of change, 173
Termination issues, 2, 9–10
Tracking response, 51
Transference, 2, 9–10
Transitional objects, 121–122
Trauma, 128
Trauma psychology, 34

U
Unconditional positive regard, 66, 73–74

V
Values in Action-Inventory of Strengths (VIA-IS),
        192, 200, 201
Verdeli, Lena, 138
Voices, hearing, 40, 43, 45–47, 48–50, 51

W
Wakefield, Georgina, 55
Walsh, Roger, 172
A Way of Being (Rogers), 55
Weissman, Myrna, 138, 140, 143
Well-being, defined, 197

Y
Yalom, Irvin, 102